Diagnostic Issues in Substance Use Disorders

Refining the Research Agenda for DSM-V

Diagnostic Issues in Substance Use Disorders

Refining the Research Agenda for DSM-V

Edited by

John B. Saunders, M.D., F.R.C.P.
Marc A. Schuckit, M.D.
Paul J. Sirovatka, M.S.
Darrel A. Regier, M.D., M.P.H.

Published by the
American Psychiatric Association
Arlington, Virginia

Note: The authors have worked to ensure that all information in this book is accurate at the time of publication and consistent with general psychiatric and medical standards, and that information concerning drug dosages, schedules, and routes of administration is accurate at the time of publication and consistent with standards set by the U.S. Food and Drug Administration and the general medical community. As medical research and practice continue to advance, however, therapeutic standards may change. Moreover, specific situations may require a specific therapeutic response not included in this book. For these reasons and because human and mechanical errors sometimes occur, we recommend that readers follow the advice of physicians directly involved in their care or the care of a member of their family.

The findings, opinions, and conclusions of this report do not necessarily represent the views of the officers, trustees, or all members of the American Psychiatric Association. The views expressed are those of the authors of the individual chapters.

11 10 09 08 07 5 4 3 2 1
First Edition

Typeset in Adobe's Frutiger and AGaramond.

American Psychiatric Association
1000 Wilson Boulevard
Arlington, VA 22209-3901
www.psych.org

Library of Congress Cataloging-in-Publication Data
Diagnostic issues in substance use disorders : refining the research agenda for DSM-V / edited by John B. Saunders ... [et al.]. — 1st ed.
p. ; cm.
Includes bibliographical references and index.
ISBN 978-0-89042-299-1 (pbk. : alk. paper)
1. Substance abuse—Diagnosis. 2. Substance abuse—Classification. 3. Diagnostic and statistical manual of mental disorders. I. Saunders, John B. II. American Psychiatric Association. [DNLM: 1. Diagnostic and statistical manual of mental disorders. 5th ed. 2. Substance-Related Disorders—diagnosis. 3. Substance-Related Disorders—classification. WM 270 D5368 2007]
RC564.D533 2007
362.29—dc22

2007001492

British Library Cataloguing in Publication Data
A CIP record is available from the British Library.

CONTENTS

CONTRIBUTORS

Thomas F. Babor, Ph.D., M.P.H.
Professor and Chairman, Department of Community Medicine and Health Care, University of Connecticut School of Medicine, Farmington, Connecticut

Alan J. Budney, Ph.D.
Center for Addiction Research, Department of Psychiatry, College of Medicine, University of Arkansas for Medical Sciences, Little Rock, Arkansas

Raul Caetano, M.D., Ph.D.
Health Science Center, University of Texas–Houston School of Public Health, Dallas, Texas

Linda B. Cottler, Ph.D.
Professor of Epidemiology and Director, Epidemiology and Prevention Research Group, Department of Psychiatry, Washington University School of Medicine, St. Louis, Missouri

Thomas J. Crowley, M.D.
Director, Division of Substance Dependence, Department of Psychiatry, University of Colorado School of Medicine, Denver, CO

Javier I. Escobar, M.D.
Professor and Chairman, Department of Psychiatry, University of Medicine and Dentistry of New Jersey, Robert Wood Johnson Medical School, Piscataway, New Jersey

Bridget F. Grant, Ph.D.
Chief, Laboratory of Epidemiology and Biometry, Division of Clinical and Biological Research, National Institute on Alcohol Abuse and Alcoholism, National Institutes of Health, Bethesda, Maryland

Sarah E. Guth
Executive Assistant, Health Behavior Research Center, Department of Psychiatry, University of Vermont College of Medicine, South Burlington, Vermont

Deborah Hasin, Ph.D.
Professor of Clinical Public Health, Columbia University, New York State Psychiatric Institute, New York, New York

Mark L. Hatzenbuehler
Departments of Epidemiology and Psychiatry, New York State Psychiatric Institute, New York, New York

John E. Helzer, M.D.
Professor and Director, Health Behavior Research Center, Department of Psychiatry, University of Vermont College of Medicine, South Burlington, Vermont

Michie N. Hesselbrock, Ph.D., M.S.W.
Zachs Professor and Director of Ph.D. Program. Department of Psychiatry and School of Social Work, University of Connecticut School of Medicine, Farmington, Connecticut

Victor M. Hesselbrock, Ph.D.
Department of Psychiatry, University of Connecticut School of Medicine, Farmington, Connecticut

John R. Hughes, M.D.
Department of Psychiatry, University of Vermont, Burlington, Vermont

Katherine Keyes
Departments of Epidemiology and Psychiatry, New York State Psychiatric Institute, New York, New York

George F. Koob, M.D.
Professor, Department of Neuropharmacology; Director, Alcohol Research Center, The Scripps Research Institute; Adjunct Professor of Psychology and Psychiatry, University of California, San Diego, La Jolla, California

Bengt Muthén, Ph.D.
Graduate School of Education and Information Studies, Social Research Methodology Division, University of California, Los Angeles, California

Edward V. Nunes, M.D.
Professor of Clinical Psychiatry, Columbia University, New York State Psychiatric Institute, New York, New York

Elizabeth Ogburn
Departments of Epidemiology and Psychiatry, New York State Psychiatric Institute, New York, New York

Nancy M. Petry, Ph.D.
Professor, University of Connecticut Health Center, Farmington, Connecticut

Marc N. Potenza, M.D.
Director, Problem Gambling Clinic, Women and Addictive Disorders Core, Women's Health Research at Yale; Associate Professor of Psychiatry, Yale University School of Medicine, New Haven, Connecticut

Darrel A. Regier, M.D., M.P.H.
Executive Director, American Psychiatric Institute for Research and Education (APIRE), American Psychiatric Association, Arlington, Virginia

Robin Room, Ph.D.
Professor and Director, Centre for Social Research on Alcohol and Drugs, Stockholm University, Stockholm, Sweden

Bruce J. Rounsaville, M.D.
Department of Psychiatry, Yale University School of Medicine, New Haven, Connecticut

John B. Saunders, M.D., F.R.C.P.
Professor of Alcohol and Drug Studies and Director of Alcohol and Drug Services, School of Medicine, University of Queensland, Royal Brisbane and Women's Hospital, Herston, Queensland, Australia

Marc A. Schuckit, M.D.
University of California, San Diego, Veterans Association Medical Center, San Diego, California

Paul J. Sirovatka, M.S.
Associate Director for Research Policy Analysis, Division of Research/American Psychiatric Institute for Research and Education, Arlington, Virginia

Wim van den Brink, M.D.
Professor, Department of Psychiatry, Academic Medical Center, University of Amsterdam, the Netherlands

William A. Vega, Ph.D.
Professor and Director, Division of Research, Behavioral Research and Training Institute, Department of Psychiatry, University of Medicine and Dentistry of New Jersey, Robert Wood Johnson Medical School, Piscataway, New Jersey

DISCLOSURE STATEMENT

The research conference series that produced this monograph is supported with funding from the U.S. National Institutes of Health (NIH), Grant No. U13-MH067855 (Principal Investigator: Darrel A. Regier, M.D., M.P.H.). The National Institute of Mental Health (NIMH), the National Institute on Drug Abuse (NIDA), and the National Institutes on Alcohol Abuse and Alcoholism (NIAAA) jointly support this cooperative research planning conference project. The Workgroup/Conference on Diagnostic Issues in Substance Use Disorders is not part of the official revision process for the *Diagnostic and Statistical Manual of Mental Disorders,* Fifth Edition (DSM-V), but rather is a separate, rigorous research planning initiative meant to inform revisions of psychiatric diagnostic classification systems. No private-industry sources provide funding for the research review.

Coordination and oversight of the overall research review, publicly titled "The Future of Psychiatric Diagnosis: Refining the Research Agenda," is provided by an Executive Steering Committee composed of representatives of the several entities that are cooperatively sponsoring the NIH-funded project. Present and former members are as follows:

- *American Psychiatric Institute for Research and Education*—Darrel A. Regier, M.D., M.P.H.; support staff: William E. Narrow, M.D., M.P.H., Maritza Rubio-Stipec, Sci.D., Paul Sirovatka, M.S., Jennifer Shupinka, Rocio Salvador, and Kristin Edwards
- *World Health Organization*—Benedetto Saraceno, M.D., and Norman Sartorius, M.D., Ph.D. (consultant)
- *National Institutes of Health*—Michael Kozak, Ph.D. (NIMH), Wilson Compton, M.D. (NIDA), and Bridget Grant, Ph.D. (NIAAA); NIMH grant project officers have included Bruce Cuthbert, Ph.D., Lisa Colpe, Ph.D., Michael Kozak, Ph.D., and Karen H. Bourdon, M.A.
- *Columbia University*—Michael B. First, M.D. (consultant)

The following contributors to this book have indicated financial interests in or other affiliations with a commercial supporter, a manufacturer of a commercial product, a provider of a commercial service, a nongovernmental organization, and/or a government agency, as listed below:

Alan J. Budney, Ph.D.—Funding from the National Institutes of Health and the National Institute on Drug Abuse only.

Linda B. Cottler, Ph.D.—Funding from the National Institutes of health only.

Thomas J. Crowley, M.D.—Consultations to CRS Associates and Wayne State University are supported by Reckitt-Benckiser Pharmaceuticals; Black Diamond Equipment Inc. pays AvaLung royalties.

John R. Hughes, M.D.—The author is currently employed by the University of Vermont and Fletcher Allen Health Care. *Research grants* (in 2006): National Institutes of Health. *Honoraria, fees, or travel expenses:* Academy for Educational Development, Atrium Healthcare, Cambridge Hospital, Celtic Pharmaceuticals/ Xenova, Concepts in Medicine, Cowen and Companies, Cygnus, Edelman Bioscience, Exchange Supplies Ltd, Fagerstrom Consulting, Free and Clear, Health Learning Systems, Healthwise, JSR, Insyght, LEK Consulting, Maine Medical Center, Nabi Pharmaceuticals, New York Association of Substance Abuse Providers, Nabi Biopharmaceuticals, National Institutes of Health, Pfizer/US; Pfizer Canada, Pinney Associates, Sanofi-Aventis, Shire Health London, Temple University of Health Sciences, University of Wisconsin, ZS Associates.

George F. Koob, M.D.—Addex Pharmaceuticals, Alkermes, Cephalon/ COGENIX, Danya, Forest Pharmaceuticals, Kadmus Pharmaceuticals.

Bengt Muthén, Ph.D.—Co-developer of the MPlus computer program used in his chapter.

Marc N. Potenza, M.D.—*Research support:* National Institute on Drug Abuse, National Institute on Alcohol Abuse and Alcoholism, U.S. Department of Veterans Affairs, Connecticut Department of Mental Health and Addictive Services, Women's Health Research at Yale, OrthoMcNeil, Mohegan Sun. *Consultant:* Boehringer Ingelheim, Somaxon. *Financial interests:* Somaxon.

Darrel A. Regier, M.D., M.P.H.—Dr. Regier, as Executive Director of American Psychiatric Institute for Research and Education (APIRE), oversees all federal and industry-sponsored research and research training grants in APIRE but receives no external salary funding or honoraria from any government or industry sources.

The following contributors to this book do not have any conflicts of interest to disclose:

Thomas F. Babor, Ph.D., M.P.H.
Raul Caetano, M.D., Ph.D.
Javier I. Escobar, M.D.
Bridget F. Grant, Ph.D.
Sarah E. Guth
Deborah Hasin, Ph.D.
Mark L. Hatzenbuehler
John E. Helzer, M.D.

Michie N. Hesselbrock, Ph.D., M.S.W.
Victor M. Hesselbrock, Ph.D.
Katherine Keyes
Elizabeth Ogburn
Nancy Petry, Ph.D.
Robin Room, Ph.D.
Bruce J. Rounsaville, M.D.
John B. Saunders, M.D., F.R.C.P.
Marc A. Schuckit, M.D.
Paul J. Sirovatka, M.S.
Wim van den Brink, M.D.
William A. Vega, Ph.D.

FOREWORD

Darrel A. Regier, M.D., M.P.H.

Diagnostic Issues in Substance Use Disorders: Advancing the Research Agenda for DSM-V continues a series of volumes that collectively summarize an international research-planning project undertaken to assess the status of scientific knowledge relevant to psychiatric classification systems and to generate specific recommendations for research to advance that knowledge base. The conference series, titled "The Future of Psychiatric Diagnosis: Refining the Research Agenda," is being convened by the American Psychiatric Association (APA), in collaboration with the World Health Organization (WHO) and the U.S. National Institutes of Health (NIH), with NIH funding.

The APA/WHO/NIH conference series and monographs represent key elements in an extensive research review process designed to set the stage for the fifth edition of the *Diagnostic and Statistical Manual of Mental Disorders* (DSM-V). In its entirety, the project entails 11 workgroups focused on a specific diagnostic topic or category. The monographs—and, in most instances, prior publication of the workgroup/conference proceedings in the peer-reviewed literature—reflect APA's efforts to ensure that information and recommendations developed as part of this process are available to scientific groups who are concurrently updating other national and international classifications of mental and behavioral disorders.

Within the APA, the American Psychiatric Institute for Research and Education (APIRE), under the direction of Darrel A. Regier, M.D., M.P.H., holds lead responsibility for organizing and administering the diagnosis research planning conferences. Co-sponsors, and members of the Executive Steering Committee for the series, include representatives of the WHO's Division of Mental Health and Prevention of Substance Abuse and of three NIH institutes that are jointly funding the project: the National Institute of Mental Health (NIMH), the National Institute on Drug Abuse (NIDA), and the National Institute on Alcohol Abuse and Alcoholism (NIAAA).

The APA published the fourth edition of the DSM in 1994 and a text revision in 2000. Although DSM-V is not scheduled to appear until 2012, planning for the fifth edition began in 1999 with a collaboration between APA and NIMH that was designed to stimulate research that would address identified opportunities in psychiatric nosology. A first product of this joint venture was preparation of six white papers that proposed broad-brush recommendations for research in key areas; topics included developmental issues, gaps in the current classification, disability and impairment, neuroscience, nomenclature, and cross-cultural issues. Each team that developed a paper included at least one liaison member from NIMH, with the intent—largely realized—that these members would integrate many of the workgroups' recommendations into NIMH research support programs. These white papers were published in *A Research Agenda for DSM-V.*[1] This volume more recently has been followed by a second compilation of white papers[2] that outline diagnosis-related research needs in the areas of gender, infants and children, and geriatric populations.

As a second phase of planning, the APA leadership envisioned a series of international research planning conferences that would address specific diagnostic topics in greater depth, with conference proceedings serving as resource documents for groups involved in the official DSM-V revision process. A prototype symposium on mood disorders was held in conjunction with the XII World Congress of Psychiatry in Yokohama, Japan, in late 2002. Presentations addressed diverse topics in depression-related research, including preclinical animal models, genetics, pathophysiology, functional imaging, clinical treatment, epidemiology, prevention, medical comorbidity, and public health implications of the full spectrum of mood disorders. This pilot meeting underscored the importance of structuring multidisciplinary research planning conferences in a manner that would force interaction among investigators from different fields and elicit a sharp focus on the diagnostic implications of recent and planned research. Lessons learned in Yokohama guided development of the proposal for the cooperative research planning conference grant that NIMH awarded to APIRE in 2003, with substantial additional funding support from NIDA and NIAAA. The conferences funded under the grant are the basis for this monograph series and represent a second major phase in the scientific review and planning for DSM-V.

Finally, a third component of advance planning has been the DSM-V Prelude Project, an APA-sponsored Web site designed to keep the DSM user community and the public informed about research and other activities related to the fifth edition of the manual. An "outreach" section of the site permits interested parties to submit comments about problems with DSM-IV and suggestions for DSM-V. All suggestions are being entered into the DSM-V Prelude database for eventual referral to the appropriate DSM-V Work Groups. This site and associated links can be accessed at www.dsm5.org.

The conferences that constitute the core activity of the second phase of preparation have multiple aims. One is to promote international collaboration among members of the scientific community in order to increase the likelihood of developing a future DSM that is unified with other international classifications. A second is to stimulate the empirical research necessary to allow informed decision making regarding deficiencies identified in DSM-IV. A third is to facilitate the development of broadly agreed upon criteria that researchers worldwide can use in planning and conducting future research into the etiology and pathophysiology of mental disorders. Challenging as it is, this last objective reflects widespread agreement in the field that the well-established reliability and clinical utility of prior DSM classifications must be matched in the future by a renewed focus on the validity of diagnoses.

Given the vision of an ultimately unified international classification system, members of the Executive Steering Committee have attached high priority to assuring the participation of investigators from all parts of the world in the project. Toward this end, each conference in the series has two co-chairs, drawn respectively from the United States and a country other than the United States; approximately half of the experts invited to each working conference are from outside the United States; and half of the conferences are being convened outside the United States. Given the breadth of issues encompassed by this conference, we were pleased to be able to invite some 35 participants, in contrast to the approximately 25 scientist/participants in other of the series' conferences.

Two leaders in the field of substance use disorders research—John B. Saunders, M.D., School of Medicine, University of Queensland, Australia, and Marc Alan Schuckit, M.D., University of California, San Diego, and Veterans Administration Medical Center, San Diego—agreed to organize and co-chair the substance use disorders workgroup and conference, which convened in Rockville, Maryland, in February 2005. The co-chairs worked closely with the APA/WHO/NIH Executive Steering Committee to identify and enlist a stellar roster of participants for the conference.

Papers from the conference on substance use disorders initially appeared in *Addiction* (Vol. 101, Suppl 1, September 2006). We wish to express our appreciation to officials at NIDA and NIAAA who made supplementary funding available to ensure publication of these papers in a premier, international journal focused on addictive disorders. In addition, a summary report of the conference is available on-line at www.dsm5.org.

The American Psychiatric Association greatly appreciates the contributions of all participants in the substance use disorders research planning workgroup and the interest of our broader audience in this topic.

References

1. Kupfer DJ, First MB, Regier DA (eds): A Research Agenda for DSM-V. Washington, DC, American Psychiatric Association, 2002.
2. Narrow WE, First MB, Sirovatka P, Regier DA (eds): Age and Gender Considerations in Psychiatric Diagnosis: A Research Agenda for DSM-V. Arlington, VA, American Psychiatric Association, 2007.

INTRODUCTION

Development of a Research Agenda for Substance Use Disorders Diagnosis in DSM-V[1]

John B. Saunders, M.D., F.R.C.P.
Marc A. Schuckit, M.D.

Categorization and classification are ways that enable us to make sense of our observations of the world and that help us communicate our findings to others. In the field of medical diagnosis, they provide a foundation for furthering our understanding of the causes of human illness and its natural history, and responses to treatment. Such clinical diagnoses and classifications provide an important basis for the effective management of people with these disorders. The clinician working with patients with substance use disorders can apply the same types of logic to identifying these conditions and as a guide to selecting treatment as apply in all other fields of medical care.

Although many different systems of diagnosis and classification have been proposed to encapsulate substance use disorders and mental health conditions, two have international recognition. These are the *Diagnostic and Statistical Manual of Mental Disorders* (DSM), currently in its fourth edition (DSM-IV),[1] which is issued by the American Psychiatric Association (APA), and the *International Classification of Diseases* (ICD), published by the World Health Organization (WHO), which is presently in its tenth revision (ICD-10).[2] The chapters in this volume, originally published in a supplement to the journal *Addiction* (Volume 101, Supplement 1), are designed to stimulate questions and help guide research related to the development of the next editions of these two international diagnostic systems, with a particular emphasis on DSM-V.

The DSM arose in the mid-twentieth century to respond to the need for a sys-

---

[1]Reprinted from Saunders JB, Schuckit MA: "The Development of a Research Agenda for Substance Use Disorders Diagnosis in the *Diagnostic and Statistical Manual of Mental Disorders*, Fifth Edition (DSM-V)." *Addiction* 101 (suppl 1):1–5, 2006. Used with permission of the Society for the Study of Addiction.

tem of mental health disease coding and classification following World War II. The first edition (DSM-I)[3] of this standardized nomenclature of disorders was published in 1952 by the APA, and DSM-IV appeared in 1994.

The ICD has its origins in lists of causes of death, morbidity, and hospitalization that first appeared in the mid-late nineteenth century. In 1946, WHO was delegated to prepare a list of diseases suitable for all countries, irrespective of culture, level of economic development, and nature of their health care system. The latest revision of the ICD, published in 1992 (ICD-10),[2] has a substantially reworked section on substance use disorders. It was strongly influenced by the development of the concept of a dependence syndrome[4] caused by the repetitive use of psychoactive substances, with subsequent adverse consequences.

Considerable effort was made during the development of DSM-IV and ICD-10 to ensure as far as possible that the major substance use diagnoses represented the same condition. The concept of substance dependence in DSM-IV is very similar to that in ICD-10, although the diagnostic labels of harmful substance use (ICD-10) and substance abuse (DSM-IV) probably address different conditions. As with all diagnostic systems, to be of optimal use in the clinic or for the needs of epidemiology and public health planning, the criteria must be both valid and straightforward, and this was foremost in the minds of those who fashioned them.

Toward DSM-V

In 2002 the APA embarked on a program of work to prepare for DSM-V, with a projected date of publication between 2012 and 2014. A core workgroup to spearhead the review of evidence relevant to the diagnosis and classification of substance use disorders was established in 2003, with Marc Schuckit and John Saunders as the co-chairs. The goals of this committee are 1) to identify important questions for discussion; 2) to stimulate review of the available scientific and clinical literature; 3) to propose analyses of existing data; and 4) to propose new research to enhance our understanding of substance use disorders. In doing so, the core workgroup was to pave the way for the formation of a DSM Substance Use Disorders Committee, which will develop and test the DSM-V criteria. Members of the current core workgroup and the steering committee formed by the APA, the National Institute on Alcohol Abuse and Alcoholism, and the National Institute on Drug Abuse are listed in the table on the next page.

To initiate the process of identifying areas of research that might be helpful to the future DSM-V Substance Use Disorders Committee, the core workgroup charged with the research agenda process and the steering committee initially met during the DSM-V Launch Conference in February 2004. Over the next year they convened through conference calls to refine the research agenda, and to plan for a more broad-based meeting through which the next draft of a potential research agenda could be developed.

Members of the current core workgroup and the steering committee formed by the American Psychiatric Association, the National Institute on Alcohol Abuse and Alcoholism, and the National Institute on Drug Abuse.

Members of the core workgroup	Country	Members of the steering committee	Country
Marc A. Schuckit (Co-chair)	USA	Darrel Regier (Chair)	USA
John B. Saunders (Co-chair)	Australia	Wilson Compton	USA
Kathleen K. Bucholz	USA	Bridget Grant	USA
Linda B. Cottler	USA	William Narrow	USA
Wilson Compton	USA	Benedetto Saraceno	Switzerland
Colin Drummond	UK	Norman Sartorius	Switzerland
Bridget Grant	USA		
Deborah Hasin	USA		
John E. Helzer	USA		
John Hughes	USA		
Bruce Rounsaville	USA		
Wim van den Brink	Netherlands		

The resulting conference, titled "Diagnostic Issues in Substance Use Disorders: Refining the Research Agenda," was held in Washington, D.C., in February 2005. Here, in addition to the core workgroup and the steering committee, approximately 50 individuals were asked to take various roles, including developing and presenting papers, serving as formal discussants, and fulfilling the role of expert advisors. Participants included individuals from the United States, Europe (including the United Kingdom, Germany, the Netherlands, Sweden, and Switzerland), Russia, the rest of the Americas (Mexico, Puerto Rico), Asia (including Thailand, Japan, and Korea), and Australia. The goal of the meeting was to expand and revise the initial tentative list of research priorities.

The meeting centered around formal presentations (ranging from 20 to 40 minutes), each of which discussed items from the preliminary research priority list, with an emphasis on suggesting how literature reviews, reanalyses of existing data sets, or new research initiatives might help address problems relevant to the DSM-V process. After each major topic, a formal discussant was asked to present his or her thoughts on the questions raised by the formal presentations as an entrée into a general discussion involving all participants.

All questions raised at the meeting of potential interest to DSM-V were recorded, and an abbreviated overview of these items was shared with participants at the end of the symposium. This large and unedited group of questions was then considered by the core workgroup and steering committee, and subsequently refined further. The more focused list presented in the final paper in the supplement (see Chapter 19) was created by eliminating redundancy among questions and placing the items into four categories: 1) questions that could be addressed immediately through secondary analyses of existing data sets; 2) items likely to require position papers to propose criteria or more focused questions with a view to subsequent analyses of existing data sets; 3) issues that could be proposed for literature reviews, but with a lower probability that these might progress to a data analytic phase; and 4) suggestions or comments that might not require immediate action but that should be considered by the DSM-V Committee as part of its deliberations, and potentially by the committee charged with producing the next edition of the ICD.

An Overview of the Contributions

The 18 articles in the original journal supplement, and reproduced in this volume, represent the written versions of the major presentations at the February 2005 meeting, which have been updated to late 2005. The final paper (see Chapter 19) comprises the recommendations for developing the research program to underpin the developments of DSM-V.

The first three articles deal with overarching issues relevant for the development of international diagnostic systems. Bengt Muthén (see Chapter 1) describes how statistical modeling techniques can be useful in addressing diagnosis-related issues, focusing on the question of whether DSM-V should use categorical and/or dimensional diagnostic approaches. Muthén reviews the relevant methods and places an emphasis on new hybrid techniques for developing and testing diagnostic concepts. John Helzer and colleagues (see Chapter 2) canvass the need for separate clinical and research-oriented diagnostic criteria and offer ideas as to how both categorical and dimensional attributes can be incorporated into the criteria sets. The biological basis of repetitive substance use is summarized by George Koob (see Chapter 3), who considers how the neurobiological changes that characterize substance dependence might impact on the diagnostic process, especially in the future.

The next two articles, by Robin Room (see Chapter 4) and Javier Escobar and William Vega (see Chapter 5), review the importance of considering cultural attributes in developing definitions of substance use disorders. The authors raise issues relevant to future research into diagnostic criteria, such as the importance of developing clear guidelines on how cultural issues are to be interpreted and considered as part of the diagnostic process. They offer thoughts on the importance of these perspectives for cross-culturally appropriate definitions of intoxication, withdrawal, patterns of harmful use, and substance dependence. The next two articles, by John Saunders (see Chapter 6) and Deborah Hasin and colleagues (see Chapter 7), describe the history of the development of diagnostic systems and identify issues that must be addressed to optimize the crosswalk between the DSM and ICD systems for clinician and researcher. These include the specific criteria offered in the two systems, the need to deal with diagnostic orphans (individuals who have substance-related problems but who do not endorse enough items to meet the criteria for dependence, while also not meeting the criteria for abuse), and challenges associated with the concepts of behaviors, such as hazardous substance use, that place an individual at high risk for subsequent substance use disorders but are not themselves part of the current diagnostic systems.

The second set of articles deals with research questions that are more specific to the substance use disorders section of DSM. Two articles, by Marc Schuckit (see Chapter 8) and Edward Nunes and Bruce Rounsaville (see Chapter 9), present information on comorbidity between substance use disorders and other psychiatric conditions. The two articles complement each other in giving an historical perspective, with an emphasis on how comorbidity was handled in DSM-III-R and the reasons for the algorithm presented in DSM-IV. Schuckit reviews data that support the importance of recognizing the relatively unique clinical course of substance-induced mental disorders and treatment approaches appropriate to them. Nunes and Rounsaville consider steps that may be needed for improving the precision of the criteria, the threshold for a diagnosis, and other relevant items.

The theme of subgroups among individuals with substance use disorders is continued in the articles by Victor and Michie Hesselbrock (see Chapter 10) and Thomas Babor and Raul Caetano (Chapter 11). In the former article, Hesselbrock and Hesselbrock review the literature on subtypes of substance use disorder and note the need for longitudinal data before final decisions are made regarding how these schemes might impact on the DSM-V system. Babor and Caetano examine the bases by which subtypes of substance use disorder have been derived and the extent to which they relate to neurobiological processes. In a related article, Caetano and Babor (see Chapter 12) address the issue of the seemingly high prevalence of alcohol dependence in young people in recent epidemiological studies. They raise the question of whether this represents the same type of alcohol dependence as seen in older people or is a feature of the questionnaire approaches used in these studies.

Thomas Crowley (see Chapter 13) then suggests research questions that might help the framers of DSM-V evaluate the application of diagnostic criteria to adolescents, especially in light of the types of substances they are more likely to consume (e.g., "club drugs") and the importance of disruptive behaviors, such as conduct disorder, regarding the onset and course of substance-related conditions. In this article, Crowley also considers the impact that specific diagnoses and criterion items, such as those related to cannabis withdrawal and for substance abuse, might have in this young population.

The final two articles in this group address specific psychoactive substances. Alan Budney (see Chapter 14) discusses the application of substance use disorder criteria to cannabis, offering thoughts on the benefits and drawbacks of developing a weighting system for different criterion items, while also offering perspectives on whether new, cannabis-specific diagnostic items should be tested for DSM-V. Similar issues are considered by John Hughes (see Chapter 15) regarding nicotine. Here, the author compares the application of dependence criteria to nicotine as compared with other substances of abuse and explores the potential appropriateness of deleting nonspecific diagnostic items while adding some nicotine-unique diagnostic criteria.

In the third section, two articles consider whether substance use disorders should be included in a broader section termed "Addictive Disorders," which encompasses various repetitive compulsive and problematic behaviors. Marc Potenza (see Chapter 16) discusses the impulse-control disorders and, with particular reference to pathological gambling, identifies research opportunities regarding their assessment and their neurocognitive and physiological bases, as well as the importance of gathering additional data on genetic components of these conditions. Nancy Petry (see Chapter 17) reviews the history and characteristics of pathological gambling. After discussing the present criteria for this syndrome, she describes the prevalence and characteristics of this syndrome and discusses the advantages as well as disadvantages of adding this condition to the current substance use disorders section.

The final two articles address the specifics of the research agenda and how it might be operationalized. Linda Cottler and Bridget Grant (see Chapter 18) summarize the existing data sets that might be appropriate for addressing the research questions generated. They set forth their thoughts on the characteristics that are likely to make such data resources optimally informative. The last paper, by Marc Schuckit and John Saunders (see Chapter 19), presents the questions that have been generated by the research agenda developmental process, identifying those that could bc addressed by secondary data analysis without delay, those that require further refinement of the issues and subsequent data analysis, and those requiring more extended thought, including further literature review, or that could be presented to the DSM-V Committee for further consideration.

Into the Future

An important purpose of publishing these articles in a supplement to *Addiction* was to seek the help of colleagues working in the substance use disorders field around the world. The research questions that are listed in the final paper have been generated through an iterative process that started with the DSM-V Launch Conference and the Substance Use Disorders Conference in February 2004 and February 2005, respectively. Incorporation of comments from the discussants and subsequent consultations among the workgroup and expert advisors have led to the research agenda set out in the final paper (see Chapter 19). However, there is still much to do in generating as complete a list as possible of key issues that need addressing in the research phase and the subsequent criteria development and field-testing phases to ensure that the substance use disorders section serves its constituency well for a generation to come.

Acknowledgments

We thank the sponsoring organizations, the American Psychiatric Association, the National Institute on Alcohol Abuse and Alcoholism, the National Institute on Drug Abuse, and the World Health Organization. Our appreciation goes to Darrel Regier, Bridget Grant, Wilson Compton, Paul Sirovatka, and William Narrow. Without their efforts, together with those of Jennifer Shupinka, this program of work and the articles that appear in the supplement on which this book is based would not have been possible. We also acknowledge the superb efforts made by the authors of the articles reprinted in this book, who have given unstintingly of their time to develop, present, and discuss these interesting ideas at the February 2005 meeting and through the articles presented here. Finally, we are grateful to you, the reader, for taking the time to think about the information offered here, and we look forward to correspondence with you in the future.

The authors would like to acknowledge the support received from the New South Wales Health Department, Sydney, Australia (J.B.S.), and the Veterans Affairs Research Service, United States (M.A.S.). Dr. Schuckit's research program is supported by NIAAA grants AA005526 and AA00840116.

References

1. American Psychiatric Association: Diagnostic and Statistical Manual of Mental Disorders, 4th Edition. Washington, DC, American Psychiatric Association, 1994.
2. World Health Organization: The ICD-10 Classification of Mental and Behavioural Disorders: Clinical Descriptions and Diagnostic Guidelines. Geneva, Switzerland, World Health Organization, 1992.
3. American Psychiatric Association: Diagnostic and Statistical Manual of Mental Disorders. Washington, DC, American Psychiatric Association, 1952.
4. Edwards G, Gross MM: Alcohol dependence: provisional description of a clinical syndrome. Br Med J 1:1058–1061, 1976.

1

SHOULD SUBSTANCE USE DISORDERS BE CONSIDERED CATEGORICAL OR DIMENSIONAL?

Bengt Muthén, Ph.D.

In this chapter I discuss the representation of diagnostic criteria based on categorical and dimensional modeling. The choice between categorical and dimensional views of disorders has created a long-standing debate in psychiatry. In the context of traditional *Diagnostic and Statistical Manual of Mental Disorders* (DSM) diagnosis, the categorical view dominates because it meets clinical needs and the needs of reporting for health care planners and insurance companies. Recent interest, however, focuses on the possibility of dimensional approaches in which a quantitative score, or scores, can be used for research purposes. This raises questions about which approach is most suitable for a particular domain of disorders and for which particular purpose, as well as if and how one can translate between categorical and continuous representations.

This research was supported by grant K02 AA00230 from NIAAA. The author thanks Tihomir Asparouhov for stimulating modeling discussions, Tom Harford for preparing the NESARC data and for advice on analysis variables, and Karen Nylund, Maija Burnett, and Danqing Yu for helpful displays of the results.

Reprinted from Muthén JB: "Should Substance Use Disorders Be Considered as Categorical or Dimensional?" *Addiction* 101 (suppl 1):6–16, 2006. Used with permission of the Society for the Study of Addiction.

To be able to answer the question posed in the title of this chapter, it is important to bring together critical thinking in areas of both psychiatric measurement and statistical analysis. In this chapter I aim to contribute to statistical analysis, presenting the research frontier in terms of psychometric modeling. To give subject-matter experts a chance to understand the current analytical possibilities, it is necessary to give an overview of relevant methods, including particularly promising novel approaches that combine categorical and dimensional representations.

The current psychiatric debate about categorical and dimensional views has a counterpart in psychometrics and statistics in general, in which the corresponding choice is between using categorical and continuous latent variables. *Categorical latent variables* (also called *latent class variables* or *finite mixture components*) are used to find homogeneous groups of individuals using latent class analysis or, with longitudinal data, to describe across time changes in group membership using latent transition analysis. *Continuous latent variables* (also called *traits, factors,* or *random effects*) are used to study underlying dimensions by explaining correlations among outcomes in item response theory and factor analysis or, with longitudinal data, to describe individual differences in development in growth modeling (also called *repeated measures analysis* or *multilevel analysis*).

Conventional modeling using categorical or continuous latent variables has limitations for the analysis of diagnostic criteria and symptom items. In latent class analysis, which uses categorical latent variables, the latent classes ignore possible within-class heterogeneity such as individual differences in severity, and the categorical nature of the latent variable causes relatively low power for genetic analysis such as linkage analysis. In factor analysis, which uses continuous latent variables, there is no model-based classification and it may be difficult to find natural cut points or thresholds for diagnostic purposes. Novel psychometric developments, using hybrids of categorical and continuous latent variable models, aim to circumvent these limitations and provide a useful bridge between the two modeling traditions. Two such hybrids will be discussed here: latent class factor analysis and factor mixture analysis.

My aim in this chapter is to present new methodology for studying categories and dimensions rather than trying to reach substantive conclusions. Readers interested in substantive aspects of the debate may consult the large set of papers in psychology and psychiatry, including those of Meehl[1]; Widiger and Clark[2]; De Boeck, Wilson, and Acton[3]; and Markon and Krueger.[4] Early methods for clustering in alcohol studies (see, e.g., references 5 and 6) are also not covered in this chapter. These methods have shortcomings[7] and are inferior to the statistically more rigorous latent class analysis approach (see reference 8 and the references therein).

This chapter begins with a brief, nontechnical overview of the two conventional models of latent class analysis and factor analysis from the perspective of analyzing diagnostic criteria and symptom items. In the context of factor analysis, I also briefly describe a reporting system used for educational achievement testing, in which issues of categories and dimensions similar to those in psychiatry have been discussed.

The section "Hybrid Latent Variable Analysis Applied to Diagnostic Criteria" introduces the hybrid models of latent class factor analysis and factor mixture analysis. The following sections provide some general considerations for the analysis of diagnostic criteria and apply the various models to recent data on DSM-IV alcohol dependence and abuse criteria in the National Epidemiologic Survey on Alcohol and Related Conditions (NESARC). I conclude the chapter with a summary of the assets and liabilities of the different analytical approaches.

Conventional Latent Variable Analysis Applied to Diagnostic Criteria

This section gives a brief overview of latent class analysis (LCA) and factor analysis (FA). LCA uses categorical latent variables, and FA uses continuous latent variables. The presentation is nontechnical, using model diagrams and examples. References to literature with both technical and application focus are provided for further studies.

CATEGORICAL REPRESENTATION: LATENT CLASS ANALYSIS

Figure 1–1 describes LCA. Figure 1–1A considers analysis results in terms of profiles for the four items listed along the *x*-axis. Here, the example of dichotomous diagnostic criteria for attention-deficit/hyperactive disorder (ADHD) is used with the first two items representing different aspects of inattentiveness and the next two items representing different aspects of hyperactivity. The picture shows four hypothetical classes of individuals who are homogeneous within classes and different across classes. The class membership is not known but is latent (unobserved) and to be inferred from data using the LCA model. In this sense, LCA has the same aim as cluster analysis. Class 1 consists of individuals who have a high probability of endorsing both types of items ("combined class"), class 2 consists of individuals who show low inattentiveness and high hyperactivity probability ("hyperactive-only class"), class 3 consists of individuals who show high inattentiveness and low hyperactivity probability ("inattentiveness-only class"), and class 4 consists of individuals who have low probabilities for all types of items ("unaffected class"). It is seen that the item profiles are distinct and even show two classes with crossing profiles. In a general population sample, the prevalence is the largest for the normative class 4, whereas it is found typically that the hyperactive-only class is the least prevalent in that hyperactivity is observed most often in conjunction with inattentiveness. The class probability may be regressed on background variables (covariates) such as family history of ADHD to estimate how elevated the prevalence is for each of the affected classes 1–3 for individuals with a positive family history as compared with having no such family history.

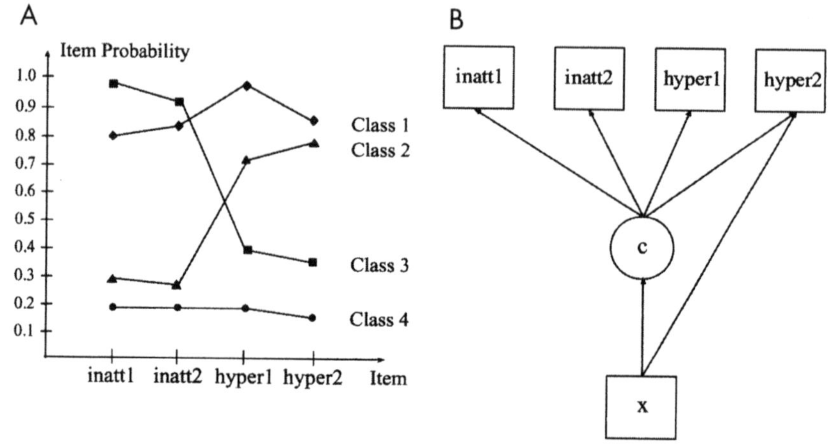

FIGURE 1–1. Latent class analysis.
(A) Item profiles. (B) Model diagram.

Figure 1–1B shows a corresponding model diagram. The boxes at the top represent the four observed items, the circle in the middle represents the categorical latent variable *c* with four classes, and the box at the bottom represents a covariate *x*, such as family history. LCA with covariates has four key sets of parameters: 1) the influence of *c* on each of the items (as shown in the left-hand picture); 2) the prevalence for the classes of *c;* 3) the influence of *x* on *c;* and 4) the direct influence of *x* on an item. The fourth type of parameter is useful in studying measurement noninvariance. As an example, consider a covariate such as gender or age. It is often the case that males and females and old and young differ in their responses on certain items, even when they belong to the same latent class. For example, in the class of combined inattentiveness and hyperactivity, expressions of hyperactivity are more common among younger individuals. A proper model needs to allow for such partial measurement noninvariance. When the covariate has a genetic content, such item noninvariance may be of particular interest in that certain criteria may show especially strong heritability. A fifth type of parameter is also possible, allowing for correlations between items within class (e.g., due to similar question wording). Such relaxation of the independence of the items within class can affect the class formation. Given an estimated model, each individual's probability of class membership can be estimated and the person may be classified into his or her most likely class.

For an overview of LCA methods and applications see, for example, the book by Hagenaars and McCutcheon.[9] In terms of statistical specifications for LCA, both the influence of *c* on an item and the influence of *x* on *c* are modeled using logistic regression and can therefore be expressed in common terms of odds, odds ratios, probabilities and logits. The decision on the number of classes to be used in the analysis is perhaps the most difficult part of LCA, but a combination of statistical and substantive consideration is usually satisfactory. Muthén[10] put LCA into a broader latent variable modeling framework. Muthén and Muthén[11] discussed several applications, including LCA of antisocial behavior items in the National Longitudinal Survey of Youth (NLSY), a survey of individuals in early adulthood, where, in addition to a normative class, they found three classes of individuals with clearly different profiles of antisocial acts: property offense, person offense and drug offense. Rasmussen et al.[12] applied LCA to DSM-IV ADHD symptoms in Australian twin data and found an eight-class solution in which only some classes were congruent with DSM-IV subtypes. While these studies did not show parallel profiles for all classes, the parallel profiles outcome is often seen in LCA with alcohol use disorder criteria—see, for example, Bucholz et al.[13] for Collaborative Study on the Genetics of Alcoholism data and Muthén[10] for NLSY data—but has also been found in other cases such as with schizophrenia.[14]

DIMENSIONAL REPRESENTATION: FACTOR ANALYSIS

Consider a different version of Figure 1–1A in which the profiles are parallel. Parallel profiles obtained by LCA may be seen as an indication that the construct under study is unidimensional. This view would suggest a factor analysis (latent trait) representation instead of LCA.

Factor analysis is described in Figure 1–2. FA is often referred to as *latent trait analysis* or *item response theory modeling,* particularly when a single factor is used. For this situation, Figure 1–2A shows how the probability of endorsing an item increases as a function of the factor *f.* Different items have different functions, represented by logistic regressions with different intercepts and slopes. Below the *f*-axis is shown the distribution of the factor, assumed typically to follow a normal distribution.

Figure 1–2B shows the corresponding model diagram. The factor *f* is assumed to describe all the correlations among the items. The model has a set of four key types of parameters similar to those of LCA: 1) the two measurement parameters for the influence of *f* on each item (logit intercept and slope); 2) the mean and variance of the factor distribution (typically standardized to 0, 1); 3) the influence of the covariate *x* on *f;* and 4) the direct influence of *x* on an item. The interpretations of the parameters are similar to those of LCA, although for the influence of *x* on *f* a regular linear regression specification, not a logistic regression, is used because the dependent variable *(f)* is continuous. A fifth type of parameter is also possible, allowing for correlations between items within class. Given an estimated factor model, each individual's factor score can be estimated. The estimated precision of this estimate, referred to typically as *information curves,* can also be assessed.

Analysis and reporting of national general population surveys is one important area of interest for DSM-V considerations. In this context it is interesting to note

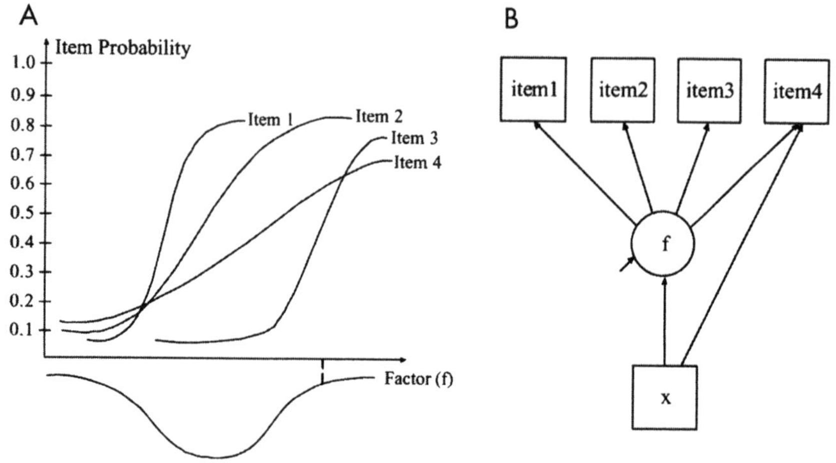

FIGURE 1–2. One-dimensional factor analysis.
(A) Item response curves. (B) Model diagram.

that FA is used routinely for reporting on national trends in educational achievement in the survey National Assessment of Educational Progress (NAEP).[15] The basis for the reporting is a dimensional model such as the one shown in Figure 1–2B, in which the items in a particular domain such as mathematics are assumed to follow a unidimensional factor model. Different sets of students are given different test forms randomly in order to cover more content domains, which implies that for a given content domain any one student responds to a limited set of items. Because the limited set of items does not produce sufficiently precise factor score estimates, it is necessary to bring in more information in the form of a large set of covariates. Although Figure 1–2B shows only one covariate, NAEP achievement analysis uses more than 100 covariates, including detailed demographic information. The dissemination of information to the public as seen in newspaper reports, however, is not in terms of scores on the factor but in terms of regions of proficiency that are easier to understand: basic, proficient, and advanced. In this way, a categorization is made of the dimensional factor. The regions are related to the percentiles of the estimated factor distribution, with current-choices levels being approximately the 30th, 80th, and 95th percentiles (Mislevy, personal communication). The factor percentiles are anchored to performance on items discriminating well at the percentile. The choice of relevant percentiles is made in special standard setting sessions, with panels of judges basing their judgment on what might be expected of students at a given grade level and subject domain. In sum, NAEP reporting has a dimensional foundation augmented by substantively based categories. This is in contrast with analyses providing model-based categories, to be discussed later.

It is interesting to consider a procedure similar to that of NAEP to be used for analysis and reporting of national trends with respect to substance use disorders. If support for dimensional modeling of substance use disorder criteria is found, it might be possible to track national trends using categories such as unaffected, abuse and dependence, where those category boundaries are anchored in FA scores.

For an overview of methods for FA in the form of unidimensional traits see, for example, the item response theory text of Hambleton and Swaminathan.[16] Muthén[17] discusses general multifactorial FA, including the use of covariates. FA in the form of both unidimensional and multidimensional models has been suggested in mental health applications at many points in time: neuroticism in Duncan-Jones, Grayson, and Moran[18]; depression in Muthén[17,19] and Gallo, Anthony, and Muthén[20]; and alcohol in Muthén,[21,22] Muthén, Grant, and Hasin,[23] Harford and Muthén,[24] and Krueger et al.[25] The experience with latent trait modeling in education has been very positive, but it remains to be seen if this methodology is the most suitable or the only one needed for mental health applications.

Hybrid Latent Variable Analysis Applied to Diagnostic Criteria

Recent methodological developments have made efforts to use a combination of categorical and continuous latent variables to understand more clearly various substantive phenomena. Two key models are latent class factor analysis and factor mixture modeling. In the following subsection I briefly describe these analyses and discuss how they relate to the conventional techniques.

LATENT CLASS FACTOR ANALYSIS

With parallel item profiles, the notion of a dimension influencing the item responses can be formalized into a latent class factor analysis model. This modeling is described in pictorial form in Figure 1–3. Figure 1–3A shows a distribution for a factor (latent trait) f, and Figure 1–3B shows a model diagram. The distribution of the factor is shown as a histogram in Figure 1–3A, indicating a strongly non-normal distribution in which most individuals are at the unaffected point. The discrete distribution makes for a very flexible description of the factor distribution and is referred to as a nonparametric representation, in that it does not assume a specific statistical distribution such as the normal. Although the points of the distribution are occupied by individuals in different latent classes, it is up to the analysis interpretations in light of auxiliary variables (correlates) and substantive theory to decide whether these classes can be seen as substantively different categories or simply represent a single, non-normal distribution.

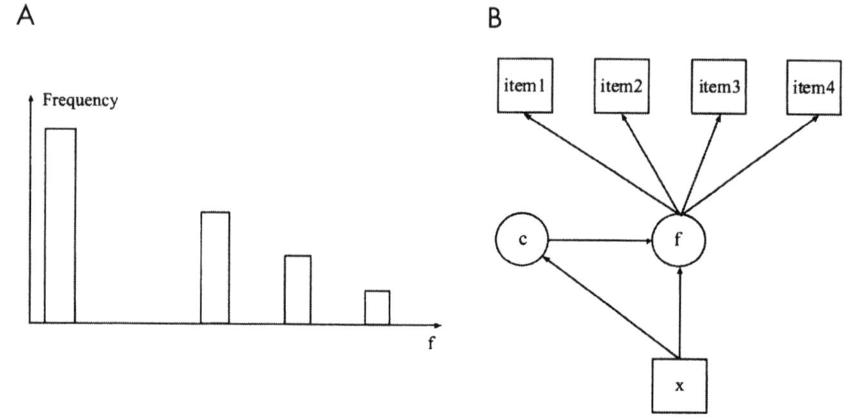

FIGURE 1–3. Latent class factor analysis.
(**B**) Factor distribution. (**b**) Model diagram.

LCFA has five key types of parameters: 1) the influence of *f* on the items is represented by logistic regressions as in the FA model, so that each item has an intercept and a slope; in line with FA, these measurement parameters do not change across the classes; 2) the influence of *c* on *f* is analogous to regression with dummy variables, so that the mean of *f* changes across the classes of *c*, giving rise to the distances between the histogram bars seen in Figure 1–3A; 3) the class probabilities give the height of the histogram bars in Figure 1–3A; 4) the influence of the covariate *x* on *c* indicates how the class probabilities change as a function of *x* (i.e., how the distribution of *f* is changed by *x*); and 5) the influence of *x* on *f* indicates that *f* may have within-class variation as a function of *x;* this within-class influence can be allowed to vary across class. In line with LCA and FA, LCFA can also have direct influence from *x* to items, and items can have residual correlations. Given an estimated model, two types of individual estimates are obtained. First, probabilities for membership in each class are provided. Second, factor score estimates are obtained, both for the most likely class and mixed over all classes.

LCFA combines the strengths of both LCA and FA, providing a categorical *and* dimensional representation. Unlike LCA, LCFA provides a factor-analytical interval-scaled dimension with quantitative scores on the factor *f*. The LCFA model is also considerably more parsimonious than LCA. Using the example of 11 dependence and abuse criteria, four classes, and no *x* variables, LCA uses 47 parameters (corresponding to 11 × four item probabilities and three class probabilities), whereas LCFA uses only 27 parameters (corresponding to 11 × two item intercepts and slopes, four factor means [of which two are fixed to set the metric], and three class probabilities). The relative parsimony of LCFA can make it more powerful in detecting the influence of covariates.

FACTOR MIXTURE ANALYSIS

A second hybrid model, factor mixture analysis (FMA), can be seen as a generalization of LCA, FA, and LCFA. FMA will be discussed only briefly but may be suitable for applications where there are reasons to believe that there is within-class variation in the item probabilities across individuals due to a common source of influence within class (e.g., representing degree of severity of alcohol dependence). This causes within-class correlation among the items because they are all influenced by this common factor. FMA can be specified to have measurement invariance or not across the latent classes for the logistic regression intercepts and slopes. With measurement invariance, the latent classes share the same dimensions; without measurement invariance, the dimensions are not comparable across classes. From an LCA perspective, FMA without measurement invariance is a more general clustering technique because it relaxes the LCA specification of zero within-class correlation (no severity variation). From an FA perspective, FMA adds latent classes corresponding to groups of individuals who behave differently. Measurement invariance may or may not be a suitable specification. With measurement invariance, FMA is a generalization of LCFA by allowing for within-class variation around the factor means represented by the *x*-axis values of the histogram bars in Figure 1–3A.

LCFA and FMA draw on statistical methods described by Asparouhov and Muthén.[26] For applications to diagnostic criteria for alcohol and tobacco disorders, see Muthén and Asparouhov[27] and Muthén, Asparouhov, and Rebollo.[28] For related modeling without covariates, see Wilson,[29] Heinen,[30] Vermunt,[31] and Formann and Kohlmann[32]; with mental health applications, see De Boeck, Wilson, and Acton[3] and Krueger et al.[33] Even without covariates, LCFA and FMA do not seem to have been used widely and seem very worthwhile to explore further in mental health contexts.

General Analysis Considerations

Although the discussion in this chapter centers on dichotomous outcomes, it should be noted that the outcomes could be of any type: dichotomous (binary), ordinal (ordered polytomous), nominal (unordered polytomous), continuous, limited-dependent (censored-normal), counts, and so forth or any combination of such outcomes. This holds true for both categorical and continuous latent variable models. In other words, the type of observed outcome does not necessarily affect the choice between categorical and continuous latent variables. The variety of observed outcome types that can be analyzed together makes it possible, for example, to combine information on dichotomous diagnostic criteria with different information such as quantitative biological measures. As one example, the Windle and Scheidt[34] analysis of alcoholic subtypes could be carried out fruitfully by LCA.

Another consideration related to variables is exemplified by the choice between analyzing symptom items and aggregating their information into diagnostic criteria. An even higher level of aggregation is considered when analyzing diagnoses of dependence for several domains, such as alcohol, tobacco, marijuana, and depression. Such different levels of aggregation may uncover different features related to categories and dimensions and the differences need to be understood.

In studying mental health phenomena, especially in general population samples, it is typically the case that a large proportion of the sample exhibits none of the symptoms. Proper modeling should include specifications that reflect this. This is possible using an added latent class, a "zero class."

Many of the models discussed here cannot be chosen based on only statistical criteria. For example, it is well known that LCA and FA models often fit the data similarly.[35] Subject-matter considerations play an important role in choosing among models used for different purposes, including considering auxiliary variables in the form of antecedents, concurrent events, and distal events (predictive validity; see reference 36). Typically, with these models, one uses maximum-likelihood estimation, in which the log likelihood (logL) can be seen as an overall assessment of the fit between the model and the data when comparing models. LogL can, however, be made larger simply by adding more parameters to the model, and therefore Bayesian information criterion (BIC) and ABIC (sample-size adjusted BIC) statistics are used to combine logL with a penalty for using many parameters. A good model has both a high logL value and low BIC and ABIC values. A likelihood ratio test referred to as LMR[37] provides testing of $k-1$ versus k classes, and bootstrapped likelihood ratio tests are also possible.[38] In models with categorical latent variables, the entropy (with a 0–1 range, 1 being optimal) gives a measure of how well the latent classes can be distinguished. This is based on individual posterior class probabilities, which can be used for classification into most likely class. The Mplus program[39] provides a very general latent variable modeling framework for maximum-likelihood estimation in which the models discussed are special cases. Some of the new models draw on techniques described in a draft paper by Asparouhov and Muthén.[26]

This method overview, by necessity, omits a host of related new and old developments, and the longitudinal data models of latent transition analysis and growth mixture modeling. An overview of these techniques is given by Muthén.[36] It also omits the work by Meehl and colleagues[40,41] on techniques for distinguishing between categories and dimensions. The taxometric approach of Meehl involves graphical displays, resulting in a useful descriptive and exploratory device. The approach is, however, limited because in line with LCA, it assumes that there is conditional independence among the items within each class, and furthermore it is applicable only to situations in which there are two latent classes.[42]

Application to NESARC Alcohol Dependence and Abuse

This section illustrates the different modeling techniques presented above using data on alcohol dependence and abuse from NESARC.[43] NESARC is a nationally representative face-to-face survey of 43,093 respondents carried out in 2001–2002. NESARC uses a complex survey design with stratification, 435 primary sampling units, and oversampling of black and Hispanic households. Within each household, one person was selected randomly for interview, with young adults (18–24 years) oversampled at the rate of 2.25.

The analyses to be presented concern a subsample of 13,067 male current drinkers (respondents who reported drinking five or more drinks on a single occasion one or more times in the past year). The analyses focus on the seven alcohol dependence criteria and the four alcohol abuse criteria, which were derived from a set of 32 past-year symptom item questions designed to operationalize DSM-IV.

The analysis steps will correspond to the order in which the methods were presented: LCA, FA, LCFA and FMA. All analyses were carried out using the Mplus program.[39] The estimation takes into account the NESARC complex survey features of stratification, clustering, and sampling weights.[44] Mplus setups are available on request from the author.

RESULTS FOR LATENT CLASS ANALYSIS

As a first step, the 11 alcohol criteria in NESARC were explored in the male current drinker sample using LCA with two to five classes. Table 1–1 shows model fit in terms of the maximum logL, BIC, ABIC, and LMR. The LCA results at the top part of the table suggest that a four-class solution is preferred. The increase in logL levels off when one goes from four to five classes, and BIC is at its optimum at four classes. Although ABIC suggests five classes, LMR points to four classes.

Figure 1–4 shows the item profiles of the regular four-class LCA model. The *x*-axis lists the seven alcohol dependence criteria and the four alcohol abuse criteria, while the *y*-axis shows the probability of endorsing an item. It is seen that this is an example of parallel profiles, suggesting an ordering among the classes from low to high. The estimated class percentages are (going from class 1 with the highest endorsement probabilities to class 4 with the lowest endorsement probabilities) 1%, 5%, 17%, and 77%. The entropy for this model is 0.83, suggesting good classification qualities.

RESULTS FOR FACTOR ANALYSIS

The model fitting results for FA are given in Table 1–1, both for a single factor and for two factors. The two-factor solution is an exploratory factor analysis solution with minimum restrictions on the factor loadings. The fit statistics of Table 1–1

TABLE 1–1. Latent class analysis, factor analysis, latent class factor analysis, and factor mixture analysis model results, NESARC, male current drinkers, *N*=13,067.

No. classes *(c)*, no. factors *(f)*	logL	No. par	BIC	ABIC	LMR
LCA					
2*c*	–25.887	23	51.993	51.590	0.0000
3*c*	–25.100	35	50.532	50.420	0.0000
4*c*	**–24.989**	**47**	**50.424**	**50.274**	**0.0025**
5*c*	–24.947	59	50.452	50.265	0.1028
FA					
1*f*	**–25.033**	**22**	**50.274**	**50.204**	—
2*f*	–24.991	32	50.285	50.183	—
LCFA					
4*c*	**–25.012**	**27**	**50.279**	**50.193**	**0.0000**
5*c*	–25.006	29	50.287	50.195	0.1520
FMA					
2*c*, 1*f*	**–24.961**	**35**	**50.254**	**50.143**	—

indicate that little is gained by adding a second factor. The second factor is measured by the last two abuse criteria, but the two factors are highly correlated (0.95), and it appears that it is not meaningful to consider two separate factors. The item slopes for the factor indicate how well an item discriminates between different levels of the factor. The one-factor model shows similar slopes for most criteria but has lower slopes for the fourth dependence criterion ("Persistent desire or unsuccessful effort to cut down or control drinking" [cut down]) and the second and third abuse criteria ("Recurrent drinking in situations where alcohol use is physically hazardous" [hazard] and "Recurrent alcohol-related legal problems" [legal]).

RESULTS FOR LATENT CLASS FACTOR ANALYSIS

Given the parallel profiles found for the four-class LCA, as well as the unidimensionality of the FA, it is natural to fit a four-class LCFA. This model adds a factor to the regular LCA in line with Figure 1–3. The model fit statistics for this model are given in Table 1–1. Although logL is worse than for the regular four-class LCA, this difference is not large, and the parsimony of the LCFA relative to the LCA is reflected by LCFA having considerably better BIC and ABIC values. It is interesting to note that the LCFA model fits better in terms of logL than the one-factor FA, although the difference is not large, and the BIC and ABIC values are rather close. LCFA does, however, have clear advantages to FA in terms of practical utility

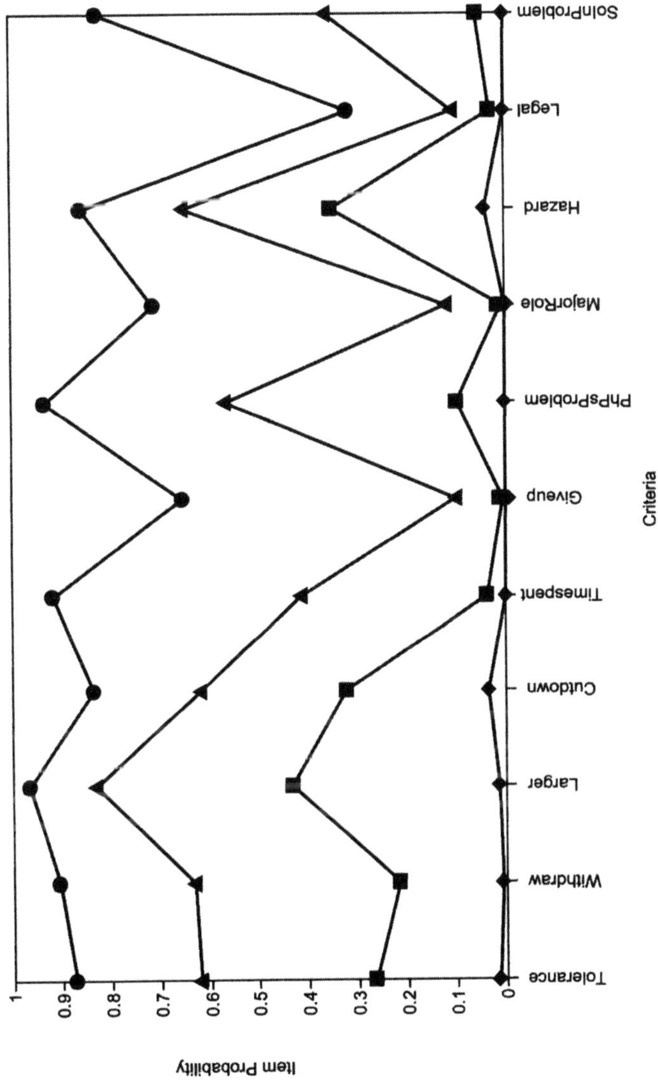

FIGURE 1–4. Latent class analysis profiles.

● Class 1, 1.1%; ▲ Class 2, 4.8%; ■ Class 3, 17.5%; ◆ Class 4, 76.6%.

as described earlier, in that it provides not only dimensional information but also a classification of individuals. The LCFA slopes in the regression of the items on the dimension have values close to those of the FA.

The LCFA estimated class percentages and entropy remain the same as for LCA. The dimensional aspect of the model is reflected in the estimated class-varying factor means, i.e., the quantitative scores on the single dimension (in the order of class 4, class 3, class 2, class 1): 0, 1, 1.5, and 1.9 (the first two values are fixed to set the metric of the scale). The 11 criteria give rise to 2,048 possible outcome patterns, of which 50 had a frequency of at least 10 in the analysis sample. The LCFA implies that the large number of response patterns for the 11 criteria has been reduced to only four significantly different types of patterns and that these types of patterns can be given these quantitative scores along a single dimension. These scores are well estimated in terms of having small standard errors. Their relative difference indicates that the last two steps are smaller than the first one.

Interpretation of the classes is aided by using the individual estimated class probabilities to classify each individual into his most likely class. For class 1, the response patterns have all dependence criteria met and have most abuse criteria met. Class 2 has mainly one abuse criterion met ("Recurrent drinking in situations where alcohol use is physically hazardous" [hazard]), and this may have to do with the high prevalence of drunken driving. Class 3 is heterogeneous. The unaffected class, class 4, consists of those responses meeting none of the criteria as well as responses with only one criterion met.

TABLE 1–2. Total number of criteria met versus latent class factor analysis diagnosis

Total	Class 1	Class 2	Class 3	Class 4	Total
11	11.27	0	0	0	11.27
10	35.93	0	0	0	35.93
9	35.76	0	0	0	35.76
8	40.52	23.07	0	0	63.58
7	8.35	91.14	0	0	99.49
6	0	129.20	0	0	129.20
5	0	197.69	0	0	197.69
4	0	134.22	175.18	0	309.39
3	0	5.32	419.43	0	424.76
2	0	0	856.16	0	856.16
1	0	0	524.40	1,195.78	1,720.18
0	0	0	0	9,183.59	9,183.59
Sum	131.83	580.63	1,975.17	10,379.37	13,067.00

ALTERNATIVE CLASSIFICATIONS: LATENT CLASS FACTOR ANALYSIS VERSUS NUMBER OF CRITERIA MET

The LCFA classification can be contrasted with DSM-IV's method of diagnosis requiring that at least three of the seven dependence criteria and at least one of the four abuse criteria be met. Basing diagnosis on the number of criteria fulfilled makes several implicit assumptions: 1) the criteria are equivalent (e.g., it does not matter which three criteria are fulfilled for a dependence diagnosis); 2) a single dimension (factor) underlies all the criteria; and 3) the same interpretation and metric can be attached to the single dimension in all parts of its range. LCFA results show that assumption 1 is not met in these data, given different logistic intercepts and slopes for the different items. The other two assumptions are, however, in line with the LCFA model.

Because LCFA specifies a unidimensional model for the 11 criteria, it is of interest to consider a classification based on the sum of all 11 criteria instead of a division into dependence and abuse criteria. Table 1–2 shows how this alternative classification relates to the LCFA classification (frequencies are computed using sampling weights). It is seen that given the LCFA model, the number of criteria met is only a crude approximation. For example, the class 1 diagnosis should be made if at least 8 of the 11 criteria are met, but 31 (8+23) individuals would be misclassified. The class 2 diagnosis should be made if between 5 and 7 of the 11 criteria are met, and the class 3 diagnosis should be made if between 2 and 4 of the 11 criteria are met, but both classifications would involve a large degree of misclassification relative to LCFA. The class 4 diagnosis should be made if 0 or 1 criterion is met, but this would include 524 individuals who are in class 3. Although a classification based on number of criteria met is possible and transparent, the classification based on the LCFA model uses more information than merely the sum of criteria and also has a statistical modeling rationale.

RESULTS FOR FACTOR MIXTURE ANALYSIS

The bottom part of Table 1–1 shows model fitting results for a two-class FMA model with one factor. This model appears to fit the data better than all the previous ones. The FMA version reported here is the one that focuses on a clustering of subjects, not a representation with measurement invariance and a single dimension for all individuals. The model has class-varying thresholds (intercepts) and factor variances, and class-invariant factor loadings. The noninvariant thresholds imply that the items measure a different construct for the two classes so that within each class, a separate dimensional representation is obtained. A class with very low probabilities of endorsing items contains 81% of the subjects. This can be compared to the 70% who do not endorse any of the 11 criteria, but the class also contains individuals who endorse 1 or 2 criteria. The high 19% class contains individuals who have varying degrees of problematic alcohol involvement. Relative to the low class, the item probability profile for this high class is characterized by especially elevated endorsement probabilities for 5 of the 7 dependence criteria (the first 4 criteria—tolerance, withdrawal, larger, cut down—and the seventh criterion—physical and psychological problems), but also for the third abuse criterion (hazard). The factor dimension for this high class may be useful for creating severity scores for this group of individuals.

Conclusion

In this chapter I describe several powerful latent variable approaches to investigating categories and dimensions of substance abuse and other mental disorders. These should be very useful techniques for investigating psychiatric measurement instruments in the process of formulating DSM-V. Some techniques have been in use for a long time and have been much explored in mental health settings—for example, latent class analysis and factor analysis (latent trait analysis) for cross-sectional data and latent transition analysis and growth modeling for longitudinal data. Methods that combine categories and dimensions—latent class factor analysis, factor mixture analysis and, with longitudinal data, growth mixture analysis (GMA)—are more recent developments that have seen little application to mental health.[11,36,45–47] LCA and LTA fit well with the need to provide categories of individuals but cannot supply dimensional assessment. FA supplies dimensional assessment but no categories. In contrast, the newer hybrid models of LCFA, FMA, and GMA provide both categories and dimensions. These techniques may be particularly promising for applications to substance use disorders in that such disorders have often been found to have dimensional aspects (see, e.g., references 22 and 25). As shown by the hybrid models, the fact that dimensions are found does not imply that categories cannot be provided as well. In sum, the answer to the question in the title of this chapter is that one does not have to choose categories *or* dimensions but can consider categories *and* dimensions.

In NESARC, data on the 11 alcohol dependence and abuse criteria were found to be fit equally well by a four-class, one-dimensional LCFA as by a one-dimensional FA (latent trait model), but the LCFA model provided a richer representation of the data. A similar four-class LCFA was also found for the 32 symptom items underlying the 11 criteria. Furthermore, three-class LCFA models were found to fit NESARC data on marijuana dependence and abuse criteria as well as tobacco dependence criteria.

The NESARC data were used to compare the LCFA classification into dependence and abuse with the number of criteria met. Instead of the DSM-IV requirement of at least three of seven dependence criteria for a dependence diagnosis and at least one of four abuse criteria for an abuse diagnosis, cut points based on the total number of criteria met were considered. They were found to provide only a crude approximation to the classification based on LCFA.

Hybrid models can be used in analyses with different aims. As opposed to FA, they can be used to produce model-based national prevalence rates in categories such as alcohol dependence and abuse. As opposed to LCA, they can be used for research analyses such as genetic analysis to attain high power due to using a more parsimonious model with a dimensional character; for ideas along these directions, see Muthén, Asparouhov, and Rebollo.[28] Translations between categories and dimensions are achieved because the categories are formed on the dimensions. Hybrid modeling with longitudinal data appears particularly powerful in uncovering different pathways of problematic development.

References

1. Meehl P: Bootstrap taxometrics: solving the classification problem in psychopathology. Am Psychol 50:266–275, 1995.
2. Widiger TA, Clark LA: Toward DSM-V and the classification of psychopathology. Psychol Bull 126:946–963, 2000.
3. De Boeck P, Wilson M, Acton GS: A conceptual and psychometric framework for distinguishing categories and dimensions. Psychol Rev 112:129–158, 2005.
4. Markon KE, Krueger E: Categorical and continuous models of liability to externalizing disorders. Arch Gen Psychiatry 62:1352–1359, 2005.
5. Morey LC, Skinner HA: Empirically derived classifications of alcohol-related problems. Recent Dev Alcohol 4:145–168, 1986.
6. Morey LC, Skinner HA, Blashfield RK: A typology of alcohol abusers: correlates and implications. J Abnorm Psychol 93:408–417, 1984.
7. Blashfield RK: The Classification of Psychopathology: Neo-Kraepelinian and Quantitative Approaches. New York, Plenum, 1984.
8. Vermunt JK, Magidson J: Latent class cluster analysis, in Applied Latent Class Analysis. Edited by Hagenaars JA, McCutcheon A. Cambridge, UK, Cambridge University Press, 2002, pp 89–106.
9. Hagenaars JA, McCutcheon A: Applied Latent Class Analysis. Cambridge, UK, Cambridge University Press, 2002.
10. Muthén B: Latent variable mixture modeling, in New Developments and Techniques in Structural Equation Modeling. Edited by Marcoulides GA, Schumacker RE. Mahwah, NJ, Lawrence Erlbaum Associates, 2001, pp 1–33.
11. Muthén B, Muthén L: Integrating person-centered and variable-centered analysis: growth mixture modeling with latent trajectory classes. Alcohol Clin Exp Res 24:882–891, 2000.
12. Rasmussen ER, Neuman RJ, Heath AC, et al: Replication of the latent class structure of attention-deficit/hyperactivity disorder (ADHD) subtypes in a sample of Australian twins. J Child Psychol Psychiatry 43:1018–1028, 2002.
13. Bucholz KK, Heath AC, Reich T, et al: Can we subtype alcoholism? A latent class analysis of data from relatives of alcoholics in a multi-center family study of alcoholism. Alcohol Clin Exp Res 20:1462–1471, 1996.
14. Nestadt G, Hanfelt J, Liang KY, et al: An evaluation of the structure of schizophrenia spectrum personality disorders. J Personal Disord 8:288–298, 1994.
15. Beaton AE, Zwick R: Overview of the National Assessment of Educational Progress. Journal of Educational Statistics 17(2):95–109, 1992.

16. Hambleton RK, Swaminathan H: Item Response Theory: Principles and Applications. Boston, MA, Kluwer Nijhoff, 1985.
17. Muthén B: Latent variable modeling in heterogeneous populations: presidential address to the Psychometric Society. Psychometrika 54:557–585, 1989.
18. Duncan-Jones P, Grayson DA, Moran PAP: The utility of latent trait models in psychiatric epidemiology. Psychol Med 16:391–405, 1986.
19. Muthén B: Dichotomous factor analysis of symptom data, in Eaton WO, Bohrnstedt GW, eds: Latent Variable Models for Dichotomous Outcomes: Analysis of Data From the Epidemiologic Catchment Area Program. Sociological Methods Research 18:19–65, 1989.
20. Gallo JJ, Anthony JC, Muthén B: Age differences in the symptoms of depression: a latent trait analysis. J Gerontol 49:251–264, 1994.
21. Muthén B: Latent variable modeling in epidemiology. Alcohol Health Res World 16:286–292, 1992.
22. Muthén B: Psychometric evaluation of diagnostic criteria: application to a two-dimensional model of alcohol abuse and dependence. Drug Alcohol Depend 41:101–112, 1996.
23. Muthén BO, Grant B, Hasin D: The dimensionality of alcohol abuse and dependence: factor analysis of DSM-III-R and proposed DSM-IV criteria in the 1988 National Health Interview Survey. Addiction 88:1079–1090, 1993.
24. Harford T, Muthén B: The dimensionality of alcohol abuse and dependence: a multivariate analysis of DSM-IV symptom items in the National Longitudinal Survey of Youth. J Stud Alcohol 62:150–157, 2001.
25. Krueger RF, Nichol PE, Hicks BM, et al: Using latent trait modeling to conceptualize an alcohol problems continuum. Psychol Assess 16:107–119, 2004.
26. Asparouhov T, Muthén B: Maximum-likelihood estimation in general latent variable modeling. Draft 2004.
27. Muthén B, Asparouhov T: Item response mixture modeling: application to tobacco dependence criteria. Addict Behav 31:1050–1066, 2006.
28. Muthén B, Asparouhov T, Rebollo I: Advances in behavioral genetics modeling using Mplus: applications of factor mixture modeling to twin data. Special Issue: Advances in Statistical Models and Methods. Twin Res Human Genet 9:313–324, 2006.
29. Wilson M: Saltus : a psychometric model for discontinuity in cognitive development. Psychol Bull 105:276–289, 1989.
30. Heinen T: Latent Class and Discrete Latent Trait Models: Similarities and Differences. Thousand Oaks, CA, Sage, 1996.
31. Vermunt JK: Log-Linear Models for Event Histories. Thousand Oaks, CA, Sage, 1997.
32. Formann AK, Kohlmann T: Three-parameter linear logistic latent class analysis, in Applied Latent Class Analysis. Edited by Hagenaars JA, McCutcheon A. Cambridge, UK, Cambridge University Press, 2002, pp 183–210.
33. Krueger RF, Markon KE, Patrick C, et al: Externalizing psychopathology in adulthood: a dimensional spectrum conceptualization and its implications for DSM-V. J Abnorm Psychol 114:537–550, 2005.
34. Windle M, Scheidt DM: Alcoholic subtypes: are two sufficient? Addiction 99:1508–1519, 2004.
35. Bartholomew DJ, Knott M: Latent Variable Models and Factor Analysis, 2nd Edition. London, England, Arnold, 1999.

36. Muthén B: Latent variable analysis: growth mixture modeling and related techniques for longitudinal data, in Handbook of Quantitative Methodology for the Social Sciences. Edited by Kaplan D. Newbury Park, CA, Sage, 2004, pp 345–368.
37. Lo Y, Mendell NR, Rubin DB: Testing the number of components in a normal mixture. Biometrika 88:767–778, 2001.
38. McLachlan GJ, Peel D: Finite Mixture Models. New York, Wiley, 2000.
39. Muthén L, Muthén B: Mplus User's Guide, 4th Edition. Los Angeles, CA, Muthén & Muthén, 1998–2006.
40. Waller NG, Meehl PE: Multivariate Taxometric Procedures. Thousand Oaks, CA, Sage, 1998.
41. Beauchaine TP: Taxometrics and developmental psychopathology. Dev Psychopathol 15:501–527, 2003.
42. McDonald RP: A review of multivariate taxometric procedures: distinguishing types from continua. Journal of Educational and Behavioral Statistics 28:77–81, 2003.
43. Grant BF, Dawson DA, Stinson FS, et al: The 12-month prevalence and trends in DSM-IV alcohol abuse and dependence: United States 1991–1992 and 2001–2002. Drug Alcohol Depend 74:223–234, 2004.
44. Asparouhov T: Sampling weights in latent variable modeling. Structural Equation Modeling 12:411–434, 2005.
45. Muthén B, Shedden K: Finite mixture modeling with mixture outcomes using the EM algorithm. Biometrics 55:463–469, 1999.
46. Muthén B, Brown CH, Masyn K, et al: General growth mixture modeling for randomized preventive interventions. Biostatistics 3:459–475, 2002.
47. Muthén B, Khoo ST, Francis D, et al: Analysis of reading skills development from kindergarten through first grade: an application of growth mixture modeling to sequential processes, in Multilevel Modeling: Methodological Advances, Issues, and Applications. Edited by Reise SR, Duan N. Mahwah, NJ, Lawrence Erlbaum Associates, 2002, pp 71–89.

2

SHOULD THERE BE BOTH CATEGORICAL AND DIMENSIONAL CRITERIA FOR THE SUBSTANCE USE DISORDERS IN DSM-V?

John E. Helzer, M.D.
Wim van den Brink, M.D.
Sarah E. Guth

Review of the Literature

CATEGORIES VERSUS DIMENSIONS

Categorical distinctions are essential to clinical decision making and efficient communication. Kraemer et al.[1] emphasize that clinicians "must decide whether to treat or not treat a patient, to hospitalize or not, to treat with drugs or with psychotherapy, to use this drug or that drug, this type of psychotherapy or that type, and thus

Reprinted from Helzer JE, van den Brink W, Guth SE: "Should There Be Both Categorical and Dimensional Criteria for the Substance Use Disorders in DSM-V?" *Addiction* 101 (suppl 1):17–22, 2006. Used with permission of the Society for the Study of Addiction.

must inevitably use a categorical approach to diagnosis. The problem is not whether to use a categorical approach, but rather which categorical approach to use."

Conversely, there is empirical evidence that dimensional approaches are advantageous for other critical goals. For example, Van Os et al.[2] conclude that dimensional assessments are superior for predicting treatment needs and clinical outcome. They also remind us that practicing clinicians are accustomed to adopting a dimensional point of view of illness in such routine activities as developing a treatment plan and assessing clinical progress.[2]

While categorical criteria may be essential for both clinical and research work, there is widespread recognition of problems of a purely categorical taxonomy. Maser and Patterson[3] argue that the issue of comorbidity may be the strongest challenge to the *Diagnostic and Statistical Manual of Mental Disorders* (DSM) and to strictly categorical approaches to diagnosis. They point out that the DSM categories do not reflect on etiology but are "symptom-based polythetic descriptors that cluster together, largely according to clinical consensus. The symptoms are not necessarily limited to a single disorder but may reappear among the criteria for other disorders."[3] This increases the likelihood that having met criteria for one diagnosis, a subject has a much greater likelihood of also meeting criteria for others. This causes serious difficulties when the goal of a taxonomy is to disaggregate the breadth of psychopathology into discrete disorders. Comorbidity is a particular problem in the substance use disorders (SUDs), in which multiple diagnoses are so common.[4] Krueger and colleagues[5,6] illustrate how more quantitative taxonomic models can help solve the "persistent puzzle" of comorbidity.

DIMENSIONS AND THE SUBSTANCE USE DISORDERS

Horn and Wanberg[7] have conducted what is perhaps the most extensive research program on the development of a dimensional model for alcohol use disorders. They derived a complex hierarchical model including 16 primary, 6 second-order and 1 general-factor "involvement with alcohol use." They have also developed related assessment instruments, including the Alcohol Use Inventory (AUI).

Tarter et al.[8] propose a taxonomy for alcohol dependence that encompasses both categorical and dimensional approaches. Their proposal has 10 domains, including measures of alcohol use, psychiatric disorder, behavioral disposition, health status, social skills, social relationships, work, school performance, family variables, and recreation and leisure. They also propose an instrument, the Drug Use Screening Inventory, a 149-item self-report questionnaire, to assess the 10 domains. Both of these dimensional approaches provide a rich set of data relating to alcohol involvement. How they might relate to the categorical diagnostic criteria in DSM or the ICD is less clear.

There are a number of dimensional tools in regular use for the identification and quantification of various aspects of alcohol use disorders. These include the Cut-down, Annoyed, Guilt, Eye-opener (CAGE) test,[9] the Alcohol Use Disorders Identification Test (AUDIT)[10] for screening and case identification, the Alcohol Dependence Questionnaire (ADQ),[11] the Addiction Severity Index (ASI),[12] and others for quantifying particular aspects of substance involvement. These and dimensional scales for other substances can be useful for both general and specific purposes, but again none necessarily relates directly to DSM categorical definitions. The Substance Abuse Module of the Composite International Diagnostic Interview (CIDI-SAM)[13] gathers clinical data necessary to diagnose the DSM-defined SUDs and also provides a quantitative score by adding the endorsed criteria within and/or across substances.

As can be seen, much work has been done to devise and test more quantitative approaches and to explore dimensional taxonomies for the SUDs. However, findings are difficult to compare across studies because of differences in overall approach, research goals, and study design. Across those studies utilizing a dimensional taxonomy there is also inconsistency in how dimensional diagnostic criteria are applied. This leaves us at a point similar to where we were in terms of categorical definitions prior to the introduction of DSM-III. The proposal discussed below for supplementing categorical substance use criteria in DSM-V with a dimensional quantitative component could help to achieve greater consistency for dimensional criteria, just as DSM-III did for the categorical taxonomy.

Specific Recommendations

Our goals in this chapter are to discuss whether DSM-V should provide both categorical and dimensional options for its diagnostic entities and to offer a model for how this could be accomplished. Categorical and dimensional illness criteria are sometimes thought of as exclusively applicable to clinical and research activities, respectively. However, as noted above, categorical "clinical" criteria have important utility for research efforts. Conversely, clinicians are likely to find a dimensional "research" component helpful to their clinical mission. Therefore, *clinical* and *research criteria* may not be the best terms to designate these two approaches. Instead, we recommend the terms *categorical* and *dimensional* as used in the model presented below and throughout this chapter.

Below we offer a series of recommendations for DSM-V. Details of our proposal follow in the subsequent subsections.

- DSM-V SUD criteria should include an option that permits a more dimensional approach to classification.
- The dimensional component should be added in a way that preserves the traditional categorical approach. Therefore, the content of the dimensional component should be determined by the categorical definition as created by the DSM-V Substance Use Disorders Revision Workgroup, a process referred to as a "top-down" approach.

- Consideration should be given to incorporating a basic level of dimensionality in the individual DSM-defined symptom items as a first step toward adding dimensional equivalents to the SUD categorical definitions.
- The dimensional diagnostic component for the DSM-V substance disorders should be constructed using these "dimensionalized" symptoms.
- The dimensional component should be created in such a way as to position the field to test empirically derived, "bottom-up" substance disorder definitions in DSM-VI.

DETAILS OF A DSM-V DIMENSIONAL COMPONENT

It is important to note that for DSM-V, this proposal preserves the categorical definition and does not alter the process by which it is to be developed. The DSM-V Diagnostic Workgroup for the SUDs would operate just as its predecessors have in the past but would expand its role to add dimensional rules into the official nomenclature. This would promote the use of quantitative scales and facilitate a more uniform approach to dimensionality of the SUDs. One simple, but inadvisable, method of adding a dimensional aspect to the categorical definitions in DSM is to simply sum the number of positive items for each disorder to obtain disorder-specific severity scores. This is not a new option and is already offered in some DSM-based structured interviews, including both the Diagnostic Interview Schedule (DIS)[14] and the CIDI,[15] which provide for both disorder-specific and global scores based on symptom counts. Although summing positive symptoms has some utility, we do not advise this approach for developing a dimensional diagnosis. It assumes a cross-symptom equivalence that is not necessarily justified. Some symptoms may be more important than others in terms of quantifying the diagnosis.

DIMENSIONALITY OF SYMPTOMS

For the dimensional component, we propose moving beyond basic symptom counts, beginning with a new element of dimensionality in the individual criterion items. We propose that each criterion item for the SUDs be ranked on a three-point scale. An example of such a scale might be 0 = not present; 1 = mild; 2 = severe.

This accomplishes two things. First, it enriches the clinical database by adding an element of quantification at the symptom level. Second, it probably reduces the patient response burden. A three-point scale that provides an intermediate between an absolute "yes" and "no" may make it easier for patients to provide accurate symptom endorsements than when they are forced to choose between two response extremes of "present" or "absent."

Going beyond a simple three-level scale may add little and could be disadvantageous. Achenbach and colleagues have studied scalar alternatives extensively in the development of the Childhood Behavior Checklist (CBCL). For example, they compared three-level scales similar to the one suggested above with a four-level option, adding a distinction for negation between "never or not at all true" and "once in a while or just a little." They found that the additional encouragement to report very mild problems introduced more statistical noise than valid variance in the identification of clinically significant problems and had significantly poorer time 1 to time 2 reliability.[16] More elaborate scales, such as five-level and visual analog scales, would significantly increase the response burden and offer little if any benefit for a basic diagnostic questionnaire. Ultimately, the type of symptom scale used is an empirical question that the DSM-V SUDs committee would have to explore. However, our recommendation would be to retain a simple three-point scale unless further exploration revealed clear advantages to more complex approaches.

DIMENSIONALITY OF DIAGNOSIS

Whatever quantification scheme for individual symptoms is used, the next step would be to design the algorithm necessary to create a dimensional diagnostic score from the symptoms in the categorical definition. The dimensional scale would be applied both to those who do and to those who do not meet the categorical definitional threshold. Muthén (see Chapter 1, this volume) offers a variety of statistical options for dimensional modeling of the alcohol use disorders, including "hybrid" approaches that provide both categorical and dimensional representations within the same model. Other approaches are also possible, including logistic regression analysis, with the categorical diagnosis as the dependent variable, or recursive partitioning methods, again with the categorical diagnosis as the dependent variable.[17] Whatever the final algorithm, we feel it is vital that the dimensional component be linked to the categorical definition. Creating a dimensional scale that is independent of the categorical definition invites taxonomic chaos. Investigators or clinicians choosing to use the dimensional equivalent must be able to identify the score on the dimensional scale that most closely reflects the diagnostic threshold in the categorical definition.

QUANTITATIVELY DERIVED TAXONOMIES

Our proposal still begins with the creation of a categorical definition by a diagnostic workgroup, just as has been carried out in the past. While this is a well-established process that has been used repeatedly in the DSM and ICD revisions, it is not a strictly empirical one. Ultimately it is based primarily on the judgment of the experts selected as members of the diagnostic workgroups. Even when such experts have abundant clinical data and secondary analyses available to guide their decisions, judgments differ and can be significantly influenced by nonempirical considerations such as personal bias and political considerations. Results may or may not closely reflect empirical reality.

Another approach is for even the categorical definitions to be derived quantitatively. This is sometimes known as a "bottom-up approach" to creating a taxonomy, in contrast to the top-down approach, the term used for the reliance on expert judgment as described above. We are not proposing consideration of a bottom-up approach for DSM-V, but we do advocate for using the DSM-V revision to position the field to at least test quantitatively derived definitions of the SUDs. If we were able even in DSM-V to directly compare expert- (top-down) and empirically (bottom-up) derived illness definitions, it would facilitate planning and subsequent revision of DSM-VI.

This latter agenda may go beyond what can be accomplished for the SUDs in isolation. Successful accomplishment would require, first, that the other diagnostic workgroups agree to work toward developing their own dimensional components for DSM-V. If each workgroup agreed to dimensionalizing symptoms for the SUDs, symptom items from all of the major diagnoses could be pooled. If each committee were to take the additional step of identifying other symptoms it felt were relevant to its diagnostic area but not included in the criteria, this enlarged symptom pool could become the basis for quantitatively derived illness definitions in the future.

ADVANTAGES OF THIS PROPOSAL

There are advantages of adding a dimensional alternative to DSM-V for the SUDs. Such quantification is already used widely, as noted in a previous section. However, there are many such scales available, and there is considerable inconsistency in the choice of scales when they are used. A uniform, officially sanctioned approach would promote consistency and improve cross-study comparability. The utility of a dimensional approach would not be confined to investigators. Even for their most basic roles, clinical providers often need to estimate and communicate a level of illness severity in addition to diagnosis. There would be other benefits as well. For example, in cases of multiple substances, comparing dimensional scores across substances would help to identify the substance(s) in most need of clinical attention; adding dimensional scores across substances could provide a score for total substance involvement.

Adding a three-level scoring format for individual symptoms, as we propose, increases the level of symptom specificity, augments the diagnostic score in a meaningful way, and probably reduces subject response burden. Additionally, even a rudimentary level of quantification increases statistical power without diminishing the utility of the categorical definitions. This is a consequence of moving the diagnostic data from the purely nominal in the categorical criteria to ordinal level data in this proposed quantitative addition. The statistical power available for hypothesis testing is reduced when restricted to categorical data.[18] In fact, conflicting conclusions may be drawn from the same data depending on where the categorical diagnostic cut point is set.[2] Signal detection methods for the optimum choice of cut points using dimensional data have been well described by Kraemer[19] and by McFall and Treat.[20]

If other DSM-V diagnostic groups adopt this quantification scheme, the potential advantages would be amplified. For example, this could give new perspectives on the perplexing taxonomic problem we face with the concept of comorbidity, the simultaneous occurrence of symptoms from more than one diagnostic category. In general we recognize that diagnosis is a convention to sort psychopathology into meaningful groups. When a single patient manifests relevant symptoms from more than one group, we often apply both diagnostic labels and then attempt to declare which of the two (or more) resulting diagnoses is "primary." However, we recognize that this is as yet an imperfect science and that our putative "categorical" groups inevitably overlap. The best we can hope for is to identify "points of rarity"[21] between diagnoses. However, studies of both clinical and population samples indicate that syndromal overlap (comorbidity) is the rule rather than the exception.[22] If utilized by other DSM-V workgroups, a quantitative system as proposed here could replace the awkwardness of categorical comorbidity with a simple severity score for each syndrome, whether or not that syndrome rises to the level of categorical diagnosis. This would disentangle the "comorbidity puzzle" and replace it with patient-specific quantitative profiles.[6] It would also help to ensure that treatment efforts address the full range of current psychopathology.

A DSM-V dimensional option is also potentially advantageous for a better understanding of public health and epidemiological data. Many concerns have been expressed about large differences in diagnostic rates in the major epidemiological studies that have been conducted in the United States and elsewhere over the past 25 years. As Regier et al.[23] point out: "Relatively small changes in diagnostic criteria and methods of ascertainment have produced substantially different results." A uniform inventory of symptoms, including both those contained in the criteria and those contained in other diagnostically relevant items, would permit comparison of the nominal categorical data to distribution scores of ordinal data. Knowing the population distribution of the clinical symptom scores also facilitates cross-population comparisons.

POTENTIAL DISADVANTAGES OF THIS PROPOSAL

There are a few potential disadvantages to this proposal. First, there would probably be resistance to and possible confusion about "a second set of diagnostic criteria." However, initial quantification would be based on whatever categorical definition the DSM-V substance use committee created and would not alter that operational definition. Enlarging the pool of symptom items as described earlier in this chapter is an additional step. However, even if this latter step were taken, diagnosis based on only the categorical symptoms would always be available.

Another possible disadvantage is that the scalar rating of individual symptoms is an added detail for clinicians. However, even at the present time there are efforts to rate symptom and syndrome severity. As noted, this is useful for both clinical and research purposes. The use of an agreed-on quantification scale, as proposed here, would provide a simple, uniform rating for individual symptoms and greatly enrich the symptom database for syndrome quantification.

Areas for Future Research

We list here three areas for additional exploration of the utility of a dimensional alternative for categorical diagnoses in DSM.

COMPARATIVE OUTCOME STUDIES OF CATEGORICAL AND DIMENSIONAL APPROACHES

In this chapter, we offer a specific proposal for dimensional criteria linked to the DSM-V categorical definition. Its adoption would offer the opportunity to compare predictive and other types of validity between these two taxonomic approaches. Does a dimensional alternative strengthen or diminish prediction of natural history outcome or treatment response?

COMPETING DIMENSIONAL MODELS

Various dimensional definitions could derive from the basic model suggested earlier in this chapter for DSM-V. For example, there are many options for how individual symptoms could be dimensionalized and for the statistical models for combining symptoms into a dimensional scale. Particular models may not work equally well across different substances. As noted earlier, symptoms that are not part of the categorical criteria could be used to create an expanded pool of items for exploring bottom-up illness definitions. Thus, a corresponding research possibility for the future would be to compare predictive validity and other parameters across top-down, expert-derived illness definitions and ones that are bottom-up, empirically derived.

There are also existing scales for measurement of substance dependence syndromes. It would be important to test how any dimensional system created for DSM compares against existing scales. We make the point above that a significant advantage of a DSM-based dimensional scale could be consistency of use across investigators and clinicians and across studies. Consistency of classificatory rules, either categorical or dimensional, is the most important reason for having a taxonomy in the first place. Currently there is little such consistency in the use of dimensional tools. However, if a DSM-based scale were found to be inferior to existing scales in terms of such important functions as predictive validity, it would be a disincentive for using the DSM-based scale.

TESTING IMPAIRMENT DEFINITIONS

While we do not necessarily recommend attempting to measure impairment at the symptom level, various definitions of impairment at the symptom, syndrome, and diagnostic level should be devised and tested. Such endeavors take on increased relevance, given the possibility that individual symptoms could be important in the search for biological markers and genetic etiologies of psychopathology.[24]

Conclusion

The long planning and preparation time being devoted to the development of DSM-V provides an opportunity for wide-ranging discussion of this next iteration of the taxonomy. The conference and subsequent articles in *Addiction* on which the chapters in this volume are based on part of that process. In this chapter, we contended that one of the most important issues to consider in the classification of the SUDs is whether and how to provide for a dimensional diagnostic component in DSM. We feel it is crucial that a dimensional approach be offered in some form in DSM-V. But we also feel it is vital that any dimensional approach be linked to the categorical definition and that any change toward a dimensional component be evolutionary, not revolutionary. There is little disagreement that a dimensional classification offers many advantages for both clinical and research efforts, but while the concept of a dimensional equivalent for the DSM-V categories is appealing, the more difficult task of working out the practical details remains. In this chapter we presented a model for how to achieve the goal; other models are possible. What is most important is to recognize the need and to capitalize on the opportunity the DSM-V planning process offers us to meet that need.

References

1. Kraemer HC, Noda A, O'Hara R: Categorical versus dimensional approaches to diagnosis: methodological challenges. J Psychiatr Res 38:17–25, 2004.
2. Van Os J, Gilvarry C, Bale R, et al: A comparison of the utility of dimensional and categorical representations of psychosis. UK700 Group. Psychol Med 29:595–606, 1999.
3. Maser JD, Patterson T: Spectrum and nosology: implications for DSM-V. Psychiatr Clin North Am 25:855–885, 2002.
4. Helzer JE, Pryzbeck TR: The co-occurrence of alcoholism with other psychiatric disorders in the general population and its impact on treatment. J Stud Alcohol 49:219–224, 1988.
5. Krueger RF, Markon KE: Reinterpreting comorbidity: a model-based approach to understanding and classifying psychopathy. Annu Rev Clin Psychol 2:111–133, 2006.
6. Krueger RF, Nichol PE, Hicks BM, et al: Using latent trait modeling to conceptualize an alcohol problems continuum. Psychol Assess 16:107–119, 2004.
7. Horn JL, Wanberg KW: Symptom patterns related to excessive use of alcohol. Q J Stud Alcohol 30:35–58, 1969.

8. Tarter RE, Moss HB, Arria A, et al: The psychiatric diagnosis of alcoholism: critique and proposed reformulation. Alcohol Clin Exp Res 16:106–116, 1992.
9. Mayfield D, McLeod G, Hall P: The CAGE questionnaire: validation of a new alcoholism screening instrument. Am J Psychiatry 131:1121–1123, 1974.
10. Saunders JB, Aasland OG, Babor TF, et al: Development of the Alcohol Use Disorders Identification Test (AUDIT): WHO Collaborative Project on Early Detection of Persons With Harmful Alcohol Consumption–II. Addiction 88:791–804, 1993.
11. Skinner HA, Allen BA: Alcohol dependence syndrome: measurement and validation. J Abnorm Psychol 91:199–209, 1982.
12. McLellan AT, Luborsky L, Woody GE, et al: An improved diagnostic instrument for substance abuse patients: the Addiction Severity Index. J Nerv Ment Dis 168:26–33, 1980.
13. Cottler LB, Robins LN, Helzer JE: The reliability of the CIDI-SAM: a comprehensive substance abuse interview. Br J Addict 84:801–814, 1989.
14. Robins LN, Helzer JE, Croughan J, et al: National Institute of Mental Health Diagnostic Interview Schedule. Arch Gen Psychiatry 38:381–389, 1981.
15. Robins LN, Wing J, Wittchen HU, et al: The Composite International Diagnostic Interview: an epidemiologic instrument suitable for use in conjunction with different diagnostic systems and in different cultures. Arch Gen Psychiatry 45:1069–1077, 1989.
16. Achenbach TA, Howell CT, Quay HC, et al: National survey of problems and competencies among four- to sixteen-year-olds: parents' reports for normative and clinical samples. Monogr Soc Res Child Dev 56:51–56, 1991.
17. Helzer JE, Kraemer HC, Krueger RF: The feasibility and need for dimensional psychiatric diagnoses. Psychol Med (in press).
18. Cohen J: The cost of dichotomization. Applied Psychological Measurement 7:249–253, 2005.
19. Kraemer HC: Evaluating Medical Tests: Objective and Quantitative Guidelines. Newbury Park, CA, Sage, 1992.
20. McFall RM, Treat TA: Quantifying the information value of clinical assessments with signal detection theory. Ann Rev Psychol 50:215–241, 1999.
21. Kendell RE: The Role of Diagnosis in Psychiatry. Oxford, England, Blackwell Scientific, 1975.
22. Helzer JE: Development of the Diagnostic Interview Schedule, in Alcoholism—North America, Europe, and Asia. Edited by Helzer JE, Canino GJ. New York, Oxford University Press, 1992, pp 13–20.
23. Regier DA, Kaelber CT, Rae DS, et al: Limitations of diagnostic criteria and assessment instruments for mental disorders: implications for research and policy. Arch Gen Psychiatry 55:109–115, 1998.
24. Van Praag HM: Two-tier diagnosing in psychiatry. Psychiatry Res 34:1–11, 1990.

3

NEUROBIOLOGY OF ADDICTION

A Neuroadaptational View Relevant for Diagnosis

George F. Koob, M.D.

Neurocircuitry of Drug Reward, Dependence, and Craving

Substance dependence is a chronically relapsing disorder characterized by 1) compulsion to seek and take the drug, 2) loss of control in limiting intake, and 3) emergence of a negative emotional state (e.g., dysphoria, anxiety, irritability) when access to the drug is prevented (defined here as dependence).[1] Addiction and substance dependence

---

Research was supported by National Institutes of Health Grants AA06420 and AA08459 from the National Institute on Alcohol Abuse and Alcoholism, DA04043 and DA04398 from the National Institute on Drug Abuse, and DK26741 from the National Institute of Diabetes and Digestive and Kidney Diseases. Research also was supported by the Pearson Center for Alcoholism and Addiction Research at The Scripps Research Institute. The author would like to thank Mike Arends for his assistance with manuscript preparation. The paper on which this chapter is based is publication number 18120-MIND from The Scripps Research Institute.

Reprinted from Koob GF: "Neurobiology of Addiction: A Neuroadaptational View Relevant for Diagnosis" *Addiction* 101 (suppl 1):23–30, 2006. Used with permission of the Society for the Study of Addiction.

(as currently defined by the *Diagnostic and Statistical Manual of Mental Disorders,* 4th Edition) will be used interchangeably throughout this text to refer to a final stage of a usage process that moves from drug use to abuse to addiction. As such, addiction can be defined by its diagnosis, etiology, and pathophysiology as a chronic relapsing disorder. Clinically, the occasional but limited use of a drug with the potential for abuse or dependence is distinct from escalated drug use and the emergence of a chronic drug-dependent state. An important goal of current neurobiological research is to understand the neuropharmacological and neuroadaptive mechanisms within specific neurocircuits that mediate the transition from occasional, controlled drug use to the loss of behavioral control over drug seeking and drug taking that defines chronic addiction.

Much of the recent progress in understanding the mechanisms of addiction has derived from the study of animal models of addiction on specific drugs, such as opiates, stimulants, and alcohol.[2] While no animal model of addiction fully emulates the human condition, animal models do permit investigation of specific elements of the process of drug addiction. Such elements can be defined by models of different systems, models of psychological constructs such as positive and negative reinforcement, and models of different stages of the addiction cycle. While much focus in animal studies has been on the synaptic sites and molecular mechanisms in the nervous system on which drugs with dependence potential act initially to produce their positive reinforcing effects, new animal models of components of the negative reinforcing effects of dependence have been developed and are beginning to be used to explore how the nervous system adapts to drug use. The neurobiological mechanisms of addiction that are involved in various stages of the addiction cycle have a specific focus on certain brain circuits and the neurochemical changes associated with those circuits during the transition from drug taking to drug addiction, and on how those changes persist in the vulnerability to relapse.[3]

A key element of drug addiction is how the brain reward system changes with the development of addiction, and one must understand the neurobiological bases for acute drug reward to understand how these systems change with the development of addiction.[1,4] A principal focus of research on the neurobiology of the positive reinforcing effects of drugs with dependence potential has been the origins and terminal areas of the mesocorticolimbic dopamine system, and there is compelling evidence for the importance of this system in drug reward. This specific brain circuit has been broadened to include the many neural inputs and outputs that interact with the ventral tegmental area and the basal forebrain, and as such has been termed by some as the mesolimbic reward system. More recently, specific components of the basal forebrain that have been identified with drug reward have focused on the "extended amygdala."[3,5] The extended amygdala comprises the bed nucleus of the stria terminalis (BNST), the central nucleus of the amygdala, and a transition zone in the medial subregion of the nucleus accumbens (shell of the nucleus accumbens). Each of these regions has certain cytoarchitectural and circuitry similarities.[6] As the neural circuits for the reinforcing effects of drugs with dependence potential have evolved, the role of neurotransmitters/neuromodulators has also evolved, and four of those systems have been identified to have a role in the acute reinforcing effects of drugs: mesolimbic dopamine, opioid peptide, γ-aminobutyric acid (GABA), and endocannabinoid.

The neural substrates and neuropharmacological mechanisms for the negative motivational effects of drug withdrawal may involve disruption of the same neural systems implicated in the positive reinforcing effects of drugs. Measures of brain reward function during acute abstinence from all major drugs with dependence potential have revealed increases in brain reward thresholds as measured by direct brain stimulation reward.[7–12] These increases in reward thresholds may reflect changes in the activity of reward neurotransmitter systems in the midbrain and forebrain implicated in the positive reinforcing effects of drugs. Examples of such changes at the neurochemical level include decreases in dopaminergic and serotonergic transmission in the nucleus accumbens during drug withdrawal as measured by in vivo microdialysis,[13,14] increased sensitivity of opioid receptor transduction mechanisms in the nucleus accumbens during opiate withdrawal,[15] decreased GABAergic and increased *N*-methyl-D-aspartate (NMDA) glutamatergic transmission during alcohol withdrawal,[16–19] and differential regional changes in nicotine receptor function.[20,21] The decreases in reward neurotransmitters have been hypothesized to contribute significantly to the negative motivational state associated with acute drug abstinence and long-term biochemical changes that contribute to the clinical syndrome of protracted abstinence and vulnerability to relapse.[3]

Different neurochemical systems involved in stress modulation also may be engaged within the neurocircuitry of the brain stress systems in an attempt to overcome the chronic presence of the perturbing drug and to restore normal function despite the presence of drug. Both the hypothalamic-pituitary-adrenal axis and the brain stress system mediated by corticotropin-releasing factor (CRF) are dysregulated by chronic administration of drugs with dependence potential, with a common response of elevated adrenocorticotropic hormone and corticosterone and amygdala CRF during acute withdrawal from all major drugs with a potential toward abuse or dependence.[22–27] Acute withdrawal from drugs also may increase the release of norepinephrine in the BNST and decrease levels of neuropeptide Y (NPY) in the central and medial nuclei of the amygdala.[28]

These results suggest that during the development of dependence, there is not only a change in function of neurotransmitters associated with the acute reinforcing effects of drugs (dopamine, opioid peptides, serotonin and GABA), but also recruitment of the brain stress system (CRF and norepinephrine) and dysregulation of the NPY brain antistress system.[3] Activation of the brain stress systems may contribute to the negative motivational state associated with acute abstinence.[29] Thus, reward mechanisms in dependence are compromised by disruption of neurochemical systems involved in processing natural rewards and by recruitment of antireward systems.[30]

The neuroanatomical entity termed the extended amygdala[6] may thus represent a common anatomical substrate for acute drug reward and a common neuroanatomical substrate for the negative effects on reward function produced by stress that help drive compulsive drug administration. The extended amygdala receives numerous afferents from limbic structures such as the basolateral amygdala and hippocampus, and sends efferents to the medial part of the ventral pallidum and a large projection to the lateral hypothalamus, thus further defining the specific brain areas that interface classical limbic (emotional) structures with the extrapyramidal motor system.[31]

Animal models of "craving" involve the use of drug-primed reinstatement, cue-induced reinstatement, or stress-induced reinstatement in animals that have acquired drug self-administration and have then been subjected to extinction from responding for the drug.[2] Most evidence from animal studies suggests that drug-induced reinstatement is localized to the medial prefrontal cortex/nucleus accumbens/ventral pallidum circuit mediated by the neurotransmitter glutamate.[32] In contrast, neuropharmacological and neurobiological studies using animal models for cue-induced reinstatement involve the basolateral amygdala as a critical substrate with a possible feed-forward mechanism through the prefrontal cortex system involved in drug-induced reinstatement.[33,34] Stress-induced reinstatement of drug-related responding in animal models appears to depend on the activation of both CRF and norepinephrine in elements of the extended amygdala (central nucleus of the amygdala and BNST).[35,36]

In summary, three neurobiological circuits have been identified that have heuristic value for the study of the neurobiological changes associated with the development and persistence of drug dependence. The acute reinforcing effects of drugs of abuse that constitute the binge/intoxication stage of the addiction cycle most probably involve actions with an emphasis on the extended amygdala reward system and inputs from the ventral tegmental area and arcuate nucleus of the hypothalamus. In contrast, the symptoms of acute withdrawal important for addiction, such as negative affect and increased anxiety associated with the withdrawal/negative affect stage, most probably involve not only decreases in function of the extended amygdala reward system but also a recruitment of brain stress neurocircuitry. The craving stage, or preoccupation/anticipation stage, involves key afferent projections to the extended amygdala and nucleus accumbens, specifically the prefrontal cortex (for drug-induced reinstatement) and the basolateral amygdala (for cue-induced reinstatement). Compulsive drug-seeking behavior is hypothesized to be driven by ventral striatal-ventral pallidal-thalamic-cortical loops (Figure 3–1).[37]

Molecular and Cellular Targets Within the Brain Circuits Associated With Addiction

With the acknowledgment that all drugs of abuse share some common neurocircuitry actions—namely, inhibition of medium spiny neurons in the nucleus accumbens through either dopamine or other G_i-coupled receptors—the search at the molecular level has led to examining how repeated perturbation of intracellular signal transduction pathways leads to changes in nuclear function and altered rates of transcription of particular target genes. Altered expression of such genes would lead to altered activity of the neurons where such changes occur, and ultimately to changes in neural circuits in which those neurons operate.

Two transcription factors in particular have been implicated in the plasticity associated with addiction: cyclic adenosine monophosphate (cAMP) response element binding protein (CREB) and ΔFosB. CREB regulates the transcription of genes that contain a CRE site (cAMP response element) within the regulatory regions and can be found ubiquitously in genes expressed in the central nervous system, such as those encoding neuropeptides, synthetic enzymes for neurotransmitters, signaling proteins, and other transcription factors. CREB can be phosphorylated by protein kinase A and by protein kinases regulated by growth factors, putting it at a point of convergence for several intracellular messenger pathways that can regulate the expression of genes.

Much work in the addiction field has shown that activation of CREB in the nucleus accumbens, one part of the brain reward circuit, is a consequence of chronic exposure to opiates, cocaine, and alcohol and deactivation in the central nucleus of the amygdala, another part of the reward circuit. The activation of CREB is linked to the activation of the "dysphoria"-inducing κ opioid receptor binding the opioid peptide dynorphin and has led one researcher, Eric Nestler, to argue,

> There is now compelling evidence that up-regulation of the cAMP pathway and CREB in this brain region (nucleus accumbens) represents a mechanism of "motivational tolerance and dependence": these molecular adaptations decrease an individual's sensitivity to the rewarding effects of subsequent drug exposures (tolerance) and impair the reward pathway (dependence) so that after removal of the drug the individual is left in an amotivational, dysphoric, or depressed-like state.[38]

In contrast, decreased CREB phosphorylation has been observed in the central nucleus of the amygdala during alcohol withdrawal and has been linked to decreased NPY function and consequently the increased anxiety-like responses associated with acute alcohol withdrawal.[39] These changes are not necessarily mutually exclusive and point to transduction mechanisms that could produce neurochemical changes in the neurocircuits outlined above as important for breaks with reward homeostasis in addiction.

The molecular changes associated with long-term changes in brain function as a result of chronic exposure to drugs of abuse have been linked to changes in transcription factors, factors that can change gene expression and produce long-term changes in protein expression and, as a result, neuronal function. While acute administration of drugs of abuse can cause a rapid (within hours) activation of members of the Fos family, such as c-fos, FosB, Fra-1, and Fra-2, in the nucleus accumbens, other transcription factors (isoforms of ΔFosB) accumulate over longer

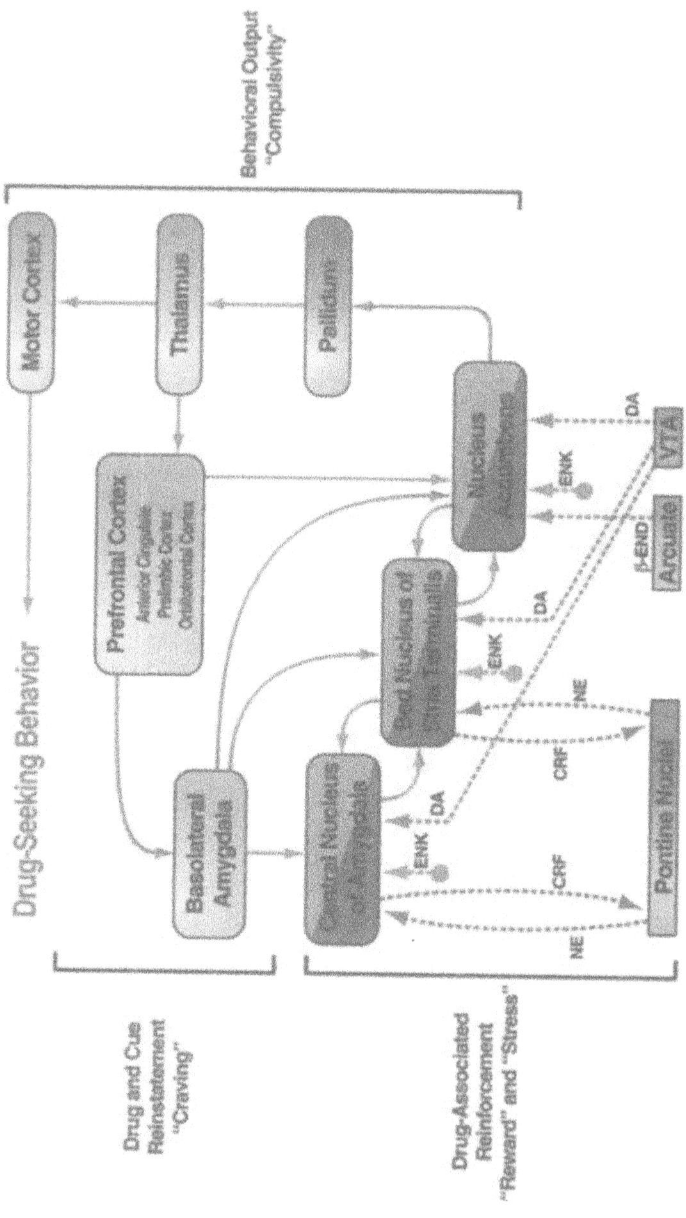
Drug-Seeking Behavior
Motor Cortex
Thalamus
Pallidum
Prefrontal Cortex
Nucleus
Basolateral Amygdala
Central Nucleus of Amygdala
Bed Nucleus of
Pontine Nuclei
Arcuate
VTA
DA
ENK
NE
CRF
β-END
Behavioral Output
"Compulsivity"
Drug and Cue
Reinstatement
"Craving"
Drug-Associated
Reinforcement
"Reward" and "Stress"

FIGURE 3–1. Key common neurocircuitry elements in drug-seeking behavior of addiction.

Three major circuits that underlie addiction can be distilled from the literature. A drug-reinforcement circuit ("reward" and "stress") comprises the *extended amygdala,* including the central nucleus of the amygdala, the bed nucleus of the stria terminalis, and the transition zone in the shell of the nucleus accumbens. Multiple modulator neurotransmitters are hypothesized, including dopamine and opioid peptides for reward and corticotropin-releasing factor and norepinephrine for stress. The extended amygdala is hypothesized to mediate integration of rewarding stimuli or stimuli with positive incentive salience and aversive stimuli or stimuli with negative aversive salience. During acute intoxication, valence is weighted on processing rewarding stimuli, and during the development of dependence-aversive stimuli come to dominate function. A drug- and cue-induced reinstatement ("craving") neurocircuit comprises the prefrontal (anterior cingulate, prelimbic, orbitofrontal) cortex and basolateral amygdala, with a primary role hypothesized for the basolateral amygdala in cue-induced craving and a primary role for the medial prefrontal cortex in drug-induced craving, based on animal studies. Human imaging studies have shown an important role for the orbitofrontal cortex in craving. A drug-seeking ("compulsive") circuit comprises the nucleus accumbens, ventral pallidum, thalamus, and orbitofrontal cortex. The nucleus accumbens has long been hypothesized to have a role in translating motivation to action and forms an interface between the reward functions of the extended amygdala and the motor functions of the ventral striatal–ventral pallidal–thalamic–cortical loops. The striatal-pallidal-thalamic loops reciprocally move from prefrontal cortex to orbitofrontal cortex to motor cortex, leading ultimately to drug-seeking behavior. Note that for the sake of simplicity, other structures, such as the hippocampus (which presumably mediates context-specific learning, including that associated with drug actions), are not included. Also note that dopamine and norepinephrine both have widespread innervation of cortical regions and may modulate function relevant to drug addiction in those structures. DA=dopamine; ENK=enkephalin; CRF=corticotropin-releasing factor; NE=norepinephrine; β-END, β-endorphin.

Source. Reproduced with permission from Koob and Le Moal.[37]

periods of time (days) with repeated drug administration. Animals with activated ΔFosB have exaggerated sensitivity to the rewarding effects of drugs of abuse. Nestler has argued that ΔFosB may be a sustained molecular "switch" that helps to initiate and maintain a state of addiction. How changes in ΔFosB that can last for days can translate into vulnerability to relapse remains a challenge for future work.[38]

Genetic and molecular genetic animal models have provided a convergence of data to support the neuropharmacological substrates identified in neurocircuitry studies. High-alcohol-preferring rats have been bred that show high voluntary consumption of alcohol, increased anxiety-like responses and numerous neuropharmacological phenotypes, such as decreased dopaminergic activity and decreased NPY activity.[40,41] In an alcohol-preferring and -non-preferring cross, a quantitative trait locus was identified on chromosome 4, a region to which the gene for NPY has been mapped. In the inbred preferring and non-preferring quantitative trait loci analyses, loci on chromosomes 3, 4 and 8 have been identified that correspond to loci near the genes for the dopamine D_2 and serotonin $5HT_{1B}$ receptors.[42]

Advances in molecular biology have led to the ability to inactivate systematically the genes that control the expression of proteins that make up receptors or neurotransmitter/neuromodulators in the central nervous system using the gene knock-out approach. Knock-out mice have a gene inactivated by homologous recombination. A knock-out mouse deficient in both alleles of a gene is homozygous for the deletion and is termed a null mutation (–/–). A mouse that is deficient in only one of the two alleles for the gene is termed a *heterozygote* (+/–). Transgenic knock-in mice have an extra gene introduced into their germ line. An additional copy of a normal gene is inserted into the genome of the mouse to examine the effects of overexpression of the product of that gene. Alternatively, a new gene not normally found in the mouse can be added, such as a gene associated with specific pathology in humans. Wild-type controls are animals bred through the same breeding strategies involving mice that received the transgene injected into the fertilized egg (transgenics) or a targeted gene construct injected into the genome via embryonic stem cells (knock-out) but lacking the mutation on either allele of the gene in question. While such an approach does not guarantee that these genes are the ones that convey vulnerability in the human population, it provides viable candidates for exploring the genetic basis of endophenotypes associated with addiction.[43]

Gene knock-out studies in mice, with notable positive results, have focused on knock-out of the μ opioid receptor, which eliminates opioid, nicotine and cannabinoid reward and alcohol drinking in mice.[44] Opiate (morphine) reinforcement as measured by conditioned place preference or self-administration is absent in mu knock-out mice, and there is no development of somatic signs of dependence to morphine in these mice. Indeed, to date, all morphine effects tested, including analgesia, hyperlocomotion, respiratory depression, and inhibition of gastrointestinal transit, are abolished in mu knock-out mice.[45]

Selective deletion of the genes for expression of different dopamine receptor subtypes and the dopamine transporter has revealed significant effects to challenges with psychomotor stimulants.[46,47] Dopamine D_1 receptor knock-out mice show no response to D_1 agonists or antagonists and show a blunted response to the locomotor-activating effects of cocaine and amphetamine. D_1 knock-out mice also are impaired in their acquisition of intravenous cocaine self-administration compared with wild-type mice. D_2 knock-out mice have severe motor deficits and blunted responses to psychostimulants and opiates, but the effects on psychostimulant reward are less consistent. Dopamine transporter knock-out mice are dramatically hyperactive but also show a blunted response to psychostimulants. Although developmental factors must be taken into account for the compensatory effect of deleting any one or a combination of genes, it is clear that D_1 and D_2 receptors and the dopamine transporter play important roles in the actions of psychomotor stimulants.[48]

Brain Imaging Circuits Involved in Human Addiction

Brain imaging studies using positron emission tomography with ligands for measuring oxygen utilization or glucose metabolism or using magnetic resonance imaging techniques are providing dramatic insights into the neurocircuitry changes in the human brain associated with the development and maintenance, and even vulnerability to addiction. These imaging results bear a striking resemblance to the neurocircuitry identified by human studies. During acute intoxication with alcohol, nicotine, and cocaine, there is an activation of the orbitofrontal cortex, prefrontal cortex, anterior cingulate, extended amygdala and ventral striatum. This activation is often accompanied by an increase in availability of the neurotransmitter dopamine. During acute and chronic withdrawal there is a reversal of these changes, with decreases in metabolic activity, particularly in the orbitofrontal cortex, prefrontal cortex and anterior cingulate, and decreases in basal dopamine activity as measured by decreased D_2 receptors in the ventral striatum and prefrontal cortex. With limited studies, cue-induced reinstatement appears to involve a reactivation of these circuits, resembling acute intoxication.[49–51] Two strongly represented markers for active substance dependence in humans across drugs of different neuropharmacological actions are decreases in prefrontal cortex metabolic activity and decreases in brain dopamine D_2 receptors that are hypothesized to reflect decreases in brain dopamine function.

Conclusion

Much progress in neurobiology has provided a heuristic neurocircuitry framework with which to identify the neurobiological and neuroadaptive mechanisms involved in the development of drug addiction. The brain reward system implicated in the development of addiction comprises key elements of a basal forebrain macrostructure, termed the *extended amygdala,* and its connections. Neuropharmacological studies in animal models of addiction have provided evidence for the dysregulation of specific neurochemical mechanisms in specific brain reward neurochemical systems in the extended amygdala (dopamine, opioid peptides, GABA, and endocannabinoids). In addition, recruitment of brain stress systems (CRF and norepinephrine) and dysregulation of brain antistress systems (NPY) provide the negative motivational state associated with drug abstinence. The changes in reward and stress systems are hypothesized to remain outside a homeostatic state and as such convey the vulnerability for development of dependence and relapse in addiction. Additional neurobiological and neurochemical systems have been implicated in animal models of relapse, with the prefrontal cortex and basolateral amygdala (and glutamate systems therein) being implicated in drug- and cue-induced relapse, respectively. The brain stress systems in the extended amygdala are directly implicated in stress-induced relapse. Genetic studies to date in animals suggest roles for the genes encoding the neurochemical elements involved in the brain reward (dopamine, opioid peptide) and stress (NPY) systems in the vulnerability to addiction, and molecular studies have identified transduction and transcription factors that may mediate the dependence-induced reward dysregulation (CREB) and chronic-vulnerability changes (ΔFosB) in neurocircuitry associated with the development and maintenance of addiction. Human imaging studies reveal similar neurocircuits involved in acute intoxication, chronic drug dependence and vulnerability to relapse.

While no exact imaging results necessarily predict addiction, three salient changes in established and unrecovered substance-dependent individuals that cut across different drugs are decreases in orbitofrontal/prefrontal cortex function, decreases in brain dopamine D_2 receptors, and overactive brain stress systems. No biochemical markers are sufficiently specific to predict a given stage of the addiction cycle, but changes in certain intermediate early genes with chronic drug exposure in animal models show promise of long-term changes in specific brain regions that may be common to all drugs of abuse. Although there are no biological markers of substance abuse disorders on the immediate horizon, there are many promising and continually evolving biological and neurobiological features of substance use disorders that eventually will aid in the specific diagnoses of substance use, misuse, and dependence.

References

1. Koob GF, Le Moal M: Drug abuse: hedonic homeostatic dysregulation. Science 278:52–58, 1997.
2. Shippenberg TS, Koob GF: Recent advances in animal models of drug addiction and alcoholism, in Neuropsychopharmacology: The Fifth Generation of Progress. Edited by Davis KL, Charney D, Coyle JT, et al. Philadelphia, PA, Lippincott Williams & Wilkins, 2002, pp 1381–1397.
3. Koob GF, Le Moal M: Drug addiction, dysregulation of reward, and allostasis. Neuropsychopharmacology 24:97–129, 2001.
4. Koob GF: Allostatic view of motivation: implications for psychopathology, in Motivational Factors in the Etiology of Drug Abuse (Nebraska Symposium on Motivation, Vol 50). Edited by Bevins RA, Bardo MT. Lincoln, University of Nebraska Press, 2004, pp 1–18.
5. Koob GF, Sanna PP, Bloom FE: Neuroscience of addiction. Neuron 21:467–476, 1998.
6. Heimer L, Alheid G: Piecing together the puzzle of basal forebrain anatomy, in The Basal Forebrain: Anatomy to Function (Advances in Experimental Medicine and Biology, Vol 295). Edited by Napier TC, Kalivas PW, Hanin I. New York, Plenum, 1991, pp 1–42.
7. Markou A, Koob GF: Post-cocaine anhedonia: an animal model of cocaine withdrawal. Neuropsychopharmacology 4:17–26, 1991.
8. Schulteis G, Markou A, Gold LH, et al: Relative sensitivity to naloxone of multiple indices of opiate withdrawal: a quantitative dose–response analysis. J Pharmacol Exp Ther 271:1391–1398, 1994.
9. Schulteis G, Markou A, Cole M, et al: Decreased brain reward produced by ethanol withdrawal. Proc Natl Acad Sci USA 92:5880–5884, 1995.
10. Epping-Jordan MP, Watkins SS, Koob GF, et al: Dramatic decreases in brain reward function during nicotine withdrawal. Nature 393:76–79, 1998.
11. Gardner EL, Vorel SR: Cannabinoid transmission and reward-related events. Neurobiol Dis 5:502–533, 1998.
12. Paterson NE, Myers C, Markou A: Effects of repeated withdrawal from continuous amphetamine administration on brain reward function in rats. Psychopharmacology (Berl) 152:440–446, 2000.
13. Parsons LH, Justice JB Jr: Perfusate serotonin increases extracellular dopamine in the nucleus accumbens as measured by in vivo microdialysis. Brain Res 606:195–199, 1993.
14. Weiss F, Markou A, Lorang MT, et al: Basal extracellular dopamine levels in the nucleus accumbens are decreased during cocaine withdrawal after unlimited-access self-administration. Brain Res 593:314–318, 1992.
15. Stinus L, Le Moal M, Koob GF: Nucleus accumbens and amygdala are possible substrates for the aversive stimulus effects of opiate withdrawal. Neuroscience 37:767–773, 1990.
16. Roberts AJ, Cole M, Koob GF: Intra-amygdala muscimol decreases operant ethanol self-administration in dependent rats. Alcohol Clin Exp Res 20:1289–1298, 1996.

17. Weiss F, Parsons LH, Schulteis G, et al: Ethanol self-administration restores withdrawal-associated deficiencies in accumbal dopamine and 5-hydroxytryptamine release in dependent rats. J Neurosci 16:3474–3485, 1996.
18. Morrisett RA: Potentiation of *N*-methyl-D-aspartate receptor-dependent afterdischarges in rat dentate gyrus following in vitro ethanol withdrawal. Neurosci Lett 167: 175–178, 1994.
19. Davidson M, Shanley B, Wilce P: Increased NMDA-induced excitability during ethanol withdrawal: a behavioural and histological study. Brain Res 674:91–96, 1995.
20. Collins AC, Bhat RV, Pauly JR, et al: Modulation of nicotine receptors by chronic exposure to nicotinic agonists and antagonists, in The Biology of Nicotine Dependence (Ciba Foundation Symposium, Vol 152). Edited by Bock G, Marsh J. New York, John Wiley, 1990, pp 87–105.
21. Dani JA, Heinemann S: Molecular and cellular aspects of nicotine abuse. Neuron 16:905–908, 1996.
22. Rivier C, Bruhn T, Vale W: Effect of ethanol on the hypothalamic-pituitary-adrenal axis in the rat: role of corticotropin-releasing factor (CRF). J Pharmacol Exp Ther 229:127–131, 1984.
23. Merlo-Pich E, Lorang M, Yeganeh M, et al: Increase of extracellular corticotropin-releasing factor–like immunoreactivity levels in the amygdala of awake rats during restraint stress and ethanol withdrawal as measured by microdialysis. J Neurosci 15:5439–5447, 1995.
24. Koob GF, Heinrichs SC, Menzaghi F, et al: Corticotropin releasing factor, stress and behavior. Seminars in Neuroscience 6:221–229, 1994.
25. Rasmussen DD, Boldt BM, Bryant CA, et al: Chronic daily ethanol and withdrawal, 1: long-term changes in the hypothalamo-pituitary-adrenal axis. Alcohol Clin Exp Res 24:1836–1849, 2000.
26. Olive MF, Koenig HN, Nannini MA, et al: Elevated extracellular CRF levels in the bed nucleus of the stria terminalis during ethanol withdrawal and reduction by subsequent ethanol intake. Pharmacol Biochem Behav 72:213–220, 2002.
27. Delfs JM, Zhu Y, Druhan JP, et al: Noradrenaline in the ventral forebrain is critical for opiate withdrawal–induced aversion. Nature 403:430–434, 2000.
28. Roy A, Pandey SC: The decreased cellular expression of neuropeptide Y protein in rat brain structures during ethanol withdrawal after chronic ethanol exposure. Alcohol Clin Exp Res 26:796–803, 2002.
29. Heinrichs SC, Koob GF: Corticotropin-releasing factor in brain: a role in activation, arousal, and affect regulation. J Pharmacol Exp Ther 311:427–440, 2004.
30. Koob GF, Le Moal M: Plasticity of reward neurocircuitry and the "dark side" of drug addiction. Nat Neurosci 8:1442–1444, 2005.
31. Alheid GF, De Olmos JS, Beltramino CA: Amygdala and extended amygdala, in The Rat Nervous System. Edited by Paxinos G. San Diego, CA, Academic Press, 1995, pp 495–578.
32. McFarland K, Kalivas PW: The circuitry mediating cocaine-induced reinstatement of drug-seeking behavior. J Neurosci 21:8655–8663, 2001.
33. Everitt BJ, Wolf ME: Psychomotor stimulant addiction: a neural systems perspective. J Neurosci 22:3312–3320, 2002 (erratum 22(16):1a, 2002).

34. Weiss F, Ciccocioppo R, Parsons LH, et al: Compulsive drug-seeking behavior and relapse: neuroadaptation, stress, and conditioning factors. Ann N Y Acad Sci 937:1–26, 2001.
35. Shaham Y, Shalev U, Lu L, et al: The reinstatement model of drug relapse: history, methodology and major findings. Psychopharmacology (Berl) 168:3–20, 2003.
36. Shalev U, Grimm JW, Shaham Y: Neurobiology of relapse to heroin and cocaine seeking: a review. Pharmacol Rev 54:1–42, 2002.
37. Koob GF, Le Moal M: Neurobiology of Addiction. London, England, Academic Press, 2006.
38. Nestler EJ: Historical review: molecular and cellular mechanisms of opiate and cocaine addiction. Trends Pharmacol Sci 25:210–218, 2004.
39. Pandey SC: The gene transcription factor cyclic AMP–responsive element binding protein: role in positive and negative affective states of alcohol addiction. Pharmacol Ther 104:47–58, 2004.
40. McBride WJ, Murphy JM, Lumeng L, et al: Serotonin, dopamine and GABA involvement in alcohol drinking of selectively bred rats. Alcohol 7:199–205, 1990.
41. Murphy JM, Stewart RB, Bell RL, et al: Phenotypic and genotypic characterization of the Indiana University rat lines selectively bred for high and low alcohol preference. Behav Genet 32:363–388, 2002.
42. Carr LG, Foroud T, Bice P, et al: A quantitative trait locus for alcohol consumption in selectively bred rat lines. Alcohol Clin Exp Res 22:884–887, 1998.
43. Koob GF, Bartfai T, Roberts AJ: The use of molecular genetic approaches in the neuropharmacology of corticotropin-releasing factor. Int J Comp Psychol 14:90–110, 2001.
44. Contet C, Kieffer BL, Befort K: Mu opioid receptor: a gateway to drug addiction. Curr Opin Neurobiol 14:370–378, 2004.
45. Gaveriaux-Ruff C, Kieffer BL: Opioid receptor genes inactivated in mice: the highlights. Neuropeptides 36:62–71, 2002.
46. Zhang J, Xu M: Toward a molecular understanding of psychostimulant actions using genetically engineered dopamine receptor knockout mice as model systems. J Addict Dis 20:7–18, 2001.
47. Uhl GR, Lin Z: The top 20 dopamine transporter mutants: structure–function relationships and cocaine actions. Eur J Pharmacol 479:71–82, 2003.
48. Caine SB, Negus SS, Mello NK, et al: Role of dopamine D2–like receptors in cocaine self-administration: studies with D2 receptor mutant mice and novel D2 receptor antagonists. J Neurosci 22:2977–2988, 2002.
49. Bonson KR, Grant SJ, Contoreggi CS, et al: Neural systems and cue-induced cocaine craving. Neuropsychopharmacology 26:376–386, 2002.
50. Breiter HC, Aharon I, Kahneman D, et al: Functional imaging of neural responses to expectancy and experience of monetary gains and losses. Neuron 30:619–639, 2001.
51. Childress AR, Mozley PD, McElgin W, et al: Limbic activation during cue-induced cocaine craving. Am J Psychiatry 156:11–18, 1999.

4

CULTURAL AND SOCIETAL INFLUENCES ON SUBSTANCE USE DIAGNOSES AND CRITERIA

Robin Room, Ph.D.

This chapter is concerned with potential variations between cultures in the meaning and meaningfulness of five different diagnostic categories in the substance use disorders: dependence, abuse, harmful use, intoxication, and withdrawal. We are thus not concerned with differences between cultures in population rates of the diagnostic categories and of their criteria, but rather with prior questions of the meaningfulness and meaning of the criteria and diagnoses in different cultures.

There are two main traditions by which the issue of such cross-cultural variations has been addressed, primarily but not solely with reference to alcohol. One tradition starts from a position of universalism and philosophical realism, presuming that there is a single underlying dependence disorder applicable, for instance,

Work on the paper reprinted in this chapter was supported by the core grant of the Swedish Council for Working Life and Social Research (FAS) to the Centre for Social Research on Alcohol and Drugs (SoRAD), Stockholm University.

Reprinted from Room R: "Taking Account of Cultural and Societal Influences on Sunstance Use Diagnoses and Criteria" *Addiction* 101 (suppl 1):31–39, 2006. Used with permission of the Society for the Study of Addiction.

to all humankind. The tradition may recognize problems in applying a diagnosis or instrument in a particular culture, but the solution to the problems lies in finding new operationalizations—the universal applicability of the underlying concept is not questioned. This has been the mainline position of American psychiatric epidemiology since the "St. Louis revolution," and it is probably difficult for many of us to set it aside and consider alternative perspectives.

The alternative tradition is more nominalist and particularistic, viewing substance use diagnoses as culturally influenced and allowing for the possibility that the cultural influence in framing the criteria or diagnoses can be strong enough that they are inherently different in different cultures. This tradition applies to the field of diagnostic concepts and instruments (e.g., ethnographic perspectives on cultural variations in the meaning of substance use and intoxication as developed for alcohol by MacAndrew and Edgerton[1]).

In his late writing about alcoholism, Jellinek was the first modern proponent of this way of thinking about substance use diagnoses. Jellinek was a thoroughgoing nominalist about what counts as a disease or disorder—more thoroughgoing than I would choose to be: for instance, when he said that "it comes to this, that a *disease is what the medical profession recognizes as such.*"[2] His late definition expanded the frame of "alcoholism" so that it lost most of its specific meaning—"any use of alcoholic beverages that causes damage to the individual or society or both"[2]—and his Greek-letter types of alcoholism within this overarching frame essentially reflected the different "species" he had heard described as alcoholism by doctors from different countries at World Health Organization (WHO) meetings: gamma alcoholism was the "Anglo-Saxon" (i.e., American) species, delta alcoholism the French, and epsilon the Finnish.[3]

Findings of Existing Studies on Cross-Cultural Equivalence and Variation

In recent decades, there has been considerable research on the cross-cultural applicability of substance use disorder criteria and diagnoses, particularly for alcohol. Many of these studies have been framed in the paradigm of the realist and universalist tradition. For example, the book by Helzer and Canino[4] on studies conducted with the Diagnostic Interview Schedule (DIS) instrument relies primarily on the fact of common methodology and that usable data could be produced as its warrants of comparability across a variety of studies,[5] but does include some side comments about issues of applicability. Another study, a side-product of the WHO collaborative project that produced the Alcohol Use Disorders Identification Test (AUDIT), performed principal-component factor analyses in each of six diverse cultures of 13 alcohol dependence items covering aspects of impaired control, salience of drinking, tolerance and withdrawal.[6] The analysis found a strong general factor in each factor analysis, with very high Cronbach alphas, and interpreted the results as support for "the hypothesis that the Alcohol Dependence syndrome has considerable cross-cultural generalizability, regardless of treatment ideology, culturally learned drinking patterns or societal response to drinking problems." However, the paper also found that the dependence score formed from the items correlated quite highly with frequency of drinking 12+ drinks on an occasion (0.67–0.86) and with a logged score of alcohol-related personal, social, and health problems (0.65–0.89). These findings are further evidence of cross-cultural commonality but raise the question: commonality in what terms? Is it specifically the alcohol dependence syndrome that serves as the engine of the cross-cultural commonalities, or might it as well be the symptomatology of frequent intoxication or the experience of alcohol-related problems?

Another study was focused more specifically on assessing the validity of *Diagnostic and Statistical Manual* (DSM) and *International Classification of Diseases* (ICD) diagnoses cross-culturally, with test–retest and cross-instrument comparisons. However, the primary weight in the main round of published analyses from this study[7,8] was on analyses combining the different sites. The main site-specific comparative analysis in this series[9] found substantial variation across sites in test–retest reliability, with Sydney, Australia, showing the highest reliability on seven of nine current alcohol dependence items (Sydney range: 0.73–0.90), and Bangalore, India, showing the lowest on all nine items (Bangalore range: 0.29– 0.53). The results in Jebel, Romania, were closer to those for Sydney than to those for Bangalore. Sydney and Jebel both also showed relatively high reliability on two alcohol abuse items, while again Bangalore showed lower reliability. Examining the patterns of discrepancies, the authors concluded that the Bangalore respondents appeared to have "difficulty understanding the constructs underlying the questions."

The alternative tradition relies on a broader range of types of evidence, reaching outside the bounds of DSM or ICD instruments. Some of the evidence comes from quantitative studies in the realist/universalist tradition, which, like that of Chatterji et al.[9] just noted, have sometimes produced findings that are problematic for the paradigm. Thus Klausner and Foulks[10] were stimulated by the outrage of their subjects at the practical impact of their study (including an abrupt fall in the market value of the community's municipal bonds) to return to their data for a kind of after-the-fact protocol analysis of what their Inuit respondents could have meant in their answers to the items of the Michigan Alcoholism Screening Test (MAST). Somewhat ruefully, the authors concluded that many of the MAST items might well have a different meaning in an Arctic indigenous culture than, for instance, in urban Michigan. Applying the Munich Alcoholism Test (MALT) developed in Germany to samples in Spain and Ecuador, Gorenc et al.[11] found that 5 of the 31 items were "relatively free of cultural differences" by their criteria, but the authors added that none of the 5 items as used in Ecuador passed the filters used to screen out items when the test was developed in Germany. Drawing on historical and anthropological studies, I argued 20 years ago[12] that perhaps alcohol dependence should be viewed as a "culture-bound syndrome," with a specific history and cultural inception that starts with the early American temperance movement.[13]

The most extensive study so far drawing on this more phenomenological tradition was the nine-site WHO study of the cross-cultural applicability of the substance use disorders.[14–16] With limited resources and time for the data collection, the study's ambitious program of key informant interviews, focus groups, and reference case interviews was only partly carried out, and the analyses rely principally on the key informant interviews with knowledgeable local professionals and laypeople—20 at each site concerning alcohol concepts and terms and 20 concerning the drug with the highest apparent rate of harmful use at the site. The study identified problems of cross-cultural applicability at the level of instrument items, at the level of criteria, and at the level of concepts and diagnoses. Some problems at the item level were easily solved: phrases such as "driving an automobile or operating a machine" obviously require adaptation. Others were less tractable: it was noted that "the diagnostic criteria and their operationalizations assume a self-consciousness about feelings, knowledge and consciousness which is foreign to the folk traditions of some cultures."[15] Thus there was no accurate translation in one or another society for words such as "feel" and "anxiety." Items and criteria "often also have built-in attributional, causal and other relational assumptions which are not customary in some languages and cultures." Thus formulations such as "trouble because of drinking," "after you had realized it had caused you," and "where it increased your chances of getting hurt" and items mentioning intentions presume "both self-consciousness and a style of causal attribution which is unrecognizable in some cultures."[15] The problems posed by such items are not merely a problem of translation. Built into the DSM and ICD criteria are formulations that reach across and connect different domains of meaning. Thus, for instance, "the substance use continued despite knowledge of having a...problem that is likely to have been caused or exacerbated by the substance" is a criterion that requires connecting together acknowledgments of use, of a problem, and of cognition about a causal relation between the two. The attribution of causality to alcohol and drug use, in particular, varies across cultures, and for that matter has varied in different periods within cultures.[16,17] The study identified several different types of difficulty with the criteria for dependence. In some cultures there was no term for the criterion; in others the meanings of two criteria overlapped; while in still others the criterion was not considered of diagnostic significance.[15]

In the context of categorical diagnoses and criteria, the issue of the threshold at which an item or criterion is considered positive becomes particularly important.[16] The WHO cross-cultural applicability study found many instances of different thresholds being applied. Where use of the substance is particularly suspect, the thresholds may be set very low. Thus in Bangalore, several reference cases qualified as positive on three or four alcohol dependence criteria on the basis of drinking a maximum of three drinks up to three times a month.[15] Conversely, in Athens and in Santander, Spain, where regular drinking is normalized, thresholds for what is problematized were set much higher.[16] We may expect the same kinds of cross-cultural variation for other drugs according to the social acceptability and familiarity of the substance. Whether and how a threshold is defined is important in distinctions between normal drinking or drug use and harmful use or intoxication,[14] and between hangover and withdrawal,[15] as well for the criteria of dependence.

Societal Framing of Diagnosis

The issue of divergent thresholds brings to the fore the fact that clinical diagnoses in the alcohol and drug area, more than most other diagnoses, usually carry a weight of moral judgment, whatever the clinician's intentions. Of course, it is not that all use is always negatively evaluated. In most human societies, one or another psychoactive substance is a valued commodity for human ingestion. Human use values for psychoactive substances are varied[18]—to ensure wakefulness, to promote sleep, to bring euphoria, to deaden pain, to pursue a transcendent experience, to quench thirst, as a nutrient, as a medium of commensality and sociability, as a signal of exclusion, and so on. The same substance often has apparently contradictory use values, sometimes simultaneously.

On the other hand, use of psychoactive substances beyond some socially defined limit (or, in some cases, at all) is commonly moralized and stigmatized. One has only to mention terms such as *drug fiend, demon rum,* and the *scourge* or *menace* of drugs to recognize the extent to which drug use is often stigmatized. In many societies a common means of derogating opponents is to label them as drunks or drug users[19]; hence, as a policy of political prophylaxis, the ban on alcohol at the December 2004 encampments of the "Orange Revolution" in Kiev.[20] Another WHO study, of the cross-cultural applicability of disability concepts and measures in 14 societies, found some variation between societies in the ranking by informants of "alcoholism" and "drug addiction" in terms of degree of stigma[21] (Table 4–1). However, the overall picture was that both conditions were ranked as among the most stigmatized of 18 conditions, roughly on a par with being "dirty and unkempt" and having a "criminal record for burglary." The moralization of drinking or drug use, beyond thresholds that vary between cultures, seems to be one commonality we can find between many modern societies.

To a certain extent, the stigmatization is built into the diagnostic terminology of DSM-IV. This is most obvious in the use of the term *abuse.* Accordingly, in 1993 the Board of the American Society of Addiction Medicine, "while recognizing that 'abuse' is part of present diagnostic terminology," recommended "that an alternative term be found for this purpose because of the pejorative connotations of the word 'abuse.'"[22] It can be argued that the term *dependence* also came with some built-in stigma; when it was adopted in the 1960s and 1970s by WHO com-

TABLE 4–1. Degree of social disapproval or stigma

Condition (ordering in total sample)	Country													
	Canada	China	Egypt	Greece	India	Japan	Luxem-bourg	Nether-lands	Nigeria	Romania	Spain	Tunisia	Turkey	UK
Wheelchair bound (1)	2	3	1	5	2	5	2	2	1	3	2	1	1	2
Blind (2)	1	5	2	2	4	9	1	1	3	1	1	2	3	1
Inability to read (3)	6	6	3	3	1	2	5	3	2	5	4	5	2	6
Borderline intelligence (4)	3	4	4	7	5	7	3	4	5	7	5	7	6	4
Obese (5)	9	1	5	1	3	1	4	7	4	4	6	3	14	11
Depression (6)	5	2	10	4	6	15	6	6	9	2	3	12	5	3
Dementia (7)	4	8	7	6	9	10	9	8	7	8	7	4	9	5
Facial disfigurement (8)	7	7	8	8	8	3	7	10	6	6	8	9	8	7
Cannot hold down a job (9)	10	11	12	10	10	4	8	9	11	10	11	11	7	10
Homeless (10)	16	9	6	9	7	12	13	15	8	16	10	8	12	8
Chronic mental disorder (11)	12	13	11	12	14	17	10	8	15	9	9	10	10	12
Leprosy (12)	11	16	9	15	13	11	11	11	18	13	14	6	13	9
Dirty and unkempt (13)	15	14	13	11	12	8	12	12	12	12	13	13	11	14

TABLE 4–1. Degree of social disapproval or stigma *(continued)*

Condition (ordering in total sample)	Country													
	Canada	China	Egypt	Greece	India	Japan	Luxem-bourg	Nether-lands	Nigeria	Romania	Spain	Tunisia	Turkey	UK
Does not take care of their children (14)	18	10	16	14	11	6	16	14	10	11	15	17	4	17
Alcoholism (15)	8	12	15	13	15	14	15	16	13	14	12	14	17	15
Criminal record for burglary (16)	13	17	17	16	16	13	17	17	17	18	16	15	15	16
HIV positive (17)	14	18	14	18	17	16	14	13	14	15	18	16	16	13
Drug addiction (18)	17	15	18	17	18	18	18	18	16	17	17	18	18	18
Number of informants	15	15	16	15	47	18	16	13	15	15	18	15	15	12

Note. Relative ordering from lowest to highest mean rating within each country (ranking of 1 indicates least stigma, ranking of 18 indicates most stigma).

Source. Room et al.[21,p.276]

mittees, it already carried a baggage of discreditable previous meanings in the United States, as in "dependent personality" or "welfare dependency."[23]

Whatever diagnostic terminology is employed, the diagnoses are used primarily in clinical settings late in a process that begins in everyday life and interactions. Typically, for a majority of the cases coming into an alcohol- or drug-specific treatment service, someone—a spouse, another family member, a judge, a social worker—has made a judgment that there is a problem needing clinical attention. In fact, of those entering alcohol treatment in a California county, over 40% had received an ultimatum from someone to enter treatment, in 24% of the cases from a family member.[24] In such circumstances, a de facto part of the diagnostic decision-tree is the threshold at which family, friends, or officials in the society notice a behavior and decide that it should be brought to professional attention. Often attached to these processes of "noticing," as Table 4–1 implies, is a great deal of stigmatization.

One decision for DSM is whether and to what extent a medical diagnostic system should build these essentially social judgments into the diagnosis and criteria, and to what extent it should seek to build diagnoses and criteria that are independent of them. This is the primary issue on which DSM-IV and ICD-10 parted company, with ICD-10's "harmful use" in principle excluding negative social consequences or reactions of others to drug use as evidence of harmful use,[25,pp.74–75] while DSM-IV's "abuse" was primarily built around them. I have noted that this divergence "reflects a long-standing difference between British and American psychiatry, with the British taking the view that social reactions and consequences do not belong in definitions of diseases and disorders."[3] Behind this difference, I believe, lie not only differences about the inclusion of stigmatizing terms in the diagnostic system, but also the very different institutional frames of British and American psychiatry. In the context of the National Health Service, British psychiatry has been in a good position to define for itself the limits of its reach, with little to lose from turning away cases that fall outside those limits. In the absence of a national health system, the social environment of American psychiatry has been more entrepreneurial and less inclined to decide collectively that cases lie outside its competence. "A health system like the American, characterized by fee-for-service and managed care," has encouraged inclusiveness in the criteria and thresholds, so it is "unlikely that a clinician will have to turn away anyone appearing for treatment on the grounds that they do not qualify for the diagnosis."[3]

To the extent this judgment is right, it underlines that cultural differences in the nature of alcohol and drug problems that are presented to the health system reflect not only cultural differences in norms and behaviors around substance use, but also societal and cultural differences in how alcohol and drug problems are defined and handled. That is, the difference between the British and American views is a reflection not so much of differences in the nature of alcohol and drug use (in a global perspective, these differences are not very great), but of differences in the way that problems from the use are handled.

DSM started as a diagnostic manual for the United States, but it has obviously taken on a much broader significance. The efforts to conform the substance use diagnoses and criteria in DSM-IV and ICD-10[3] exemplify the fact that DSM has a global reach. In this context, it seems important to take into account that problem definitions and social handling systems for alcohol and drug problems differ considerably in different societies. For instance, to include "abuse" within the competence of psychiatrists and other clinicians may make sense in the context of the U.S. system, with its strong interlinkage with the criminal justice system, but may make less sense elsewhere.

To take one example, in Sweden, where the general lay term for those with alcohol or drug problems translates as "misusers," the primary institutional frame for alcohol and drug treatment (accounting for two-thirds of it) has long been the social welfare system, with the health-based system taking on specific tasks such as detoxification and opiate maintenance.[26] The Swedish system thus does not need a medical diagnosis of "abuse" to function. It is not that Swedish doctors ignore alcohol and drug problems; in fact, there has been a long tradition of concern by Swedish doctors about alcohol problems, but the fairly consistent theme for a century has been that, while there are medical aspects such as cirrhosis, the problem is primarily social in nature.[27]

What Might Be Done?

For the following discussion, I take as one of my cues the comments by Marc Schuckit at a symposium on the validity of DSM-IV dependence, including the possibility of moving toward a dimensional approach.[28] Another cue is the fact that by international treaty, national diagnostic systems must be based on the ICD, which means that a DSM classification has to be fitted within the frame of ICD diagnoses. The other cues for the discussion come from the findings of the studies of cross-cultural comparability:

- The wording should avoid, as far as possible, causally attributive language; reference to feeling and affect states; combining different conceptual domains in the same item; and culturally specific circumstances or activities (except as examples); and
- The threshold of any application should be specified; and in the case of a dimensional approach, the degrees of severity should be specified.

It is recognized that reference to feeling and affect states cannot be avoided for one of the diagnoses, dependence, discussed below.

My suggestions for directions of work are specified in terms of five current diagnoses (three shared by ICD-10 and DSM-IV, and harmful use from ICD-10 and abuse from DSM-IV).

INTOXICATION

The current DSM-IV criteria for intoxication are focused around behavior rather than around extent of intake of the substance per se. It is clear from the anthropological literature[29] and from the qualitative cross-cultural studies[15] that there are substantial cultural differences in what are regarded as signs of alcohol intoxication, reflecting differences both in amounts of drinking equated with intoxication and in cultural expectations and norms on behavior while intoxicated.[30] Similar variations can be expected for other psychoactive substances.

One clear choice here would be to move toward setting the intoxication diagnosis on a physiological basis, as a measure of recent ingestion of substantial amounts of the substance (or, in a dimensional approach, as a quantified measure of recent ingestion). In the case of alcohol, consideration for standard measurements to use should include not only interview questions[31] and the familiar blood-alcohol measure but also a diversity of biological measures that give quantified evidence of recent alcohol use.[32–34] The extent to which such measures are available or can be developed also for other substances should be considered. The development of useful interview questions on quantity of intake of controlled substances has already been identified as a priority for the United States.[35]

A quantitative threshold or scale of intoxication is potentially a culture-free measure that is clinically relevant. There will, of course, be individual and culturally mediated differences in the behavior associated with the intoxication. As required, these could be measured separately, and then correlated to the intoxication measure.

WITHDRAWAL

The DSM criteria start with cessation or reduction of use of the substance, and a requirement of at least two (alcohol, amphetamines, cocaine, sedatives), three (opioids) or four (nicotine) physical or psychological signs, depending on the substance group. But there is also a third criterion, of "clinically significant distress or impairment in social, occupational or other important areas of functioning." The "impairment" alternative in this criterion C obviously opens the door to a great deal of variation by culture and circumstance. Is it really desirable to have a particular state qualify as withdrawal on a working day, for instance, but not on a holiday, or not for a pensioner, as the "occupational functioning" subcriterion would imply?

In the WHO cross-cultural applicability study, withdrawal was as subject to cultural variation as the psychological symptoms.[16] The main issue was cultural variation in thresholds of severity, with those in the "wet" wine cultures inclined to set relatively low thresholds and no clear distinction from hangovers, and informants in cultures in which drinking was viewed more problematically tending to give rather grave signs. Work is needed on developing specifications for thresholds for the different withdrawal signs that would reduce to a minimum cultural variation in the thresholds. It seems that, in principle, it should also be possible to develop biological measures of withdrawal that would presumably further reduce the role of cultural variation.

HARMFUL USE (ICD-10)

Harmful use is defined as "a pattern of substance use that is causing damage to health" (physical or mental). The "diagnostic criteria for research" specify that "there must be clear evidence that the substance use was responsible for (or substantially contributed to) physical or psychological harm, including impaired judgment or dysfunctional behavior, which may lead to disability or have adverse consequences for interpersonal relationships," that "the nature of the harm should be clearly identifiable (and specified)" and that "the pattern of use has persisted for at least 1 month or has occurred repeatedly within a 12-month period."

Harmful use has generally not performed very well in the test–retest studies,[36] and informants in the cross-cultural applicability study gave diverse characterizations of harm, often ranging well outside the limits of physical and mental health.[16] One problem with ascertaining harmful use from questions to patients or clients is that of all types of harm, health harms are the most difficult for non-specialists to report validly.[37]

The best use of this diagnostic category, in my view, would be as a measure of patterns of heavy use over time (sporadic or continuous, say in the last 12 months) that carry a high risk of physical or mental harm. Heavy use may eventually be amenable to biological testing, but in the meantime it could be captured by questions on patterns of heavy consumption.[31] Again, there will be a need to specify threshold and levels.

Intoxication and harmful use would thus be a complementary pair, with intoxication measuring short-term (event-related) consumption, and harmful use measuring patterning of consumption over recent time.

It must be recognized that what is being proposed here is a version of hazardous use,[38] which was rejected as a diagnostic category in the ICD-10 decision process because it was not in itself a disorder. A partial way past this objection would be to specify levels of consumption at which physical or psychological damage is measurable.

SUBSTANCE ABUSE (DSM-IV)

The category of substance abuse has also generally not performed very well in test–retest studies.[36] It also does not hang together very well in terms of scaling,[8] although in my view there is no reason to expect the criteria that compose it to be held together more than by the fact of at least occasional heavy use of the substance involved.

The criteria for substance abuse deal with the realms of social roles and social and societal reactions to the substance user's behavior. Deciding on what would be the equivalents in terms of failure in work role for a shepherd and an airline pilot in a way that is culture-free seems difficult, to say the least. Furthermore, the criteria build in the societal reaction to the behavior—for instance, in the "legal problems" of the third criterion, "expulsion from school" in the first criterion, and the "social or interpersonal problems" of the fourth criterion. An ambition to construct a measure of or criteria for "abuse" that will not be culture-bound thus seems fruitless. A further difficulty for cross-cultural comparisons is that causal connections are built into the criteria ("resulting in" in the first criterion, and "caused or exacerbated" in the third), and such conceptualizations caused difficulties in the cross-cultural applicability study.

A logical solution would be to transfer the recording of the phenomena now measured as abuse to Axes III and IV of the DSM system (mental problems would be coded elsewhere in Axis I). This would reflect the reality that the problems covered by the abuse criteria are mainly not health conditions in the usual sense. An alternative would be to retain a version of the substance abuse criteria with a notation that these criteria are developed for application only in U.S. society, and other societies should develop their own culturally appropriate measures in this area. This alternative still begs the question, however, of whether such an "unwise" behavior as driving after drinking, which accounted for half the alcohol abuse cases in a U.S. community sample, is treated appropriately as "a psychiatric disorder."[39]

DEPENDENCE

The criteria for dependence received the most attention in the cross-cultural applicability study,[15,16] as noted above. The study found a number of problems in their cross-cultural applicability. Essentially, the criteria bring together three conceptually different domains: physical dependence (tolerance and withdrawal), loss or impairment of self-control over substance use, and consequences of use. The consequences are explicit in the seventh criterion, which corresponds roughly to harmful use in ICD-10, and implicit to a varying extent in several others, most notably in the fifth: "a great deal of time spent in activities" around the substance, and the sixth: "important social, occupational or recreational activities given up or reduced because of substance use."

My suggestion, in the light of the suggestions for the other diagnoses discussed earlier, would be to "unpack" the present diagnosis and center it around the related experiences of craving, feelings of compulsion and loss or impairment of control. That is, the core of the diagnosis would be composed from the third and fourth criteria in DSM-IV and the first in ICD-10 ("a strong desire or sense of compulsion to take the substance").

Such a diagnosis, while still including a range of content, would be located solidly in the realm of the user's experiences and evaluations of his or her use. The greater conceptual coherence of the diagnosis would strengthen our ability to analyze the interrelations and contingencies of different aspects of substance use. It might thus give biological researchers a better target for their animal and other modeling. It would certainly map more readily onto public conceptions of addiction, alcoholism, or dependence.[40]

Withdrawal would still be measured as a separate diagnosis. Tolerance turned out to be a difficult criterion in the cross-cultural applicability study[15,16]; a number of different meanings were assigned to it, and in several places it was not considered to be associated with addiction. But if it were desired to keep tolerance diagnostically, it could perhaps be added in with withdrawal in a diagnosis of "physiological dependence" (although the term is now problematic, ironically in view of the term's history).

The fifth and sixth criteria (combined in a single criterion in ICD-10) are conditioned substantially by the social and cultural circumstances. Where the substance is readily and widely available (tobacco everywhere; wine in Spain), the issue of "time spent" seemed irrelevant to informants in the cross-cultural applicability study. The notion of "time spent" is also, to some degree, culturally conditioned; in Bangalore, "time was not viewed as a scarce or expendable commodity." Giving up activities for drinking seemed irrelevant in Romania; it was remarked that "almost all pleasures are related to alcohol consumption."[15] It is difficult to see how these criteria could be reformulated to be more culture-free.

In one sense, it can certainly be argued that a dependence diagnosis reformulated around the experience of impairment or loss of control and related concepts would also be culturally conditioned. Certainly, the argument that addiction concepts have a specific temporal and cultural history[12] implies that there are times and places where such concepts would not be meaningful. Here, for example, are Kunitz and Levy[41] describing the change in Navaho culture by which an addiction concept became meaningful:

> 19th century Navaho drinkers did not for the most part define themselves as sick in the same way as health professionals do. As the society changes, however, these behaviors increasingly come to be seen as maladaptive to the new world where people are expected to be at work on time; where no network of kin is available to help when a husband is out drinking; where bills must be paid; and where all sorts of obligations the dominant society takes for granted must be fulfilled.... In the new society that is emerging, older patterns of behavior are increasingly defined as in some way deviant. The drinker's behavior comes to be defined as sick. He is no longer a man who drinks a lot; he is an alcoholic. (pp. 254–255)

By now, however, an addiction or dependence concept is broadly used in much of the world, although there are certainly culturally specific nuances in its meaning. The criteria suggested here for the diagnosis are not directly dependent on interpersonal and social reactions. The desire to cut down or the intention to limit use may indeed be influenced by the wishes or mandates of others, but the wishes or mandates are not built into the criteria themselves. Instead, the criteria are organized around the user's own cognitive and affective experiences with respect to his or her use.

In revising the actual criteria for the diagnosis, attention might be paid to experience not only with the diagnostic instruments but also with various relevant assessment measures, such as the Alcohol Craving Questionnaire and the Impaired Control Scale.[42]

Conclusion

While there is much in the existing literature to draw upon, a substantial program of research and developmental work would be required to move in the directions recommended here. Reanalyses of existing data sets, both qualitative and quantitative, can contribute to the refinement of conceptualizations and measures. But if diagnoses, criteria, and instruments are to be truly cross-culturally applicable, there is a need for cross-cultural testing in the developmental phase, with a substantial program of work using such methods as key informant interviews and reference case or protocol analysis studies. Quantitative studies of test–retest reliability and convergent validation, for instance, should follow, but the purpose of these studies is more negative than positive: to establish that the measures meet acceptable standards across a range of societies, rather than establishing validity in any absolute sense. The possibility should be held open that some diagnoses or criteria should be specified as having a bounded applicability: to apply in a specified range of societies but not necessarily outside them.

References

1. MacAndrew C, Edgerton RB: Drunken Comportment: A Social Explanation. Chicago, IL, Aldine, 1969.
2. Jellinek EM: The Disease Concept of Alcoholism. New Brunswick, NJ, Hillhouse Press, 1960.
3. Room R: Alcohol and drug disorders in the International Classification of Diseases: a shifting kaleidoscope. Drug Alcohol Rev 17:305–317, 1998.
4. Helzer JE, Canino GJ (eds): Alcoholism in North America, Europe, and Asia. New York, Oxford University Press, 1992.
5. Helzer J: A wealth of data and experience on which it will be essential to capitalize. Addiction 91:223–225, 1996.
6. Hall W, Saunders JB, Babor TF, et al: The structure and correlates of alcohol dependence: WHO collaborative project on the early detection of persons with harmful alcohol consumption–III. Addiction 88:1627–1636, 1993.
7. Cottler LB, Hasin D, Grant BF (eds): WHO study on the reliability and validity of the alcohol and drug use disorder instruments (thematic section). Drug Alcohol Depend 47:159–226, 1997.
8. Nelson CB, Rehm J, Üstün TB, et al: Factor structures for DSM-IV substance disorder criteria endorsed by alcohol, cannabis, cocaine and opiate users: results from the WHO reliability and validity study. Addiction 94:843–855, 1999.
9. Chatterji S, Saunders JB, Vrasti R, et al: Reliability of the alcohol and drug modules of the Alcohol Use Disorder and Associated Disabilities Interview Schedule—Alcohol/Drug—Revised (AUDADIS-ADR): an international comparison. Drug Alcohol Depend 47:171–185, 1997.
10. Klausner SZ, Foulks EF: Eskimo Capitalists: Oil, Politics and Alcohol. Totowa, NJ, Allanheld, Osmun, 1982.

11. Gorenc K-D, Bruner CA, Nadelsticher A, et al: A cross-cultural study: a comparison of German, Spanish and Ecuadorian alcoholics using the Munich Alcoholism Test (MALT). Am J Drug Alcohol Abuse 10:429–446, 1984.
12. Room R: Dependence and society. Br J Addict 80:133–139, 1985. Available online at http://www.bks.no/dep-soc.pdf. Accessed July 5, 2006.
13. Levine HG: The discovery of addiction: changing conceptions of habitual drunkenness in America. J Stud Alcohol 39:143–174, 1978.
14. Bennett L, Janca A, Grant BF, et al: Boundaries between normal and pathological drinking: a cross-cultural comparison. Alcohol Health Res World 17:190–195, 1993.
15. Room R, Janca A, Bennett LA, et al: WHO cross-cultural applicability research on diagnosis and assessment of substance use disorders: an overview of methods and selected results. Addiction 91:199–220, 1996.
16. Schmidt L, Room R: Cross-cultural applicability in international classifications research on alcohol dependence. J Stud Alcohol 60:448–462, 1999.
17. Levine HG: The good creature of God and demon rum: colonial American and 19th century ideas about alcohol, crime and accidents, in Alcohol and Disinhibition: Nature and Meaning of the Link. NIAAA Research Monograph No 12, DHHS Publ No (ADM) 83–1246. Edited by Room R, Collins G. Washington, DC, National Institute on Alcohol Abuse and Alcoholism, 1983, pp 111–171.
18. Mäkelä K: The uses of alcohol and their cultural regulation. Acta Sociol 26:21–31, 1983.
19. Bielewicz A, Moskalewicz J: Temporary prohibition: the Gdansk experience, August 1980. Contemp Drug Probl 11:367–381, 1982.
20. Holley D: Snowy tent city holds soul of Ukraine protest. Los Angeles Times, November 28, 2004.
21. Room R, Rehm J, Trotter RT II, et al: Cross-cultural views on stigma valuation parity and societal attitudes towards disability, in Disability and Culture: Universalism and Diversity. Edited by Üstün TB, Chatterji S, Bickenbach JE, et al. Seattle, WA, Hofgrebe & Huber, 2001, pp 247–291.
22. Graham AW, Schultz TK (eds): Principles of Addiction Medicine, 2nd Edition. Chevy Chase, MD, American Society of Addiction Medicine, 1998.
23. Fraser N, Gordon L: A genealogy of dependency: tracing a keyword of the US welfare state. Signs (Chic)19:309–336, 1994.
24. Polcin DL, Weisner C: Factors associated with coercion in entering treatment for alcohol problems. Drug Alcohol Depend 54:63–68, 1999.
25. World Health Organization: The ICD-10 Classification of Mental and Behavioral Disorders: Clinical Descriptions and Diagnostic Guidelines. Geneva, Switzerland, World Health Organization, 1992.
26. Room R, Palm J, Romelsjö A, et al: Kvinnor och män i svensk missbruksbehandling. Bescrivning av en studie i Stockholms län [Women and men in alcohol and drug treatment: an overview of a Stockholm County study]. Nord Alkohol & Narkotikatidskr 20:91–100, 2003. English version available at http://nat.stakes.fi/nr/exeres/bf3172eb-97fb-4964-94b8-3bf185497813.htm. Accessed July 5, 2006.
27. Fleming R: The management of chronic alcoholism in England, Scandinavia and central Europe. N Engl J Med 216:279–289, 1937.

28. Hasin DS, Schuckit MA, Martin CS, et al: The validity of DSM-IV alcohol dependence: what do we know and what do we need to know? Alcohol Clin Exp Res 27:244–252, 2003.
29. Room R: Intoxication and bad behaviour: understanding cultural differences in the link. Soc Sci Med 53:189–198, 2001.
30. Room R, Bullock S: Can alcohol expectancies and attributions explain western Europe's north–south gradient in alcohol's role in violence? Contemp Drug Probl 29:619–648, 2002.
31. Gmel G, Rehm J: Measuring alcohol consumption. Contemp Drug Probl 31:467–540, 2004.
32. Helander A, Eriksson CJP: Laboratory tests for acute alcohol consumption: results of the WHO/ISBRA Study on State and Trait Markers of Alcohol Use and Dependence. Alcohol Clin Exp Res 26:1070–1077, 2002.
33. Wurst M, Metzger J: The ethanol conjugate ethyl glucuronide is a useful marker of recent alcohol consumption. Alcohol Clin Exp Res 26:1114–1119, 2002.
34. Allen JP, Sillanaukee P, Strid N, et al: Biomarkers of heavy drinking, in Assessing Alcohol Problems: A Guide for Clinicians and Researchers, 2nd Edition. NIH Publication No 03–3745. Edited by Allen JP, Wilson VB. Bethesda, MD, National Institute on Alcohol Abuse and Alcoholism, 2003, pp 37–53. Available online at http://pubs.niaaa.nih.gov/publications/Assesing%20Alcohol/index.pdf.
35. Manski C, Pepper J, Petrie C (eds): Informing America's Policy on Illegal Drugs: What We Don't Know Keeps Hurting Us. Washington, DC, National Academy of Sciences, 2001.
36. Üstün B, Compton W, Mager D, et al: WHO study on the reliability and validity of the alcohol and drug use disorder instruments: overview of methods and results. Drug Alcohol Depend 47:161–169, 1997.
37. Greenfield TK: What's in a problem? Type and seriousness of harmful effects of drinking on health, based on a pilot U.S. national telephone survey. Presented at the 21st Annual Alcohol Epidemiology Symposium, Kettil Bruun Society for Social and Epidemiological Research on Alcohol, Porto, Portugal, June 1995.
38. Babor TB, Campbell R, Room R, et al: Lexicon of Alcohol and Drug Terms. Geneva, Switzerland, World Health Organization, 1994. Available online at http://www.who.int/substance_abuse/terminology/who_lexicon/en. Accessed July 5, 2006.
39. Hasin D, Paykin A, Endicott J, et al: Validity of DSM-IV alcohol abuse: drunk drivers versus all others. J Stud Alcohol 60:746–755, 1999.
40. Room R: Drugs, consciousness and self-control: popular and medical conceptions. International Review Journal of Psychiatry 1:63–70, 1989.
41. Kunitz SJ, Levy JE: Changing ideas of alcohol use among Navaho Indians. Q J Stud Alcohol 35:243–259, 1974.
42. Maisto SA, McKay JR, Tiffany ST: Diagnosis, in Assessing Alcohol Problems: A Guide for Clinicians and Researchers, 2nd Edition. NIH Publication No 03–3745. Edited by Allen JP, Wilson VB. Bethesda, MD, National Institute on Alcohol Abuse and Alcoholism, 2003, pp 55–73. Available online at http://pubs.niaaa.nih.gov/publications/Assesing%20Alcohol/index.pdf. Accessed July 5, 2006.

5

CULTURAL ISSUES AND PSYCHIATRIC DIAGNOSIS

Providing a General Background for Considering Substance Use Diagnoses

Javier I. Escobar, M.D.
William A. Vega, Ph.D.

The goal of this review is to establish a general context on the topic of cross-cultural diagnosis and suggest how it can be applied to substance use disorders.

Psychiatric diagnosis has advanced considerably since the development of the third edition of the *Diagnostic and Statistical Manual for Mental Disorders* (DSM-III), and there is a good deal of confidence among researchers and practitioners about their ability to make psychiatric diagnoses that seem valid and reliable. Thus, in the last two decades, psychiatric diagnosis has attained an aura of respectability in North America and many other countries of the world. Although reliability of research diagnoses elicited with structured diagnostic instruments is reasonably good, this does not appear to be the case in day-to-day practice. Although developed for a North American population, DSM has been exported to the rest of the world—a fact that raises a number of issues about its cross-cultural applicability.

Reprinted from Escobar JI, Vega WA: "Cultural Issues and Psychiatric Diagnosis: Providing a General Background for Considering Substance Use Diagnoses." *Addiction* 101 (suppl 1): 40–47, 2006. Used with permission of the Society for the Study of Addiction.

The cross-cultural limitations of the DSM system have been raised by many authors, particularly those trained in a sociological or anthropological tradition who practice in North America.[1]

Despite questions raised about its cross-cultural equivalence, DSM is used widely across the world, particularly for research purposes by investigators who seek publication in North American journals. Albeit imperfect, the DSM system appears to offer a rational, criteria-based framework suitable for research and clinical practice, at least according to anecdotal reports of colleagues from Europe and Latin America.

In the following sections, we highlight relevant issues related to ethnicity and psychiatric diagnoses in efforts to provide a general background that may inform the reexamination of substance use diagnostic categories and their applications. We conclude the chapter with a few specific recommendations on this topic as part of the development of DSM-V.

Key Definitions

RACE

The use of race as a way to classify humans originated with Linnaeus, in his 1758 *Systema Naturae.* Blumenbach, a German anthropologist, outlined five divisions of race (Caucasian, Mongolian, Ethiopian, American, and Malay). However, population and genetic studies have questioned the use of racial divisions for humans as lacking a scientific foundation. Indeed, hundreds of human races have been proposed using anthropological criteria, and the U.S. 1990 census elicited more than 300 races in questionnaire responses.[2] In 1999, the Institute of Medicine (IOM), in its report *The Unequal Burden of Cancer,*[3] recommended that the National Institutes of Health (NIH) reevaluate the use of *race,* defined as "a construct of human variability based on perceived differences in biology, physical appearance and behavior." According to the IOM, the traditional conception of race rests on the false premise that there are natural distinctions grounded in significant biological and behavioral differences but actually rooted in physical features characteristic of diverse continental origins. Therefore this concept lacks any biogenetic or anthropological justification in cancer surveillance and other population research. The IOM advised using the term *ethnic group* instead of *race* in future endeavors.

ETHNICITY

The concept of *ethnicity* defines the ways in which one sees oneself and how one is seen by others as part of a group on the basis of cultural background and shared historical experience. Common elements often associated with a given ethnic group include skin color, religion, language, ancestry, customs, and occupational or regional features. Ethnicity boundaries are dynamic and imprecise, and further confounded with nationality. For proper clinical or research use, the concept should be defined and operationalized precisely.

PROBLEMS WITH THE "ETHNICITY" CONCEPT

While the IOM report suggested that *ethnicity* is a more neutral, less pejorative term than *race*, the former is difficult to define operationally, and often individuals responding to queries do not endorse unambiguously the choices offered in census gathering and other surveys. The "Hispanic" or "Latino" ethnicity group, in particular, is too broad and heterogeneous and it is not possible to draw inferences that universally apply to Hispanics given their diverse origins (traced to more than 20 countries), various phenotypic admixtures, divergent historical origins, and diverse social and educational levels. One consequence of this is that Hispanics were the ethnic group most likely to endorse "mixed race" in the latest U.S. census.

RACE AND ETHNICITY ISSUES IN THE UNITED STATES

Historically, there has been a long-standing preoccupation in the United States with race and ethnicity issues, particularly a need to label ethnic and racial groups for operational reasons such as population enumeration and health assessments. Interestingly, since 1997 the U.S. Office of Management and Budget (OMB), the agency that ultimately determines NIH's population taxonomy, has recognized only two categories of "ethnicity." These are "Hispanic" or "Latino" versus neither. However, despite the IOM report, OMB continues to recognize five categories of "race"—namely, Asian, American Indian or Alaska Native, Native Hawaiian or other Pacific Islander, black or African American, and white—and these continue to be used in the literature. An essential point is that the U.S. ethnic and race categories, which are growing more inaccurate with the passage of time in the United States, are even less useful when used in other nations. Thus, while many countries in western Europe, the Pacific and even Latin America have their own immigrant sets and minority groups, ethnic categories are not articulated the way they are in the United States. International studies have shown that U.S. ethnic categories have little meaning elsewhere. For example, a study of depression and painful symptoms in several Latin American countries reported that a great majority of people in Mexico and Argentina did not identify themselves as "Hispanics."[4] Also, according to reports from the Fogarty International Center, U.S. ethnic and racial categories cannot be properly applied to international research projects funded by NIH (personal communication, 2004).

ETHNICITY AND MEDICINE

In U.S. clinical medicine, references to race are standard in clinical rounds and medical records and continue to be an integral part of clinical patient documentation. For example, a medical history or a clinical presentation invariably starts as the "...-year-old Hispanic, African American, Asian or white male or female presenting with such and such a symptom," possibly reflecting the historical importance in the pregenomic era of racial background for diagnosing disorders such as sickle cell anemia, Tay-Sachs disease, thalassemia, and cystic fibrosis, among others. Unfortunately, used in such a fashion the concept of "ethnicity" is imperfect as it is too often inferred by the examiner on the basis of observed traits. For obvious reasons, the use of ethnic identification and concerns about cultural orientation have had significantly more influence in psychiatry and psychology compared with the rest of medicine. For example, anthropologically and socially oriented psychiatrists continue to insist on the formal use of the "cultural formulation," a process that takes into account the person's cultural identity and background for formulating diagnosis and treatment plans. Indeed, a review in the traditional series updating progress in psychiatry in North America stated that "a consideration of culture is essential in the process of the interview, case formulation, diagnosis and treatment of culturally diverse individuals."[5]

The relevance of ethnic or cultural formulation has gained visibility following the recent Surgeon General's report on "health disparities" (which in psychiatry have only applied to access and treatment quality issues rather than disorder phenomenology or diagnosis). This has led to positive developments such as the requirement that "cultural competence standards" (ensuring practitioners' awareness on such issues as culturally related attitudes, symptoms, language and interpretation of clinical data) be developed in state systems in efforts to improve access and quality of care. However, it has been difficult to define with any precision the key ethnic issues, or a modus operandi, to be taken into account for making valid psychiatric diagnoses. Also, specific applications of this to the area of substance use disorders are not documented clearly.

COUNTRY OF ORIGIN AND IMMIGRANT STATUS

In our view, country of origin and immigrant status are less ambiguous items, are easier to define, and elicit precisely and have proven less controversial and transferable for international use. For example, epidemiological studies in the United States have shown that these variables, and related markers such as age at arrival and time in country among immigrants, have utility for demarcating important differences in levels of psychopathology and general health. The observation that immigrants from Latin America have better health and mental health status than those born in the United States[6–8] was coined the "Latino paradox" by Scribner,[6] who suggested that much could be gained from identifying the determinants of these differences. These findings illustrate the utility of carefully constructed demographic descriptors for deriving subgroup comparisons. Regarding issues of self-report veracity about substance use, and potential variations among and within ethnic groups, it has yet to be demonstrated that these problems have resulted in serious underreporting or systematic biasing of substance use information.

"RELATIVISTIC" VERSUS "UNIVERSALISTIC" PERSPECTIVES

In cultural psychiatry, the terms *emic* and *etic* illustrate, respectively, relativistic and universalistic perspectives in diagnosis. The concept of *emic* (from *phonemics*) refers to culture-specific patterns of psychopathology, while the concept of *etic* (from *phonetics*) presupposes that psychopathology is universal. Kraepelin was perhaps the first to use the universalistic (etic) approach to psychopathology. This approach signified a departure from a system of classification based on etiological assumptions and was representative of philosophical realism or positivism that was ultimately incorporated into diagnostic classifications in North America by the pioneering research group at Washington University in St. Louis. These criteria, known as the St. Louis or Feighner criteria, set the pace for the new diagnostic developments that would evolve into the Research Diagnostic Criteria (RDC) and then the DSM-III classification. The emic, or "relativistic," point of view observes psychiatric disorders within their respective cultural context and argues that the content of psychiatric diagnosis will vary to some degree inherently by cultural context. This is the position adopted by anthropologically, socially oriented psychiatrists, particularly in North America. In the case of alcohol disorders, this tradition is represented in the subtypes of alcoholism.[10] There is evidence that intra-ethnic group variance in emic perspectives exists in self-rated health among Latinos, underscoring the difficulty of applying specific criteria of illness and dysfunction with acceptable precision.[11] To the extent that normative definitions of severity or of ambiguous symptoms are inferred by individuals of differing cultural backgrounds during psychiatric evaluations, some cultural variance can be anticipated in applying diagnostic criteria. Strategies for overcoming these challenges to diagnostic accuracy are not readily available for practitioners.

EVOLUTION OF PSYCHIATRIC DIAGNOSIS

Diseases cause symptoms, and these are experienced and expressed by patients and elicited by physicians. Obviously, unpleasant physical symptoms are easier to define and recognize than psychological or behavioral manifestations. Physical characteristics such as sweating or trembling are not necessarily symptomatic of a disorder just because they are "physical." A.J. Lewis[12] coined the term "psychological dysfunction," which he defined as a deviation from a standard of normal psychological functioning. With scientific progress, the hope was that these "psychological dysfunctions" would be linked eventually to abnormalities of biological functioning.[13] Relevant examples of these are symptoms such as obsessions and other psychological dysfunctions that can be defined precisely, may have biological underpinnings and can be separated clinically from one another (e.g., phobias, thought insertion). In traditional psychopathology, there has been an effort to utilize well-defined symptoms as much as possible and a tendency to avoid the inclusion of purely social or experiential factors in criteria and definitions. The more exclusive the social component in defining deviance, the less applicable is the symptom label. For example, undesirable behaviors defined in purely social terms, such as drug addiction, shoplifting, and vandalism, are relatively easy to define reliably. However, while biological theories can be invoked to help explain some aspects of these behaviors in some people, they are highly unlikely to account for a useful proportion of the variance or to offer a comprehensive explanation.[13] As disease theories become more successful in providing a solid basis of knowledge about abnormalities of psychological and biological functioning, the dimensional aspects of measurement within and between clinical syndromes become apparent. According to Wing et al.,[13] a system of clinical measurement cannot be purely categorical or purely dimensional. The most obvious example of the dimensional approach is in defining severity of symptom types (be it for investigation, treatment purposes or assessment of outcomes), but the symptoms themselves have to be defined first.

In the last two decades, there has been a mushrooming of the type and number of psychiatric diagnoses. Thus, the very few classical psychiatric syndromes refined over one and a half centuries, such as mania, melancholia, hysteria and hypochondriasis, rose to 14 in the Washington University Criteria, exceeded 100 in DSM-III, and topped the 300 mark in DSM-IV. Despite the progress made, and the revolutionary process of building diagnoses, official additions to the DSM books often reflect capricious actions of committees or opinions of single individuals.[14]

LANGUAGE AND TRANSLATION ISSUES

Considering sociolinguistic implications is a critical step in adapting diagnostic instruments and criteria to other countries. Equivalence has to be attained in a number of dimensions (semantic, conceptual and technical). Even words such as *depression* and *anxiety* are difficult to translate precisely into some languages. Also, certain somatic or mental experiences that are clearly a sign of disease in some cultures may be very important to patients from these specific cultural backgrounds, but others pay little attention to them ("loss of semen" is viewed as a significant problem in India but is given little or no attention in other countries). Embarrassment or loss of face may be a reason for suicide in some cultures, while it may be irrelevant in others. Symptoms such as tremor, a common physical symptom and a sign of pathology in most cultures, may be advantageous in Mali, where "trembling hands" is a sign of virility.[15]

HEURISTIC MODELS FOR PSYCHIATRIC DIAGNOSIS

The definition of *disease, disorder,* or *abnormality* is a critical element for classification systems. There are several models for psychological abnormalities in the literature. A biological model defines *abnormality* on the basis of biological criteria; a statistical model defines it as deviation from the norm; a subjective discomfort model as suffering experienced by an affected individual; and a subjective value model defines it as what is viewed as undesirable for society. Because all these models are incomplete, Wakefield[16] posited that the definition of *abnormality* requires both social and biological criteria. He proposed "harmful dysfunction analysis" as a model for developing meaningful diagnoses in psychiatry and psychology. This model uses a "Darwinian" principle, of failure of systems to function as designed by natural selection, and, according to Wakefield, applies to both physical and mental diseases. Key elements of the model are 1) subjective value that a condition is harmful or undesirable and 2) objective identification of a malfunctioning internal mechanism.[16] This proposal has stimulated lengthy philosophical, epistemological, and methodological debates.[17]

Key Questions Related to Ethnicity and Psychopathology

A critical issue is to examine whether or not symptoms and syndromes can be reliably elicited and recognized, not only as part of research collaborations launched to confirm the "universality" of psychiatric syndromes and the reliability of structured diagnostic instruments, but in "real world" day-to-day clinical practice. That the system is far from perfect in this particular instance can be deduced from a recent statement by the system's pioneer, Robert Spitzer, who was quoted as saying that "to say that we've solved the reliability problem is just not true. It has been improved. But if you are in a situation with a general clinician, it's certainly not very good."[14] Even the fidelity of clinical research interviews with field interviews using fully structured diagnostic interviews for case ascertainment is inconsistent, although substance use disorders have been the most likely to achieve adequate "procedural validity" compared with nonaddictive disorders.

WORLD HEALTH ORGANIZATION INTERNATIONAL STUDIES

International studies sponsored by the World Health Organization (WHO) have provided strong support for the universal presence of major mental disorders such as depression and schizophrenia.

In depression, the weight of somatic and affective dimensions and narrative context may differ from culture to culture.[18] For example, major depression is conceptualized differently in Native American populations and involves at least five illness categories.[19] In anxiety syndromes there is significant cross-cultural variation in type of specific fears as well as associated somatic, dissociative and affective symptoms.[20] Obviously, culture "colors" these syndromes, and their basic elements may not be elicited or recognized everywhere. A few syndromes have been designated as "culture-bound," indicating their exclusive presence in some countries. Nevertheless, if proper training is provided and structured instruments are used to elicit the symptoms, an acceptable level of comparability is usually possible in international clinical and epidemiological studies.[21]

WHO CLASSIFICATIONS AND CULTURE

WHO endorses a universalistic view of psychiatric disorders. Curiously, in international settings, there seems to be much less preoccupation with cultural psychiatry in clinical practice than is the case in the United States. Thus, international classifications have been much less concerned about cross-cultural issues. There have been a few exceptions: the tenth revision of the *International Classification of Diseases* (ICD-10) incorporated an international psychiatric lexicon that contains a description of culture-bound syndromes as well as an international casebook.[21] Also, the more recent ICD-10 Diagnostic Criteria for Research included an appendix on cross-cultural issues.[21]

CONTRIBUTION OF EPIDEMIOLOGY TO CROSS-CULTURAL DIAGNOSIS

Comparative studies in the United States and abroad have supported the "universalistic" view of psychiatric diagnosis by showing that major disorders can be elicited in many countries and various ethnic groups through the use of structured interviews such as the Diagnostic Interview Schedule (DIS) and the Composite International Diagnostic Interview (CIDI). The WHO World Mental Health Surveys, using population samples with rigorous epidemiological designs, reported wide international variability in rates of DSM-IV disorders and in related impairments, especially for drug dependence.[22] Similar population differences were reported in the United States. Two epidemiological studies showed lower prevalence rates for psychiatric disorders in Mexico-born Mexican Americans compared with non-Hispanics and found that years in the United States influenced these trends.[23,24] This was particularly salient for substance use disorders, a finding validated with anonymous urine toxicology screening.[25] While instruments appeared to work well in these studies, it is not clear if these low rates were influenced by such factors as differential reporting of symptoms due to misunderstanding or social desirability, or nonequivalence of certain symptoms or syndromes. However, the prevalence rates in Mexico-born Mexican Americans were very similar to those found in Mexico City using the same instrument.[26] These results have been replicated in at least one other large national survey in the United States.[27]

A recently published study on American Indians[28] found that alcohol disorders and posttraumatic stress disorder were more common in American Indian populations compared to other populations. Interestingly, the prevalence of depression was low, a finding the authors attribute to cultural factors. Diagnoses of major depression were based on the endorsement of at least five of the nine major depressive episode symptoms and yielded low prevalence. Patients with disorders sought help primarily from traditional healers, not physicians. Diagnoses such as psychoses are excluded from studies of Native American populations because of cultural concerns (seeking of "visions" is a trait traditionally nurtured in those cultures). Also, cognitive dysfunction elicited with the Mini-Mental State Examination could not be used in the Epidemiologic Catchment Area study because of educational and linguistic issues.[29]

SOMATIC PRESENTATIONS

In most cultures, the presentation of personal/social "distress" in the form of somatic complaints appears to be the norm.[30]

Dominant cultural tendencies influence the expression of "proper" behavioral displays for each society, reciprocally influenced by the culture of current medical practice.[31] Thus, patients tend to develop symptoms that are "medically correct" (what doctors expect and understand) and cluster commonly into recognizable patterns. Moreover, a great majority of these patients present to primary care, and a large proportion of them are found to have psychiatric disorders, including substance abuse/ dependence.[32,33] Tien et al.[34] reported that high levels of unexplained physical symptoms predicted "extreme alcohol use" in an epidemiological sample, and concluded that self-reported somatization symptoms could add to the detection of severe substance abuse. Because somatic presentations appear to be more common in developing societies, and the symptoms themselves may differ across cultures,[31] they need to be incorporated in diagnostic formulations.

DIAGNOSTIC DISPARITIES

A number of clinical reports have documented that clinicians are more likely to give a diagnosis of psychosis, or to prioritize signs of substance abuse over other primary disorders, in minority patients, particularly African Americans.[35–37] A recent study using a large data set in a mental health system found that clinicians in a large mental health system diagnose psychosis in African Americans and depression in Latinos disproportionately.[38] The reasons for this, although unclear, potentially include information variance, deficiencies in patient–clinician communication and inadequate diagnostic criteria. The frequent presentation of psychotic symptoms by certain ethnic groups with common mental disorders and medical conditions (e.g., Latinos and African Americans) contributes to diagnostic ambiguities and misdiagnoses, yet empirically supported guidelines to assist clinicians are not available.[39]

DSM-IV's Cultural Appendix

The increased visibility and enhanced political voice of some minority psychiatrists within the American Psychiatric Association (APA) would eventually bring awareness on culture to the official diagnostic manual. In 1988 the APA appointed a task force, one of whose subcommittees addressed the area of cultural issues in psychiatric diagnosis. While a specific proposal for a "cultural axis" never came forward, there were ambitious recommendations, including a complementary cultural formulation, cultural statements in the introduction to the manual, annotations under each diagnostic category, and a glossary of culture-specific terms. However, the major piece related to culture in DSM-IV is a brief appendix placed at the end of the rather massive manual. This section outlines the relevance of culture and provides an exhaustive list of "culture-bound syndromes." Many of those entities included in the appendix are rare, uncommon conditions, some poorly defined and others that can be classified in areas of general psychopathology. As a result they have limited practical relevance, as they are encountered infrequently by a majority of practicing psychiatrists in the United States and other countries.

It is our impression that in its current state the appendix is of limited utility in the absence of additional technical information and supporting research to provide guidance to clinicians. Many of the general recommendations provided are based on anecdotal, "commonsense" observations. They are, of necessity, very broad because inadequate research is available to develop guidelines for practitioners working with ethnically diverse patients. A major challenge is that given the heterogeneity of these groups, research is not easily generalized. On the biological side, there are only a few pharmacogenetic clues from recent research, and these appear to be practically relevant only to certain Asian American groups; we await research advances for other ethnic groups. Other than endorsing and promoting "cultural competency" (a field that is struggling to define its clinical domain aside from language), the cultural appendix does not offer either an adequate framework or clinical guidelines for the scope of applications originally envisioned. Regrettably, the research envisioned as an essential step in implementing the cultural formulation into clinical practice has not been advanced adequately, resulting in inadequate empirical validation.

Recommendations for DSM-V and ICD-11 Regarding Cultural and Ethnic Issues

Beyond the general recommendations already made by Alarcon et al.,[40] regarding culture/ethnicity issues in DSM-V, we wish to add the following caveats:

1. Define cultural/ethnic issues in clear terms that lend themselves to operational definitions.
2. Define the "ethnicity" concept much more precisely. Demographic descriptors are needed that coincide with ethnic subgroup variations in prevalence of substance use disorders and related patterns of patient presentation of disorders, including beliefs and behaviors that have value for refining cultural aspects of DSM-V. For example, Mexican Americans, Puerto Ricans, Cubans, South Americans, and other Latino populations should not continue to be

blended into a "Hispanic" group for the sake of convenience, as research is showing significant differences among these groups in prevalence of DSM-IV disorders and use of services. Moreover, behavioral genetics research involving even one Latin American nationality of mixed historical ancestry (Indian, African, and European) must contend with complex genetic heterogeneity.

3. Enter more specific ethnicity elements as variables rather than one overarching "ethnic group" variable in analyses of ethnic influences on substance use symptoms and syndromes. Ethnicity can be characterized according to a) the ethnic group to which that person most closely relates; b) his or her ethnic ancestry, which may range from one to four categories; c) the language spoken by his or her parents; and d) the language most commonly spoken at home. In this regard, there is a need for nationally representative surveys that either are larger than those conducted so far or oversample populations of interest.
4. Make recommendations that are research-based and testable. The necessary research in this area should be articulated in a more practical, hierarchical fashion so that these goals can become attainable in stages.
5. Develop a well-defined research program to support and justify a cultural axis with practical utility or scientific validation.
6. Provide crisp, practical examples, including illustrative clinical vignettes in key areas. The use of brief, precise, illustrative appendices may be helpful.
7. Provide meaningful cultural annotations and a glossary of cultural terms that are applicable in daily clinical practice and not limited to less frequently encountered syndromes (culture-bound). Of high value for practitioners would be explanations of terms used in different cultures to express signs and symptoms of specific DSM disorders, and information about cultural assumptions regarding substance use problems and related behaviors and impairments. This may include a dictionary with key words in several languages.

References

1. Lewis-Fernandez R, Kleinman A: Cultural psychiatry: theoretical, clinical and research issues. Psychiatr Clin North Am 18:433–448, 1995.
2. Witzig R: The medicalization of race: scientific legitimization of a flawed social construct. Ann Intern Med 125:675–679, 1996.
3. Hayes MA, Smedley D (eds): The Unequal Burden of Cancer: An Assessment of NIH Research and Programs for Ethnic Minorities and the Medically Underserved. Washington, DC, Institute of Medicine, National Academy Press, 1999.
4. Munoz RA, McBride ME, Brnabic AJM, et al: Major depressive disorder in Latin America: the relationship between: depression severity, painful somatic symptoms, and quality of life. J Affect Disord 86:93–98, 2005.

5. Lu FG, Lim RF, Mezzich JE: Issues in the diagnostic assessment and diagnosis of culturally diverse individuals, in American Psychiatric Press Review of Psychiatry, Vol 14. Edited by Oldham JM, Riba MS. Washington, DC, American Psychiatric Press, 1995, pp 477–510.
6. Scribner R: Paradox as paradigm: the health outcomes of Mexican Americans. Am J Public Health 86:303–305, 1996.
7. Vega WA, Kolody B, Aguilar-Gaxiola S, et al: Lifetime prevalence of DSM-III-R psychiatric disorders among urban and rural Mexican-Americans in California. Arch Gen Psychiatry 55:771–778, 1998.
8. Escobar JI: Immigration and health: why are immigrants better off? Arch Gen Psychiatry 55:781–782, 1998.
9. Escobar JI, Hoyos-Nervi C, Gara M: Immigration and mental health: the case of Mexican-Americans. Harv Rev Psychiatry 8:64–72, 2000.
10. Room R, Janca A, Bennett LA, et al: WHO cross-cultural applicability research on diagnosis and assessment of substance use disorders: an overview of methods and selected results. Addiction 91:199–230, 1996.
11. Finch BK, Hummer RA, Reindl M, et al: Validity of self-rated health among Latinos. Am J Epidemiol 155:755–759, 2002.
12. Lewis AJ: Health as a social concept. Br J Sociol 4:109–124, 1953.
13. Wing JK, Sartorius N, Üstün TB: Diagnosis and Clinical Measurement in Clinical Psychiatry. Cambridge, UK, Cambridge University Press, 1998.
14. Spiegel A: The dictionary of disorder. The New Yorker, January 3, 2005, pp 56–63.
15. Sartorius N: SCAN translation, in Diagnosis and Clinical Measurement in Clinical Psychiatry. Edited by Wing J, Sartorius N, Üstün TB. Cambridge, United Kingdom, Cambridge University Press, 1998, pp 44–57.
16. Wakefield J: Disorder as harmful dysfunction: a conceptual critique of DSM-III-R's definition of mental disorder. Psychol Rev 99:322–347, 1992.
17. Murphy D, Woolfolk R: The Harmful Dysfunction Analysis of Mental Disorders: Philosophy, Psychiatry and Psychology, Vol 7, No 4. Baltimore, MD, Johns Hopkins University Press, 2000, pp 242–252.
18. Manson S: Culture and major depression, in Cultural Psychiatry, Vol 18, No 3. Edited by Alarcon RD. Philadelphia, PA, WB Saunders, 1995.
19. Manson SM, Shore JH, Bloom JD: The depressive experience in American Indian communities: a challenge for psychiatric theory and diagnosis, in Culture and Depression: Studies in the Anthropology and Cross-Cultural Psychiatry of Affect and Disorder. Edited by Kleinman A, Good B. Berkeley, University of California Press, 1985, pp 331–368.
20. Kirmayer LJ, Young A, Hayton BC: The cultural context of anxiety disorders, in Cultural Psychiatry, Vol 18, No 3. Edited by Alarcon RD. Philadelphia, PA, WB Saunders, 1995, pp 503–521.
21. World Health Organization: The ICD-10 Classification of Mental and Behavioural Disorders. Geneva, Switzerland, World Health Organization, 1992.
22. WHO World Mental Health Survey Consortium: Prevalence, severity, and unmet need for treatment of mental disorders in the World Health Organization World Mental Health Surveys. JAMA 291:2581–2590, 2004.

23. Burnam MA, Hough RH, Karno M, et al: Acculturation and lifetime prevalence of psychiatric disorders among Mexican Americans in Los Angeles. J Health Soc Behav 28:89–102, 1987.
24. Vega WA, Sribney WM, Aguilar-Gaxiola S, et al: 12-Month prevalence of DSM-III-R psychiatric disorders among Mexican Americans: nativity, social assimilation, and age determinants. J Nerv Ment Dis 192:532–541, 2004.
25. Vega W, Kolody B, Hwang J, et al: Prevalence and magnitude of perinatal substance exposure in California. N Engl J Med 329:850–854, 1993.
26. Medina-Mora ME, Borges G, Lara C, et al: Prevalence of mental disorders and use of services: results from the Mexican National Survey of Psychiatric Epidemiology. Salud Mental 26:1–16, 2003.
27. Grant BF, Stinson FS, Hasin DS, et al: Immigration and lifetime prevalence of DSM-IV psychiatric disorders among Mexican-Americans and non-Hispanic whites in the United States: results from the National Epidemiologic Survey on Alcohol and Related Conditions. Arch Gen Psychiatry 61:1226–1233, 2004.
28. Beals J, Manson SM, Whitesell NR, et al: Prevalence of major depressive episode in two American Indian reservation populations: unexpected findings with a structured interview. Am J Psychiatry 162:1713–1722, 2005.
29. Escobar JI, Karno M, Burnam A, et al: Use of the Mini Mental State Examination (MMSE) in a community population of mixed ethnicity: cultural and linguistic artifacts. J Nerv Ment Dis 174:607–614, 1986.
30. Kleinman A: Anthropology and psychiatry. Br J Psychiatry 151:447–454, 1987.
31. Shorter E: From the Mind Into the Body: The Cultural Origin of Psychosomatic Symptoms. New York, Free Press, 1994, pp 90–117.
32. Kroenke K, Spitzer RL, Williams JBW, et al: Physical symptoms in primary care. Arch Fam Med 3:774–779, 1994.
33. Feder A, Olfson M, Gameroff M, et al: Medically unexplained symptoms in an urban general medicine practice. Psychosomatics 42:261–268, 2001.
34. Tien AY, Schlaepfer TE, Fisch H: Self-reported somatization symptoms associated with risk for extreme alcohol use. Arch Fam Med 7:33–37, 1998.
35. Lawson WB, Hepler N, Holladay J, et al: Race as a factor in inpatient and outpatient admissions and diagnosis. Hosp Community Psychiatry 45:72–74, 1994.
36. Strakowski SM, Keck PE, Arnold LM, et al: Ethnicity and diagnosis in patients with affective psychosis. J Clin Psychiatry 64:747–754, 2003.
37. Minsky S, Vega WA, Miskimen T, et al: Diagnostic patterns in Latino, African American and European American psychiatric patients. Arch Gen Psychiatry 60:637–644, 2003.
38. Vega WA, Sribney WM, Miskimen TM, et al: Putative psychotic symptoms in the Mexican American population: prevalence and co-occurrence with psychiatric disorders. J Nerv Ment Dis 194:471–477, 2006.
39. Olfson M, Feder A, Fuentes M, et al: Psychotic symptoms in an urban general medicine practice. Am J Psychiatry 159:1412–1419, 2002.
40. Alarcon RD, Alegria M, Bell CC, et al: Beyond the funhouse mirrors: research agenda on culture and psychiatric diagnosis, in A Research Agenda for DSM-V. Edited by Kupfer D, First MB, Regier DA. Washington, DC, American Psychiatric Publishing, 2003, pp 219–281.

6

SUBSTANCE DEPENDENCE AND NONDEPENDENCE IN DSM AND THE ICD

Can an Identical Conceptualization Be Achieved?

John B. Saunders, M.D., F.R.C.P.

This chapter has a threefold purpose. The first is to examine the various historical conceptualizations of substance use disorders, in particular as they are represented in the *Diagnostic and Statistical Manual of Mental Disorders* (DSM) and the *International Classification of Diseases* (ICD). The second is to appraise how the core substance use disorders currently listed in these two systems perform psychometrically and in terms of clinical utility. The third is to explore to what extent the needs of a clinically oriented system such as DSM can be reconciled with the requirements of systems that primarily serve the fields of epidemiology, health service management, and morbidity and mortality analysis, and suggest a research agenda for this purpose.

Reprinted from Saunders JB: "Substance Dependence and Nondependence in the *Diagnostic and Statistical Manual of Mental Disorders* (DSM) and the *International Classification of Diseases* (ICD): Can an Identical Conceptualization Be Achieved?" *Addiction* 101 (suppl 1):48–58, 2006. Used with permission of the Society for the Study of Addiction.

Background

Systems of diagnosis and classification are optimally based on an understanding of the symptomatology, pathophysiology, and natural history of human conditions, which allows us to identify discrete disorders that can be distinguished to a fair degree from others. In the fields of mental health and substance use disorders, our understanding has not advanced to the stage that this can be achieved. In all current diagnostic and classification systems, these disorders are defined and delineated on a phenomenological basis. In the substance use disorders field, there is the additional difficulty that there have been many alternative, indeed competing, schools of thought about the nature of these conditions.

Before presenting the recent history of diagnostic and classification systems that cover substance use disorders, I briefly summarize the history of the competing conceptualizations. In retrospect, these different philosophies may be seen to contribute a piece of understanding as to the nature of these conditions. However, the interpretation of proponents of a particular tradition is often that the tradition represents the totality of our understanding. This has been a cause of controversy and a significant limitation to a broadly based understanding of substance use disorders and to the development of a common language for communication. Hence, the history of conceptual developments in this field can be seen as a series of parallel pathways of thought, with little attempt at synthesis until recent years.

Different Conceptualizations

In the nineteenth century the popular conception of alcoholism was that it represented a failure of morals or character.[1] In early formulations of DSM, alcoholism and drug addiction were, as will be described below, grouped within the personality disorders. A different tradition saw these problems as reflecting a disease process that was biologically determined, resulted in the individual having some type of idiosyncratic reaction to alcohol or a drug, and had a relatively predictable natural history. This conceptualization influenced and was subsequently embraced by the self-help movements, such as Alcoholics Anonymous. The concept of an underlying disease reached its apotheosis with the work of Jellinek in the 1940s and 1950s, although in his later work he increasingly recognized the role of environmental influences.[2]

A third tradition may be described as the epidemiological and public health one. In this view, as enunciated by Ledermann,[3] alcohol- and drug-related problems are envisaged as occurring fundamentally because of the overall level of use of a psychoactive substance in society. The level of use is, in turn, influenced by cultural traditions, the availability of that particular substance, its ease of manufacture and distribution, and its price. Inherent in these conceptualizations was the idea that individual pathology is considered of secondary importance and that there is no special phenomenology of pathological substance use. The social constructionist school viewed substance use problems as, essentially, being disaggregated, with no special relationship among them. This school of thought was concerned about the stigma attributable to diagnostic labels and the potential of treatment as a form of social control.[4]

The 1970s saw the rise of social cognitive theory[5] as an influential paradigm to explain the development and resolution of alcohol and drug problems. This school of thought taught that the (many) influences that determined any behavior applied to the uptake of substance use and the development of disordered use. A positive consequence would encourage repeated use, whereas a negative outcome would encourage the opposite. Patterns of substance use behavior could become entrenched in this way but, equally, repetitive substance use could be "unlearned." This led to the development of a range of cognitive-behavioral therapies, which included some aimed at moderated or "controlled" substance use.[6,7]

During the 1960s and 1970s, the concept that substance use disorders might represent a disease process was dismissed by many observers. Similarly, the role of genetic predisposition was thought to be inconsequential. Kessel and Walton stated firmly that "alcoholism is passed on in the same way that money is inherited, not in the way that, say, eye colour is."[8] This created a huge gulf between many professionally trained therapists (including those from the socio-cognitive school) and those, many of whom were members of the self-help movement, who understood these disorders to be biologically driven.

Perhaps the major recent development in our understanding of the basis of substance use disorders has been the burgeoning of knowledge about neurobiological processes and findings from associated genetic research. Briefly, there is increasing evidence that psychoactive substance use activates mesolimbic dopamine reward pathways, which in turn results in reinforcement of such use.[9] Dopamine release leads to neuronal plasticity that underpins learning and a set of feelings (such as craving) and memories that perpetuate substance use and favor the development of dependence. Thus, dependence may be construed as an "internal driving force" that results from repeated exposure to a psychoactive substance and that leads in turn to repetitive substance use that is self-perpetuating and typically occurs even in the face of harmful consequences. A recent publication on the neuroscience of addiction by the World Health Organization (WHO) summarizes the key developments in biomedical research over this period.[10]

The Dependence Syndrome

The needs of many groups—practitioners, health service administrators, and policy makers, for example—were not well served by these competing models of substance use. Could substance use disorders be defined in a practically useful and empirically supported way? A pivotal development was the publication in 1976 of a "provisional description" of the "alcohol dependence syndrome" by Edwards and Gross.[11] This depicted a syndrome in which certain experiences, behaviors, and symptoms related to repetitive alcohol use tended to cluster in time and occur repeatedly. Unlike many previous conceptualizations, this conceptualization was essentially descriptive in nature rather than etiological. This offered an advantage over previous models, which were based predominantly on particular theoretical concepts or represented the influence of a particular school of thought.

The concept of the dependence syndrome has been adopted successively for most other psychoactive substances that have the potential for reinforcement of use. These include benzodiazepines,[12–14] illicit and prescribed opioids,[13–15] cannabis,[13,16,17] inhalants,[18] psychostimulants such as cocaine[13] and the amphetamines and their derivatives,[19,20] nicotine,[21] caffeine,[22] and anabolic steroids.[23] It may also apply to repetitive behaviors that do not involve self-administration of a psychoactive substance. These include pathological gambling, compulsive shopping, and compulsive exercise.[24]

The dependence syndrome concept has formed the basis of the classification system of psychoactive substance use disorders in the tenth revision of the ICD (ICD-10), published in 1992,[25] and in recent revisions of DSM, namely DSM-III-R,[26] published in 1987, and DSM-IV,[27] which appeared in 1994.

Dependence in Context

In the work undertaken by a WHO expert group in the late 1970s and early 1980s, the dependence syndrome was complemented by four other conditions that also reflected repetitive substance use.[28] These conditions, termed "unsanctioned use," "dysfunctional use," "hazardous use," and "harmful use," may be regarded as forms of repetitive substance use that do not fulfill the criteria for the dependence syndrome but that nonetheless may result in significant harm to the individual or to society. These terms are defined in Table 6–1. In summary, *unsanctioned use* is defined as substance use that does not conform to traditional practices or societal mores. *Dysfunctional use* is repetitive use that causes social problems. *Hazardous use* is repetitive substance use that confers the risk of harmful consequences. It has been operationalized for alcohol consumption in several countries (e.g., in Australia) as the repeated daily consumption of more than 40 g of alcohol for a man or more than 20 g for a woman.[29] However, its operationalization for other substances has lagged behind. *Harmful use* is repeated use that has actually caused adverse physical (medical) and/or mental health consequences.

There was also a set of conditions termed "substance-related disabilities" or "substance-related problems" that were conceptualized as the consequences of repetitive substance use. These include substance-induced psychotic disorder, substance-induced amnesic syndrome, substance-induced mood disorders, and a raft of physical complications.

TABLE 6–1. WHO nomenclature and definitions of repetitive substance use

Unsanctioned use

Use of a substance that is not approved by a society or by a group within that society. The term implies that this disapproval is accepted as a fact in its own right, without the need to determine or justify the basis of the disapproval.

Dysfunctional use

Substance use that is leading to impaired psychological or social functioning (e.g., loss of employment or marital problems).

Hazardous use

A pattern of substance use that increases the risk of harmful consequences for the user. Some would limit the consequences to physical and mental health (as in harmful use); some would also include social consequences. In contrast to harmful use, *hazardous use* refers to patterns of use that are of public health significance despite the absence of any current disorder in the individual user. The term is used currently by WHO but is not a diagnostic term in ICD-10.

Harmful use

A pattern of psychoactive substance use that is causing damage to health. The damage may be physical (e.g., hepatitis following injection of drugs) or mental (e.g., depressive episodes secondary to heavy alcohol intake). Harmful use commonly, but not invariably, has adverse social consequences; social consequences in themselves, however, are not sufficient to justify a diagnosis of harmful use. [Harmful use] supplanted "non-dependent use" as a diagnostic term.

Source. Edwards et al. 1981.[28]

The Diagnostic and Statistical Manual

The need to respond to major public health problems (largely infectious diseases) in the late nineteenth century spawned the development in the United States of systems of disease coding and classification. In the mental health field there was an additional requirement, to ensure that patients admitted to institutions were there for legitimate medical reasons and to allow uniform statistics to be collected. In 1917 a standardized nomenclature for mental disorders was developed. It was adopted by the American Psychiatric Association,[30] which also contributed to the development of an international standardized nomenclature of diseases.

The first edition of DSM was published in 1952[31] and included a standard nomenclature, definitions of terms and a statistical classification. Substance use disorders were grouped under personality disorders, where alcoholism was defined as "well-established addiction to alcohol without recognized underlying disorder." Drug addiction was not defined specifically, but there was a statement that "addiction is usually symptomatic of a personality disorder. The proper personality classification is to be made as an additional diagnosis." Alcohol intoxication was called a "nondiagnostic term," in the same league as being a boarder in an institution or a malingerer.

The second edition, published in 1968,[32] still had substance use disorders classified within the personality disorders. There were no specific definitions or criteria and little description of the conditions was provided. For alcoholism there was a statement that "the best direct evidence for alcoholism is the appearance of withdrawal symptoms." The diagnosis of drug dependence required "evidence of habitual use or a clear sense of a need for the drug."

The third edition, DSM-III,[33] represented a major advance. For the first time diagnostic criteria were included, an expanded description of the disorders was given, and a multiaxial approach to evaluation was employed. This reflected what was considered to be the growing importance of diagnosis in clinical practice and research, and the need for clinicians and researchers to have a common language. Clear definitions of diagnostic terms were provided, and consistency with research findings was considered of paramount importance, together with field-testing of diagnostic concepts and criteria.

Substance use disorders were, for the first time, classified separately. In developing descriptions of the various disorders, the authors of DSM-III adopted a generally atheoretical perspective, believing that basing a system on one conceptual model would impede its use by clinicians of different theoretical orientations. A distinction was made between substance abuse and dependence. Substance abuse had three criteria: a pattern of pathological use, impairment in social or occupational functioning, and duration of 1 month or more. Dependence for most substances had only one criterion—namely, evidence of tolerance or withdrawal. However, the criteria for alcohol and cannabis also had impairment in social or occupational functioning and a pattern of pathological use.

The next revision, DSM-III-R,[26] was published in 1987. The central syndrome of dependence was influenced strongly by the Edwards and Gross conceptualization. The definition was broadened considerably, indeed to an extent that it was thought it might incorporate the entire spectrum of repetitive damaging substance use. Prior to publication, the diagnostic term *substance abuse* was restored, but it was regarded as a residual diagnosis that would be applied only to individuals who did not fulfill even this broad definition of dependence.

The next edition, DSM-IV,[27] refined and to some extent narrowed the definition of the dependence syndrome. This narrowing might have led to dependence being based on physiological criteria—namely, a mandatory requirement for tolerance and/or withdrawal symptoms. However, the data analyses did not support restricting dependence to this extent, although there is a fifth-digit specifier that indicates whether or not there are physiological features. The lack of insistence on a physiological component was considered to accommodate more readily syndromes of dependence on substances in which withdrawal is not prominent or had been difficult to define, such as the hallucinogens, psychostimulants, cannabis, and the inhalants. Overall, DSM-IV dependence has proved at least as robust a diagnosis, and it captures more people than the corresponding DSM-III version.[34]

In DSM-IV, substance abuse is understood as a less severe condition than dependence. The two diagnoses cannot coexist in the same time period, as substance abuse is preempted by a diagnosis of dependence. Substance abuse is defined as repeated substance use that leads to one or more social or occupational problems. It is envisaged as one axis of a biaxial conceptualization of substance use disorders that separates the inner core syndrome (dependence) from the consequences (abuse). Substance abuse is therefore related orthogonally to dependence, rather than being a *forme fruste* of it. The extent to which the biaxial relationship applies remains controversial, with some studies finding a one-factor solution that covers the spectrum of abuse and dependence as being the optimal one.[17,35,36]

The International Classification of Diseases

The ICD is the principal international coding system of diseases, injuries, and causes of death. It is overseen by WHO, which is mandated to issue periodic revisions. The ICD has its origins in the International List of Causes of Death, which was developed in the mid-nineteenth century. The list was extended to cover causes of hospitalization and then causes of morbidity in the general population. By the mid-twentieth century, there were several competing national disease classification systems, and in 1946 WHO was entrusted with preparing a revision that would be suitable for all countries, irrespective of their level of economic development and the nature of their health care system. The ninth and tenth revisions, published in 1978[37] and 1992,[25] respectively, represented substantial revisions. The aim of the tenth revision was to produce a "stable and flexible" classification system that would serve the needs of morbidity and mortality statistical systems worldwide for 10–20 years. Presently WHO is mandated to publish the next revision, the 11th, in 2011. Mental health disorders are listed in Chapter V of the ICD and are allocated codes in the form FXx.x. Substance use disorders are in the second section of Chapter V and are coded F1x.x. Thus alcohol dependence is F10.2. Fifth-digit codes are used for subtypes of disorder or as course specifiers.

ICD-10, influenced strongly by the work of the WHO Expert Committee, accepted the dependence syndrome as the central diagnosis.[25,38] It has six criteria, compared with DSM-IV's seven, and includes a cognitive item (craving) that does not appear in DSM-IV. While complementary nondependence conditions were considered for inclusion, only one, "harmful use," survived to appear in ICD-10. Hazardous use appeared in early drafts of ICD-10 but was omitted from the published version following the results of field trials that revealed an inter-rater reliability (kappa) coefficient of only 0.4.[39] Because of the difficulty in operationalizing it, the diagnosis was considered to be open to misuse. The decision to omit hazardous substance use was also influenced by doubts as to whether it represented a disease process, in many people's minds a prerequisite for inclusion in a classification system of diseases.

For epidemiological and public health purposes, having a term that defines various levels or patterns of substance use as conferring risk is advantageous. At the same time, examining relationships between use patterns and consequences without considering whether a diagnosable substance use disorder is present is limiting. The reduction in all-causes mortality among people with moderate levels of alcohol consumption is not seen in those with a previous diagnosis of alcohol dependence.[40] In support of including hazardous use in a diagnostic system is the evidence that such use can be defined and responds to therapy, with the evidence base for the effectiveness of interventions for hazardous alcohol consumption being particularly strong.[41] Thus, in a comprehensive diagnostic system, there are grounds for having a dependence category, a nondependence disorder that is of clinical consequence, and a "subthreshold" disorder that indicates risk to individuals and populations.

Experience With DSM-IV Substance Use Diagnoses

The dependence syndrome in DSM-IV (see Table 6–2) has proved to be a robust and clinically useful construct, applicable to a range of psychoactive substances,[13] arising from a distinct set of predisposing factors,[21,42–44] and having a symptom profile and a natural history that are more severe and progressive than substance abuse and other forms of repetitive substance use.[45–47] Dependence syndromes tend to be chronic disorders with a relatively severe course.[46] A subdiagnosis suggested in DSM-IV, dependence with physiological features, has a worse natural history, being associated with more alcohol (and drug) problems over a 5-year follow-up.[48]

Substance abuse is a less severe disorder than substance dependence and is characterized essentially by recurrent use that leads to social problems. Psychometrically, it performs less well than DSM-IV dependence, with kappa reliability coefficients of around 0.6–0.7.[49,50] When subjects who fulfill the criteria for dependence are excluded, the diagnosis of alcohol abuse is uncommon in some populations,[51] but this may be an artifact of the hierarchical exclusion rules. In some populations, alcohol abuse appears to be part of a continuum with dependence.[51,52] When considered separately, alcohol abuse is a more heterogeneous condition than dependence, at least in young people.[53] It is associated less commonly with mental health disorders, suicidal behavior, being assaulted, malnutrition, and treatment-seeking than dependence.[42] How persistent it is depends partly on the demographics of the population studied. In young people remission is more common than persistence of the diagnosis or progression to dependence.[36] In older age groups it tends to per-

TABLE 6–2. Dependence criteria for ICD-10 and DSM-IV, with corresponding elements from Edwards and Gross's original description of the syndrome,[11] and sample questions from the CIDI 1.1. alcohol and drug sections

ICD-10[25] (Flx.2)	DSM-IV[27]	Edwards and Gross[11]	Sample questions
Evidence of tolerance, such that increased doses of the psychoactive substance are required in order to achieve effects originally produced by lower doses	Tolerance, as defined by either of the following: a) a need for markedly increased amounts of the substance to achieve intoxication or desired effect; b) markedly diminished effect with continued use of the same amount of substance	Increased tolerance to alcohol	Found that you began to need to [use] much more than before to get the same effect? Found that [using] your usual amount began to have less effect on you?
A physiological withdrawal state when substance use has ceased or been reduced, as evidenced by the characteristic withdrawal syndrome for the substance or use of the same (or a closely related) substance with the intention of relieving or avoiding withdrawal symptoms	Withdrawal, as manifested by either of the following: (a) the characteristic withdrawal syndrome for the substance (b) the same (or a closely related) substance is taken to relieve or avoid withdrawal symptoms	Repeated withdrawal symptoms Relief or avoidance of withdrawal symptoms by further drinking	Did stopping or cutting down on your [use] ever cause you problems such as…[list withdrawal symptoms]? Ever [used substance] to keep from having problems or to make any of these problems go away?

TABLE 6–2. Dependence criteria for ICD-10 and DSM-IV, with corresponding elements from Edwards and Gross's original description of the syndrome,[11] and sample questions from the CIDI 1.1. alcohol and drug sections *(continued)*

A strong desire or sense of compulsion to take the substance	No equivalent criterion; mentioned in text	Subjective awareness of compulsion to drink, incorporating "loss of control"	Felt such a strong desire or urge to [use substance] that you could not resist it?
No equivalent criterion, but text states that "the subjective awareness of compulsion to use drugs is most commonly seen during attempts to stop or control substance use"	There is a persistent desire or unsuccessful efforts to cut down or control substance use		Wanted to stop or cut down on your [use] but couldn't? More than once try unsuccessfully to stop or cut down on your [use]?
Difficulties in controlling substance-taking behavior in terms of its onset, termination or levels of use	The substance is often taken in larger amounts or over a longer period than was intended		Used much more than you expected to when you began, or for a longer period of time than you intended to? Started [using] and found it difficult to stop before you became [intoxicated]?
Progressive neglect of alternative pleasures or interests because of psychoactive substance use	Important social, occupational, or recreational activities are given up or substance use reduced because of substance use	Salience of drink-seeking behavior	Given up or greatly reduced important activities in order to [use]…like sports, work, or associating with friends and relatives?

TABLE 6–2. Dependence criteria for ICD-10 and DSM-IV, with corresponding elements from Edwards and Gross's original description of the syndrome,[11] and sample questions from the CIDI 1.1. alcohol and drug sections *(continued)*

Increased amount of time necessary to obtain or take the substance or to recover from its effects	A great deal of time is spent in activities necessary to obtain the substance, use the substance, or recover from its effects		A period when you spent a great deal of time [using substance] or getting over the effects of [substance]?
Persisting with substance use despite clear evidence of overtly harmful consequences. Efforts should be made to determine that the user was actually, or could be expected to be, aware of the nature and extent of the harm	The substance use is continued despite knowledge of having a persistent or recurrent physical or psychological problem that is likely to have been caused or exacerbated by the substance		Has [substance use] ever caused you any physical/psychological problems? If yes,... Did you continue to [use] after you realized that it caused [state problem]?
No equivalent criterion; mentioned in text	No equivalent criterion	Narrowing of the drinking repertoire	[Using substance] became so regular that you would not change when you [used] or how much you [used], no matter what you were doing or where you were?
No equivalent criterion; mentioned in text	No equivalent criterion	Reinstatement after abstinence	

sist, with more than one-third fulfilling the diagnosis at a 5-year follow-up.[54] The extent to which alcohol abuse represents a prodromal phase of alcohol dependence is controversial.[55,56] In two studies 10% or fewer of respondents diagnosed with alcohol abuse developed alcohol dependence over 3- and 5-year follow-up periods.[46,54] Substance abuse applied to other drugs is also generally less severe than dependence but, upon factor analysis, is less clearly distinguished from it.[17] For alcohol and cannabis it may be a prodromal condition, but less so for opiates and cocaine, possibly because dependence on these substances develops more rapidly.[57]

A key question is whether dependence accompanied by substance abuse affects different people or has a natural history or treatment response that is different from dependence without abuse. In a recent analysis, the latter was found to be more common in women and in ethnic minorities.[58]

A third category, termed "diagnostic orphans," has been the subject of recent investigations. These are substance users who report some symptoms of DSM-IV dependence but do not meet diagnostic criteria for either dependence or substance abuse. In a sample of young men, 16% were labeled as diagnostic orphans for alcohol use, compared with 15% who were alcohol-dependent, 18% who had alcohol abuse, and 51% who had no diagnosis.[59] In terms of natural history, the diagnostic orphans fell between individuals with a dependence syndrome and individuals with no alcohol use disorders. They were most similar to individuals with alcohol abuse,[60] although had fewer alcohol-related problems at follow-up.[59] Cannabis users who were diagnostic orphans reported use patterns that were more similar to those among users who fulfilled the criteria for cannabis abuse.[61] However, they did not have higher rates of illicit drug use or mental health disorders than non–cannabis users.

Experience With ICD-10 Substance Use Diagnoses

Although the ICD is the world's primary disease coding system, and large-scale surveys using ICD-10 substance use diagnostic criteria have been undertaken, the number of published studies that report on the validity and usefulness of ICD-10 diagnoses is, to date, much lower than the number of such studies for DSM-IV. Given that the ICD-10 definition and criteria for dependence are almost identical to those in DSM-IV (Table 6–2), it may be assumed that the same comments apply, and indeed it proves to be a psychometrically robust diagnosis[49,62] that defines a relatively severe disorder that is persistent. In a large study that formed part of the WHO–National Institutes of Health Joint Project, Üstün and colleagues found that test–retest reliability of ICD-10 dependence for a variety of psychoactive substances was high (kappa coefficients of 0.7–0.9).[49] Validity against clinical data was also high.

ICD-10 harmful use, on the other hand, has proved to be much less reliable psychometrically.[49,50,62,63] In the original field trials, the test–retest reliability coefficient was only 0.3–0.4,[39] and in the Joint Project study both reliability and validity were substantially lower than for dependence.[49] Similarly, in a sample of probands and relatives from the Collaborative Study on the Genetics of Alcoholism (COGA), kappa coefficients for harmful use rarely exceeded 0.10.[62] Harmful use also seems to be an uncommon condition: in an analysis of U.S. population data, Grant found negligible rates of harmful alcohol use after excluding individuals who also fulfilled the criteria for dependence.[64] Concordance with DSM-IV substance abuse is essentially nonexistent.[65]

Summary of the Issues

1. The DSM-IV and ICD-10 dependence syndromes hold up well. They are both psychometrically robust, and the differences are minimal. The main conceptual difference is that ICD-10 dependence includes craving, whereas DSM-IV does not. These diagnoses represent the majority of contacts for treatment service providers. There is a clear distinction between the natural history of substance dependence (whether defined by DSM-IV or ICD-10) and nondependence. There are clear differences in family history and early childhood experiences between those with a dependence syndrome and those with nondependent substance use disorders.
2. In aggregate, the nondependence substance use disorders in DSM-IV and ICD-10 represent less severe conditions. Progression to dependence occurs in the minority of cases, the level of substance use is more variable, and the condition tends to be intermittent. They are less psychometrically robust conditions than dependence, and indeed it may be argued that the very constructs are unsatisfactory. ICD-10 harmful substance use (where there is no concurrent diagnosis of dependence) performs poorly as a diagnostic entity and is rare in both clinical and general population samples. DSM-IV substance abuse is more satisfactory, at least in North American populations, but it has the disadvantage of being defined essentially by social criteria, which are highly culture-dependent.
3. There exists a substantial proportion of people in the general community who have some dependence symptoms but who are not captured by either of these diagnoses ("diagnostic orphans").
4. There also exists a large section of the general community whose repetitive substance use puts them at risk of harm, be it physical, mental, or social. They are not embraced by either diagnostic system.

Looking Ahead

At the time of writing, DSM-V is expected to be published in 2012–2014. WHO is mandated to publish the eleventh revision of the ICD by 2011. This period provides an opportunity for the two systems to develop in parallel, as was achieved to a great extent with DSM-IV and ICD-10. No other international disease classification and coding systems are contemplated to the best of the author's knowledge, although national and regional systems may emerge.

While the process by which ICD-11 will be developed will become clear shortly, it is useful to examine the comparative needs of a clinically oriented system such as DSM and an international system of morbidity and mortality statistics. This leads naturally to the identification of a research agenda, summarized as follows, to underpin the development of the two systems.

1. A simple conceptualization of substance use disorders would be helpful in portraying the nature of these conditions. The concept of an acquired underlying "driving force" to continued substance use (without the need for external reinforcement) might serve such a role. At the more severe end of the spectrum, this force would be represented by the dependence syndrome.
2. The dependence syndrome provides a sufficient foundation for the years ahead. The differences in current DSM and ICD formulations are small and could probably be reconciled. The comparative performance of the respective diagnostic criteria in data sets derived from different populations is a key research question.
3. The less severe end of the substance use disorder spectrum would encompass repetitive forms of substance use leading to adverse consequences but having a less predictable course, and emotional or environmental triggers are important in perpetuating the condition.
4. Whatever conceptualization of nondependent substance use disorders is adopted, there has to be a clear rationale for subdividing it. Whether harmful use and substance abuse can be combined should be subjected to empirical testing. Minimum criteria for nondependent use need to be established.
5. There remains the issue of enhancing the value of the classification systems for epidemiological and public health purposes. Describing repetitive patterns and levels of substance use that confer risk is necessary for epidemiological and public health purposes. A condition termed "hazardous" or "risky" use would fulfill these requirements and could be subtyped according to whether it represented periodic intoxication, exposure to continual high levels of psychoactive substance, or other patterns. The psychometric performance of hazardous substance use and its various subtypes is a key part of the research agenda. Whether hazardous use should be included in a clinically oriented diagnostic system such as DSM will need to be debated.

6. Examining to what extent concepts used to describe substance use disorders apply to other repetitive behaviors will form an additional challenge. Candidate conditions include pathological gambling, Internet addiction, compulsive shopping, and potentially certain eating disorders.
7. Although not the focus of the present chapter, it will be important to delineate addictive disorders from those disorders characterized by repetitive behaviors but with ego-dystonic thoughts.
8. Within the realm of dependence, there is a particular need for
   - Defining the role of family history and genetic factors in the delineation of subtypes of the dependence syndrome;
   - Defining whether there are sufficient commonalities in the psychophysiological mechanisms of the dependence syndrome that such criteria could form part of the diagnostic criteria for dependence; and
   - Defining whether subtypes based on other than family history and genetic factors can be identified and whether they are sufficiently useful for understanding the natural history of different types of dependence and their response to intervention.

References

1. Krabman PB, Saunders JB: Diagnostic criteria for substance misuse and dependence. Baillière's Clinical Psychiatry 21:375–404, 1996.
2. Jellinek EM: The Disease Concept of Alcoholism. New Brunswick, NJ, Hillhouse Press, 1960.
3. Ledermann S: Alcool, alcoolism, alcoolisation: données scientifiques de caractère physiologique, économique et social. Cahier 29. Paris, France, Presses Universitaires de France, Institut National d'Etudes Démographiques, 1960.
4. Room R: Drugs, consciousness and self-control: popular and medical conceptions. Int Rev Psychiatry 1:63–70, 1989.
5. Bandura A: Social Learning Theory. Englewood Cliffs, NJ, Prentice Hall, 1977.
6. Sobell MB, Sobell LC: Problem Drinkers: Guided Self-Change Treatment. New York, Guilford, 1993.
7. Sobell LC, Cunningham JA, Sobell MB: Recovery from alcohol problems with and without treatment: prevalence in two population surveys. Am J Public Health 86:966–972, 1996.
8. Kessel N, Walton H: Alcoholism. London, Penguin, 1969, p 71.
9. Self D: Drug dependence and addiction: neural substrates. Am J Psychiatry 161:223, 2004.
10. World Health Organization: Neuroscience of Psychoactive Substance Use and Dependence (Summary). Geneva, Switzerland, World Health Organization, 2004.
11. Edwards G, Gross MM: Alcohol dependence: provisional description of a clinical syndrome. Br Med J 1:1058–1061, 1976.

12. Owen RT, Tyrer P: Benzodiazepine dependence: a review of the evidence. Drugs 25:385–398, 1983.
13. Feingold A, Rounsaville B: Construct validity of the dependence syndrome as measured by DSM-IV for different psychoactive substances. Addiction 90:1661–1669, 1995.
14. Ashton H: Benzodiazepine dependence, in Adverse Syndromes and Psychiatric Drugs. Edited by Haddad P, Dursun S, Deakin B. Oxford, England, Oxford University Press, 2004, pp 239–260.
15. Sproule BA, Busto UE, Somer G, et al: Characteristics of dependent and non-dependent regular users of codeine. J Clin Psychopharmacol 19:367–372, 1999.
16. Swift W, Hall W, Teesson M: Cannabis use and dependence among Australian adults: results from the National Survey of Mental Health and Wellbeing. Addiction 96:737–748, 2001.
17. Teesson M, Lynskey M, Manor B, et al: The structure of cannabis dependence in the community. Drug Alcohol Depend 68:255–262, 2002.
18. Wu L-T, Pilowsky DJ, Schlenger WE: Inhalant abuse and dependence among adolescents in the United States. J Am Acad Child Adolesc Psychiatry 43:1206–1214, 2004.
19. Topp L, Darke S: The applicability of the dependence syndrome to amphetamine. Drug Alcohol Depend 48:113–118, 1997.
20. Cottler LB, Womack SB, Compton WM, et al: Ecstasy abuse and dependence among adolescents and young adults: applicability and reliability of DSM-IV criteria. Hum Psychopharmacol 16:599–606, 2001.
21. Lessov CN, Martin NG, Statham DJ, et al: Defining nicotine dependence for genetic research: evidence from Australian twins. Psychol Med 34:865–879, 2004.
22. Hughes JR, Oliveto AH, Liguori A, et al: Endorsement of DSM-IV dependence criteria among caffeine users. Drug Alcohol Depend 52:99–107, 1998.
23. Copeland J, Peters R, Dillon P: Anabolic–androgenic steroid use disorders among a sample of Australian competitive and recreational users. Drug Alcohol Depend 60:91–96, 2000.
24. Lejoyeux M, McLoughlin M, Ades J: Epidemiology of behavioral dependence: literature review and results of original studies. Eur Psychiatry 15:129–134, 2000.
25. World Health Organization: The ICD-10 Classification of Mental and Behavioural Disorders: Clinical Descriptions and Diagnostic Guidelines. Geneva, Switzerland, World Health Organization, 1992.
26. American Psychiatric Association: Diagnostic and Statistical Manual of Mental Disorders, 3rd Edition, Revised. Washington, DC, American Psychiatric Association, 1987.
27. American Psychiatric Association: Diagnostic and Statistical Manual of Mental Disorders, 4th Edition. Washington, DC, American Psychiatric Association, 1994.
28. Edwards G, Arif A, Hodgson R: Nomenclature and classification of drug- and alcohol-related problems: a WHO memorandum. Bull World Health Organ 59:225–242, 1981.
29. National Health and Medical Research Council: Is There a Safe Level of Daily Consumption of Alcohol for Men and Women? Canberra, Australia, Australian Government Publishing Service, 1992.
30. American Psychiatric Association: Statistical Manual for the Use of Hospitals for Mental Diseases, 10th Edition. Utica, NY, New York State Hospitals Press, 1942.

31. American Psychiatric Association: Diagnostic and Statistical Manual of Mental Disorders. Washington, DC, American Psychiatric Association, 1952.
32. American Psychiatric Association: Diagnostic and Statistical Manual of Mental Disorders, 2nd Edition. Washington, DC, American Psychiatric Association, 1968.
33. American Psychiatric Association: Diagnostic and Statistical Manual of Mental Disorders, 3rd Edition. Washington, DC, American Psychiatric Association, 1980.
34. Hasin D, Li Q, McCloud S, et al: Agreement between DSM-III, DSM-III-R and ICD-10 alcohol diagnoses in US community-sample heavy drinkers. Addiction 91:1517–1527, 1996.
35. Fulkerson JA, Harrison PA, Beebe TJ: DSM-IV substance abuse and dependence: are there really two dimensions of substance use disorders in adolescents? Addiction 94: 495–506, 1999.
36. Nelson CB, Rehm J, Üstün TB, et al: Factor structures for DSM-IV substance disorder criteria endorsed by alcohol, cannabis, cocaine and opiate users: results from the WHO reliability and validity study. Addiction 94:843–855, 1999.
37. World Health Organization: International Classification of Diseases, 9th Revision Clinical Modification (ICD-9-CM). Ann Arbor, MI, Commission on Professional and Hospital Activities, 1978.
38. Babor TF, Campbell R, Room R, et al: A Lexicon of Alcohol and Other Drug Terms. Geneva, Switzerland, World Health Organization, 1994.
39. Sartorius N, Kaelber CT, Cooper JE, et al: Progress toward achieving a common language in psychiatry. Results from the field trial of the clinical guidelines accompanying the WHO classification of mental and behavioral disorders in ICD-10. Arch Gen Psychiatry 50:115–124, 1993.
40. Dawson DA: Alcohol consumption, alcohol dependence and all-cause mortality. Alcohol Clin Exp Res 24:72–81, 2000.
41. Bertholet N, Daeppen J-B, Wietlisbach V, et al: Reduction of alcohol consumption by brief alcohol intervention in primary care. Arch Intern Med 165:986–995, 2005.
42. Hasin D, Van Rossem R, McCloud S, et al: Alcohol dependence and abuse diagnoses: validity in community sample heavy drinkers. Alcohol Clin Exp Res 21:213–219, 1997.
43. Harford T, Muthén BO: The dimensionality of alcohol abuse and dependence: a multivariate analysis of DSM-IV symptoms in the National Longitudinal Survey of Youth. J Stud Alcohol 62:150–157, 2001.
44. De Bellis MD: Developmental traumatology: a contributory mechanism for alcohol and substance use disorders. Psychoneuroendocrinology 27:155–170, 2002.
45. Hasin D, Paykin A: Alcohol dependence and abuse diagnoses: concurrent validity in a nationally representative sample. Alcohol Clin Exp Res 23:144–150, 1999.
46. Schuckit MA, Smith TL, Danko GP, et al: Five-year clinical course associated with DSM-IV alcohol abuse or dependence in a large group of men and women. Am J Psychiatry 158:1084–1090, 2001.
47. Hoffmann NG, Hoffmann TD: Construct validity for alcohol dependence as indicated by the SUDDS-IV. Subst Use Misuse 3:293–306, 2003.
48. Schuckit MA, Danko GP, Smith TL, et al: A 5-year prospective evaluation of DSM-IV alcohol dependence with and without a physiological component. Alcohol Clin Exp Res 27:818–825, 2003.

49. Üstün B, Compton W, Mager D, et al: WHO study on the reliability and validity of the alcohol and drug use disorder instruments: overview of methods and results. Drug Alcohol Depend 47:161–169, 1997.
50. Pollock NK, Martin CS, Langenbucher JW: Diagnostic concordance of DSM-III, DSM-III-R, DSM-IV and ICD-10 alcohol diagnoses in adolescents. J Stud Alcohol 61:439–446, 2000.
51. Hasin DS, Grant B: Nosological comparisons of DSM-III-R and DSM-IV alcohol abuse and dependence in a clinical facility: comparison with the National Health Interview Survey results. Alcohol Clin Exp Res 18:272–279, 1994.
52. Hasin D, Hatzenbuehler M, Smith S, et al: Co-occurring DSM-IV drug abuse in DSM-IV drug dependence: results from the National Epidemiologic Survey on Alcohol and Related Conditions. Drug Alcohol Depend 80:117–123, 2005.
53. Martin CS, Kaczynski NA, Maisto SA, et al: Patterns of DSM-IV alcohol abuse and dependence symptoms in adolescent drinkers. J Stud Alcohol 56:672–680, 1995.
54. Schuckit MA, Smith TL, Danko GP, et al: Prospective evaluation of the four DSM-IV criteria for alcohol abuse in a large population. Am J Psychiatry 162:350–360, 2005.
55. Langenbucher JW, Chung T: Onset and staging of DSM-IV alcohol dependence using mean age and survival-hazard methods. J Abnorm Psychol 104:346–354, 1995.
56. Grant BF, Stinson FS, Harford T: The 5-year course of alcohol abuse among young adults. J Subst Abuse 13:229–238, 2001.
57. Ridenour TA, Cottler LB, Compton WM, et al: Is there a progression from abuse disorders to dependence disorders? Addiction 98:635–644, 2003.
58. Hasin DS, Grant BF: The co-occurrence of DSM-IV alcohol abuse in DSM-IV alcohol dependence: results of the National Epidemiologic Survey on Alcohol and Related Conditions on heterogeneity that differ by population subgroup. Arch Gen Psychiatry 61:891–896, 2004.
59. Eng MY, Schuckit MA, Smith TL: A five-year prospective study of diagnostic orphans for alcohol use disorders. J Stud Alcohol 64:227–234, 2003.
60. Sarr M, Bucholz KK, Phelps DL: Using cluster analysis of alcohol use disorders to investigate "diagnostic orphans": subjects with alcohol dependence symptoms but no diagnosis. Drug Alcohol Depend 60:295–302, 2000.
61. Degenhardt L, Lynskey M, Coffey C, et al: "Diagnostic orphans" among young adult cannabis users: persons who report dependence symptoms but do not meet diagnostic criteria. Drug Alcohol Depend 67:205–212, 2002.
62. Schuckit MA, Hesselbrock V, Tipp J, et al: A comparison of DSM-III-R, DSM-IV and ICD-10 substance use disorders diagnoses in 1922 men and women subjects in the COGA study. Addiction 89:1629–1638, 1994.
63. Hasin D: Classification of alcohol use disorders. Alcohol Res Health 27:5–17, 2003.
64. Grant BF: ICD-10 harmful use of alcohol and the alcohol dependence syndrome: prevalence and implications. Addiction 88:413–420, 1993.
65. Grant BF: DSM-IV, DSM-III-R and ICD-10 alcohol and drug abuse/harmful use and dependence, United States 1992: a nosological comparison. Alcohol Clin Exp Res 20: 1482–1488, 1996.

7

SUBSTANCE USE DISORDERS

DSM-IV and ICD-10

Deborah Hasin, Ph.D.
Mark L. Hatzenbuehler
Katherine Keyes
Elizabeth Ogburn

Two major nomenclatures define substance use disorders for broad audiences of users with different training, experience, and interests. The *Diagnostic and Statistical Manual of Mental Disorders,* 4th Edition (DSM-IV), was developed in the United States by the American Psychiatric Association. DSM-IV is used in the United States and elsewhere. It includes only psychiatric disorders, including substance use disorders. The *International Classification of Diseases,* 10th Revision (ICD-10), was developed and published by the World Health Organization, is used mainly outside the United States, and covers the entire range of medical disorders, of which one specific section covers psychiatric disorders. The ICD-10 section on psychiatric disorders includes substance use disorders.

This research was supported in part by grants from the National Institute on Alcoholism and Alcohol Abuse (K05 AA014223) and the National Institute on Drug Abuse (RO1 DA018652) and support from the New York State Psychiatric Institute. The authors wish to thank Valerie Richmond, M.A., for editorial assistance and manuscript preparation.

Reprinted from Hasin D, Hatzenbuehler ML, Keyes K, Ogburn E: "Substance Use Disorders: DSM-IV and ICD-10." *Addiction* 101 (suppl 1):59–75, 2006. Used with permission of the Society for the Study of Addiction.

Users of the substance use disorders sections of DSM-IV and ICD-10 include medically and behaviorally trained clinicians, neuroscientists, geneticists, investigators conducting clinical trials, epidemiologists, policy makers, insurance companies, and others. Both DSM-IV and the research version of ICD-10 enable these diverse groups to arrive at common definitions of disorders by providing specific, generally observable criteria for each disorder. Specifically for substance use disorders, DSM-IV and ICD-10 diagnostic criteria define two disorders, *dependence* and a secondary category, called *abuse* in DSM-IV and *harmful use* in ICD-10. DSM-IV and ICD-10 also provide substance-specific intoxication and withdrawal symptoms, as well as methods for diagnosing substance-induced psychiatric disorders. Considerable evidence is available to answer many questions about the reliability and validity of the substance use disorders as defined in DSM-IV and ICD-10, although some questions remain unanswered and require additional research.

Background of DSM-IV and ICD-10 Definitions of Dependence and Abuse/Harmful Use

The basis for the substance use disorders originated in a paper on the alcohol dependence syndrome (ADS).[1] The ADS was presented as a combination of psychological and physiological processes occurring on a continuum of severity, leading to heavy drinking increasingly unresponsive to adverse consequences. ADS was considered one axis of alcohol problems, while social, legal, and other adverse consequences of heavy drinking were considered another axis ("biaxial").[2] The biaxial concept was generalized to all drugs of abuse.[3] The distinction between dependence and its conceptually distinct but empirically correlated medical, psychological, legal, or social consequences has been interpreted as meaning that the consequences are independent or orthogonal.[4] The environmental and neurobiological processes leading to dependence may differ from the processes leading to development of some of the consequences of heavy use, potentially causing confusion in etiological research if these consequences are considered part of dependence. However, increasing severity of dependence is unlikely to be independent of the probability or severity of its consequences, leading to separate but correlated dimensions.

The biaxial concept forms the basis of the definitions and distinction between dependence and abuse in DSM-III-R and DSM-IV and harmful use in ICD-10.[4,5] DSM-IV criteria for dependence are similar to DSM-III-R and agree highly, although small changes in DSM-IV slightly elevated the threshold for dependence. The DSM-III-R workgroup considered omitting a secondary disorder, but concerns arose that individuals having alcohol or drug problems without a dependence syndrome could not be characterized for treatment or reimbursement if a secondary condition were not included. The problem was how to define such a condition. Because of the different emphasis on cross-cultural applicability, the systems resolved the issue of the secondary disorder in somewhat different ways in DSM-IV and ICD-10,[4] as discussed below.

Criteria for Dependence and Abuse/Harmful Use in DSM-IV and ICD-10

DEPENDENCE

As shown in Table 7–1, DSM-IV and ICD-10 criteria for substance dependence are similar, with criteria for tolerance, withdrawal, continued use despite problems, and various indicators of impaired control. Each system requires at least three criteria to diagnose dependence, and co-occurrence of criteria within a 12-month period. The main difference between the two diagnoses is that "a strong desire or sense of compulsion to drink" is an ICD-10 criterion but is not stated directly in DSM-IV. Further, "difficulties controlling use in terms of onset, termination, or levels of use" is stated explicitly in ICD-10, whereas DSM-IV does not use the specific language of "onset" and "termination" but rather includes "drinking more or longer than intended" and "a great deal of time spent getting, using or getting over the effects of the substance." Despite these differences, if these two criteria sets describe the same underlying condition, then small differences between them should not produce large differences in their reliability, validity, or concordance. We address this below.

Both DSM-IV and ICD-10 dependence criteria include "continued use despite physical or psychological problems caused or exacerbated by the substance." If one attends to the "continued use despite…" portion of the criterion, it indicates a process motivating continued use despite consequences that would cause nondependent individuals to cease use, consistent with Edwards and Gross.[1] If one attends to the "physical or psychological problems" portion, then the criterion indicates consequences. In DSM-IV and ICD-10, negative consequences are limited to physical or psychological problems and are not extended to social or interpersonal problems.

ABUSE/HARMFUL USE

ICD-10 and DSM-IV both treat abuse and dependence hierarchically—only individuals without dependence are diagnosed with abuse or harmful use. Otherwise, the criteria differ (Table 7–1). In DSM-IV, one of four abuse criteria is required. One of these criteria is hazardous use—that is, use that elevates the risk of physical harm. In contrast, ICD-10 has only one criterion, harmful use, indicating physical or psychological harm has actually taken place. ("Hazardous use" of a substance was included in a prepublication version of ICD-10 and in the World Health Organization's 1994 *Lexicon of Alcohol and Drug Terms*[6] but was not

TABLE 7–1. Substance dependence and abuse/harmful use criteria: DSM-IV and ICD-10

Dependence	ICD-10	DSM-IV
Clustering criterion	a) Three or more of the following six symptoms occurring together for at least 1 month, or if < 1 month, occurring together repeatedly within a 12-month period	a) A maladaptive pattern of substance use, leading to clinically significant impairment or distress as manifested by three or more of the following seven symptoms occurring in the same 12-month period
Tolerance	Need for significantly increased amounts of substance to achieve intoxication or desired effect or markedly diminished effect with continued use of the same amount of substance	Need for markedly increased amounts of substance to achieve intoxication or desired effect; or markedly diminished effect with continued use of the same amount of substance
Withdrawal	A physiological withdrawal state of the characteristic withdrawal syndrome for the substance, or use of the substance (or closely related) to relieve or avoid symptoms	The characteristic withdrawal syndrome for the substance or the same (or a closely related) substance is taken to relieve or avoid withdrawal symptoms
Impaired control	Difficulties controlling use in terms of onset, termination, or levels of use; using in larger amounts or over a longer period than intended; or a persistent desire or unsuccessful efforts to reduce or control use	Persistent desire or one or more unsuccessful efforts to cut down or control use Using in larger amounts or over a longer period than the person intended
Neglect of activities	Important alternative pleasures or interests given up or reduced because of use; or	Important social, occupational, or recreational activities given up or reduced because of use

TABLE 7–1. Substance dependence and abuse/harmful use criteria: DSM-IV and ICD-10 *(continued)*

Time spent in substance-related activity	A great deal of time spent in activities necessary to obtain or use or to recover from its effects	A great deal of time spent in activities necessary to obtain, to use or to recover from the effects of use
Continued use despite problems	Persisting with use despite clear evidence and knowledge of harmful physical or psychological consequences	Continued use despite knowledge of having a persistent or recurrent physical or psychological problem that is likely to be caused or exacerbated by use
Compulsion	Strong desire or sense of compulsion to use	None
Abuse	a) (Harmful use) Clear evidence that substance use contributed to physical or psychological harm, which may lead to disability/adverse consequences b) The nature of harm should be clearly identifiable (and specified) c) The pattern of use has persisted for at least 1 month or has occurred repeatedly within a 12- month period d) Symptoms do not meet criteria for any other mental or behavioral disorder related to substance in the same time period (except for acute intoxication)	a) A maladaptive pattern of substance use, leading to clinically significant impairment or distress as manifested by at least one of the following occurring within a 12-month period: Recurrent use of substance resulting in a failure to fulfill major role obligations at work, school, or home (e.g., repeated absences or poor work performance related to substance use; related absences, suspensions, or expulsions from school; neglect of children or household) Recurrent use in situations in which it is physically hazardous (e.g., driving an automobile or operating a machine when impaired by substance use) Recurrent substance-related legal problems (e.g., arrests for related disorderly conduct) Continued substance use despite having persistent or recurrent social or interpersonal problems caused by or exacerbated by the effects of substance (e.g., arguments with spouse about consequences of intoxication) b) Symptoms have never met criteria for substance dependence

included as a diagnostic criterion in the final version of ICD-10.) The time frame for symptom expression in the two classifications is similar. DSM-IV explicitly includes "clinically significant impairment or distress" for both dependence and abuse, whereas ICD-10 does not.

In DSM-IV, continued use despite social/interpersonal problems is an abuse criterion. Despite wording suggesting the dependence process ("continued use despite…"), the criterion is usually understood as social consequences. ICD-10 omits this criterion entirely, on the grounds that social or legal reactions to substance use vary across times and cultures (e.g., drug use leads to legal problems in some areas or countries but not in others; heavy drinking leads to more criticism and marital conflict in some cultures than in others). Given the variability in reactions to substance use, these reactions were considered poor cross-cultural disorder indicators.[4] The rationale for continued use despite some problems but not others as a dependence indicator is questioned below in the subsection on animal models, and the general idea of consequences is considered in the section on alternative systems.

It is worth noting that the term *abuse* in DSM-IV creates some confusion because it is also commonly used, although with different connotations, for abuse of people (child abuse and/or spouse abuse, experiences that commonly co-occur with heavy use of alcohol or drugs). In future versions of DSM, changing the name of "abuse" to a more explicitly substance-related term such as *dysfunction* may alleviate such confusion.

Withdrawal Criteria: DSM-IV and ICD-10

WITHDRAWAL CRITERIA BY SUBSTANCE

In DSM-IV and ICD-10, physical withdrawal is a dependence criterion for every substance except cannabis and hallucinogens. There are general criteria for withdrawal across substances, and substance-specific criteria.

In DSM-IV, general withdrawal criteria include 1) development of substance-specific syndrome due to cessation of (or reduction in) heavy and prolonged substance use; 2) syndrome causes clinically significant distress or impairment in social, occupational, or other important areas of functioning; and 3) syndrome is not due to general medical condition and not better accounted for by other mental disorder. In ICD-10, the first and third criteria are similar to DSM-IV. However, ICD-10 does not require clinically significant distress or impairment. ICD-10 states that symptoms and signs must be compatible with known features of withdrawal from the particular substance.

Substance-specific withdrawal criteria (Table 7–2) overlap considerably. The most common difference is that "craving the same substance" (opiate, cocaine, nicotine, stimulants), present in ICD-10, is absent in DSM-IV. "Headache" is included for ICD-10 but not DSM-IV alcohol and sedative withdrawal. DSM-IV and ICD-10 include "malaise" as a symptom for cocaine and stimulant withdrawal, but ICD-10 also includes "malaise" for alcohol, sedatives and nicotine. ICD-10 generally requires fewer symptoms than DSM-IV for withdrawal to be diagnosed. Relative validity of the differences is unknown.

CANNABIS AND HALLUCINOGEN WITHDRAWAL

Accumulating evidence from animal, laboratory, and clinical studies (reviewed by Budney et al.[7]) supports the validity of cannabis withdrawal. New epidemiological evidence from a U.S. national survey (Hasin et al., under review) also supports a cannabis withdrawal syndrome: among 1,119 frequent cannabis users who never abused other substances, a two-factor model was found. One factor was characterized by weakness, hypersomnia, and psychomotor retardation (factor loadings range: 0.65–0.88). A second factor was characterized by anxiety symptoms (factor loadings range: 0.55–1.00). The two factors were moderately correlated (0.59). Cannabis withdrawal should be considered as an addition to DSM-V and ICD-11. To our knowledge, no corresponding syndrome has emerged for hallucinogens.

Test–Retest Reliability of Alcohol Abuse and Dependence Diagnoses

Many test–retest studies of DSM-IV and ICD-10 drug and alcohol dependence and abuse have been conducted in a range of samples, settings, and diagnostic interviews. Results for DSM-IV (Table 7–3) consistently show good to excellent reliability for dependence. In fact, this is one of the most reliable diagnoses in DSM-IV. The limited exceptions occur for cannabis, hallucinogen, and nicotine or for substances that were rare in the samples. When the dependence and abuse categories are combined, reliability is high but lower than dependence alone. The reliability of abuse is more variable and generally lower than dependence. The range was from no better than chance agreement to excellent, with many studies showing poor to low–fair values.

Test–retest results for ICD-10 (Table 7–4) were similar to those for DSM-IV, with reliability of alcohol and drug dependence or a combined abuse/dependence diagnosis ranging from good to excellent. In fact, only two drugs (sedatives and cocaine) were below the good range in any time frame. Given the diversity in study designs, the consistent findings on the reliability of dependence indicate its robustness. Similar to DSM-IV, the reliability of ICD-10 harmful use was generally lower than that of dependence.

To understand more clearly the lower reliability of abuse/harmful use, recall that a diagnosis of abuse is not given to an individual who meets criteria for dependence. Some reliability studies[8,9] further examined the reliability of abuse criteria when considered independently from dependence. These indicated that the reliability of abuse or its symptoms was considerably improved when the condition

TABLE 7–2. Comparison of substance withdrawal symptoms

	Symptoms																													
Substance	1	2	3	4	5	6	7	8	9	10	11	12	13	14	15	16	17	18	19	20	21	22	23	24	25	26	27	28	29	30
Alcohol																														
DSM-IV	✓	✓	✓	✓	✓		✓	✓	✓	✓																				
ICD-10	✓	✓	✓	✓	✓	✓	✓	✓	✓	✓																				
Opiates																														
DSM-IV		✓	✓				✓						✓	✓	✓		✓	✓	✓	✓	✓	✓								
ICD-10			✓	✓			✓					✓	✓	✓	✓		✓	✓	✓	✓										
Sedative-Hypnotics																														
DSM-IV	✓		✓	✓	✓		✓		✓	✓	✓																			
ICD-10	✓		✓	✓	✓	✓	✓	✓	✓	✓													✓	✓						
Cocaine																														
DSM-IV					✓		✓	✓																	✓	✓				
ICD-10					✓		✓	✓				✓													✓	✓				
Nicotine																														
DSM-IV							✓									✓					✓				✓		✓			✓
ICD-10							✓	✓		✓	✓										✓				✓		✓	✓	✓	✓
Stimulants* (includes amphetamines†)																														
DSM-IV					✓		✓	✓																		✓	✓			
ICD-10					✓		✓	✓				✓														✓	✓			

TABLE 7–2. Comparison of substance withdrawal symptoms *(continued)*

*ICD-10 criteria; †DSM-IV criteria.

1. Tremor of the tongue, eyelids or outstretched hands.
2. Sweating.
3. Nausea, retching or vomiting, or abdominal cramps.
4. Tachycardia or hypertension/autonomic hyperactivity.
5. Psychomotor agitation/retardation.
6. Headache.
7. Sleep disturbance.
8. Malaise or weakness/lethargy and fatigue.
9. Transient visual, tactile, or auditory hallucinations or illusions.
10. Grand mal convulsions.
11. Anxiety.
12. Craving for same substance.
13. Rhinorrhea or sneezing.
14. Lacrimation.
15. Muscle aches or cramps.
16. Decreased heart rate.
17. Diarrhea.
18. Papillary/pupillary dilation.
19. Piloerection or recurrent chills.
20. Yawning.
21. Dysphoric mood.
22. Fever.
23. Postural hypotension.
24. Paranoid ideation.
25. Increased appetite.
26. Bizarre or unpleasant dreams.
27. Irritability or restlessness.
28. Increased cough.
29. Mouth ulceration.
30. Difficulty in concentrating.

TABLE 7–3A. DSM-IV test–retest reliability[1] of alcohol abuse and dependence diagnoses, Part 1

	ALCOHOL		CANNABIS		COCAINE		NonA DRUG		HALLUCINOGENS		HEROIN	
Study	Current	Life	Current	Life	Current	Life	Current	Life	Current	Life	Current	Life
AUDADIS[+]												
Canino et al. 1999, $n=169$; Hispanic primary care patients: Puerto Rico												
Dependence	0.79	0.66					—	—				
Abuse	−0.01	0.20					—	—				
Dependence or abuse	0.75	0.72					0.56	0.59				
Nonhierarchical	0.66	0.64					—	—				
AUDADIS[+]												
Chatterji et al. 1997, $n=495$; general and substance treatment patients: India, Romania, Australia												
Dependence	0.75	0.71	0.71	0.65	–	0.75			—	0.49		
Abuse	0.49	0.47	0.70	0.54	–	0.44			0.72	0.55		
AUDADIS[+2]												
Grant et al. 1995, $n=664$; urban community: USA												
Dependence	0.75	0.63	0.94	0.70	0.99	0.89	—	—			0.73	0.81
Abuse	0.73	0.73	0.86	0.65	0.81	0.86	—	—			0.87	0.83
Dependence or abuse	0.76	0.73	0.78	0.71	0.91	0.68	0.79	0.66			0.66	0.80

TABLE 7–3A. DSM-IV test–retest reliability[1] of alcohol abuse and dependence diagnoses, Part 1 *(continued)*

	ALCOHOL		CANNABIS		COCAINE		NonA DRUG		HALLUCINOGENS		HEROIN	
Study	Current	Life	Current	Life	Current	Life	Current	Life	Current	Life	Current	Life
AUDADIS[+]												
Grant et al. 2003, *n*=2,657; general population: USA												
Dependence												
Dependence or abuse	0.74	0.70										
AUDADIS[+]												
Hasin et al. 1997, *n*=296; substance and psychiatric treatment patients: USA												
Dependence	0.76	0.75	0.63	0.66	0.72	0.72					0.86	0.80
Abuse	0.27	0.43	0.24	0.25	0.10	0.23					0.01	0.16
Nonhierarchical	0.79	0.79	0.70	0.68	0.76	0.76					0.83	0.79
AUDADIS-ADR[+3]												
Vrasti et al. 1998, *n*=149; substance and general care patients: Romania												
Dependence	0.66	0.68										
Abuse	0.45	0.49										

TABLE 7–3A. DSM-IV test–retest reliability[1] of alcohol abuse and dependence diagnoses, Part 1 *(continued)*

	ALCOHOL		CANNABIS		COCAINE		NonA DRUG		HALLUCINOGENS		HEROIN	
Study	Current	Life	Current	Life	Current	Life	Current	Life	Current	Life	Current	Life
CIDI-SAM+++												
Horton et al. 2000, n=various[4]; white/black alcohol drinkers: USA												
Dependence	0.80	0.78	0.69	0.50	0.67	0.63						
Nonhierarchical (individual criteria)	0.55–0.90/ 0.68–0.82		0.46–0.69/ 0.41–0.66		0.59–0.77/ 0.52–0.64							
CIDI-SAM+++												
Langenbucher et al. 1994, n=201; substance use patients: northeast USA												
Dependence			—	0.71	—	0.61						
M-CIDI+												
Wittchen et al. 1998, n=60; community residents, age 14–28: Germany												
Dependence												
Dependence or abuse	—	0.78					—	0.64				

TABLE 7–3A. DSM-IV test–retest reliability[1] of alcohol abuse and dependence diagnoses, Part 1 *(continued)*

	ALCOHOL		CANNABIS		COCAINE		NonA DRUG		HALLUCINOGENS		HEROIN	
Study	Current	Life	Current	Life	Current	Life	Current	Life	Current	Life	Current	Life
PRISM+												
Hasin et al. 1996a, $n=172$; substance and dual-diagnosis patients: USA												
Dependence	0.81	0.69	0.80	0.63	0.92	0.88			0.49	0.53	0.94	0.95
Abuse	0.32	0.18	0.51	0.50	–0.01	0.28			–0.01	0.40	1.00	0.49
PRISM+												
Hasin et al. 2006, $n=285$; substance and dual-diagnosis patients: USA												
Dependence	0.82	0.76	0.73	0.63	0.90	0.87			0.54	0.51	0.94	0.96
Abuse	0.56	0.52	0.42	0.48	0.50	0.33			–0.01	0.28	—	0.33
Nonhierarchical	0.80	0.77	0.66	0.69	0.88	0.88			0.54	0.95	0.90	0.95
SCAN++												
Easton et al. 1997, $n=287$; community residents, substance treatment and general care patients: USA, Turkey												
Dependence	0.80	0.76	0.77	0.88	0.69	0.74						
Abuse	0.53	0.63	0.57	0.65	—	—						

+Test–retest reliability using different interviewers; ++between-site reliability; +++6-month follow-up.

1. Each subject evaluated with the same diagnostic interview by at least two independent interviewers at different times. Reliability represented by the kappa statistic, indicating chance-corrected agreement between independent assessments. Kappa values of 0.75 and higher indicate excellent reliability, values of 0.60–0.74 represent good reliability, values of 0.40–0.59 indicate fair reliability and values of 0.39 or lower indicate poor reliability (Fleiss 1981).
2. This study did not report lifetime rates; table includes kappas for "prior to last year" instead.
3. Only alcohol users are included in analysis.
4. There were 10 different sample sizes in the study, ranging from 31 subjects to 191 subjects; a different sample for each drug category in both race categories.

TABLE 7–3B. DSM-IV test–retest reliability[1] of alcohol abuse and dependence diagnoses, Part 2

	NICOTINE		OPIATES		OPIATES (LICIT)		SEDATIVES		STIMULANTS	
Study	Current	Life	Current	Life	Current	Life	Current	Life	Current	Life
AUDADIS[+]										
Canino et al. 1999, $n=169$; Hispanic primary care patients: Puerto Rico										
Dependence										
Abuse										
Dependence or abuse										
Nonhierarchical										
AUDADIS[+]										
Chatterji et al. 1997, $n=495$; general and substance treatment patients: India, Romania, Australia										
Dependence			0.96	0.94			0.95	0.86	0.92	0.84
Abuse			0.36	0.26			0.74	0.63	0.74	0.53
AUDADIS[+2]										
Grant et al. 1995, $n=664$; urban community: USA										
Dependence										
Abuse										
Dependence or abuse										

TABLE 7–3B. DSM-IV test–retest reliability[1] of alcohol abuse and dependence diagnoses, Part 2 *(continued)*

	NICOTINE		OPIATES		OPIATES (LICIT)		SEDATIVES		STIMULANTS	
Study	Current	Life	Current	Life	Current	Life	Current	Life	Current	Life
AUDADIS[+]										
Grant et al. 2003, *n*=2,657; general population: USA										
Dependence	0.63	0.60								
Dependence or abuse										
AUDADIS[+]										
Hasin et al. 1997, *n*=296; substance and psychiatric treatment patients: USA										
Dependence					0.59	0.59	0.66	0.57	0.80	0.77
Abuse					0.00	0.14	0.00	0.41	0.00	0.33
Nonhierarchical					0.62	0.56	0.42	0.67	0.80	0.78
AUDADIS-ADR[+3]										
Vrasti et al. 1998, *n*=149; substance and general care patients: Romania										
Dependence										
Abuse										

TABLE 7–3B. DSM-IV test–retest reliability[1] of alcohol abuse and dependence diagnoses, Part 2 *(continued)*

	NICOTINE		OPIATES		OPIATES (LICIT)		SEDATIVES		STIMULANTS	
Study	**Current**	**Life**	**Current**	**Life**	**Current**	**Life**	**Current**	**Life**	**Current**	**Life**
CIDI-SAM+++										
Horton et al. 2000, n=various[4]; white/black alcohol drinkers: USA										
Dependence			0.71	0.77						
Nonhierarchical (individual criteria)			0.47–0.63	0.42–0.75						
CIDI-SAM+++										
Langenbucher et al. 1994, n=201; substance use patients: northeast USA										
Dependence			—		0.73					
M-CIDI+										
Wittchen et al. 1998, n=60; community residents, age 14–28: Germany										
Dependence	—	0.64								
Dependence or abuse										
PRISM+										
Hasin et al. 1996a, n=172; substance and dual-diagnosis patients: USA										
Dependence					0.85	0.85	0.81	0.69	0.66	0.68
Abuse					–0.01	0.26	0.20	0.36	—	0.39

TABLE 7–3B. DSM-IV test–retest reliability[1] of alcohol abuse and dependence diagnoses, Part 2 *(continued)*

	NICOTINE		OPIATES		OPIATES (LICIT)		SEDATIVES		STIMULANTS	
Study	Current	Life	Current	Life	Current	Life	Current	Life	Current	Life
PRISM⁺										
Hasin et al. 2006, *n*=285; substance and dual-diagnosis patients: USA										
Dependence			0.62		0.66		0.74	0.76	0.66	0.51
Abuse			0.44		0.44		0.42	0.36	—	0.20
Nonhierarchical			0.61		0.61		0.72	0.73	0.39	0.60
SCAN⁺⁺										
Easton et al. 1997, *n*=287; community residents, substance treatment and general care patients: USA, Turkey										
Dependence			0.97		0.96					
Abuse			—		—					

⁺Test–retest reliability using different interviewers; ⁺⁺between-site reliability; ⁺⁺⁺6-month follow-up.

1. Each subject evaluated with the same diagnostic interview by at least two independent interviewers at different times. Reliability represented by the kappa statistic, indicating chance-corrected agreement between independent assessments. Kappa values of 0.75 and higher indicate excellent reliability, values of 0.60–0.74 represent good reliability, values of 0.40–0.59 indicate fair reliability and values of 0.39 or lower indicate poor reliability (Fleiss 1981).
2. This study did not report lifetime rates; table includes kappas for "prior to last year" instead.
3. Only alcohol users are included in analysis.
4. There were 10 different sample sizes in the study, ranging from 31 subjects to 191 subjects; a different sample for each drug category in both race categories.

TABLE 7–4A. ICD-10 test–retest reliability[1] of alcohol abuse and dependence diagnoses, Part 1

	ALCOHOL		CANNABIS		COCAINE		NonA DRUG		HALLUCINOGENS		HEROIN	
Study	Current	Life	Current	Life	Current	Life	Current	Life	Current	Life	Current	Life
AUDADIS+												
Chatterji et al. 1997, *n*=495; general population and substance treatment patients: India, Romania, Australia												
Dependence	0.77	0.73	0.69	0.69	—	0.60			0.72	0.70		
Abuse	0.37	0.15	0.67	0.41	—	0.19			0.75	0.49		
AUDADIS+2												
Grant et al. 1995, *n*=664; urban community participants: USA												
Dependence	0.76	0.64	0.95	0.70	0.98	0.89	—	—			0.74	0.81
Abuse	0.63	0.66	0.92	0.87	0.93	0.64	—	—			0.71	0.77
Dependence or abuse	0.62	0.68	0.82	0.69	0.93	0.60	0.80	0.56			0.67	0.79
AUDADIS-ADR+3												
Vrasti et al. 1998, *n*=149; substance and general care patients: Romania												
Dependence	0.71	0.73										
Abuse	0.48	0.38										
CIDI-Auto+												
Rubio-Stipec et al. 1999, *n*=286; treated alcohol drinkers: Australia and Puerto Rico												
Dependence	0.71	0.71	0.79	0.71	0.92	0.83						
Abuse	0.36	0.58	0.62	0.45	0.54	0.46						

TABLE 7–4A. ICD-10 test–retest reliability[1] of alcohol abuse and dependence diagnoses, Part 1 *(continued)*

	ALCOHOL		CANNABIS		COCAINE		NonA DRUG		HALLUCINOGENS		HEROIN	
Study	Current	Life	Current	Life	Current	Life	Current	Life	Current	Life	Current	Life
CIDI[+]												
Üstün et al. 1997, *n*=288; general population and substance treatment patients: San Juan and Sydney												
Dependence	—	0.75	—	0.69	—	0.76			—	0.79		
Abuse	—	0.60	—	0.41	—	0.50			—	0.72		
SCAN[++]												
Easton et al. 1997, *n*=287; community residents, substance treatment and general care patients: USA, Turkey												
Dependence	0.85	0.79	0.77	0.78	0.69	0.74						
Abuse	0.20	0.36	0.57	0.40	—	—						
SDSS[+4]												
Miele et al. 2001, *n*=137 (alc), 68 (can), 92 (coc), 74 (her); treated substance users: USA												
Dependence	0.78	—	0.73	—	0.54	—					0.71	—
Abuse	0.61	—	0.43	—	0.49	—					0.47	—

[+]Test–retest reliability using different interviewers; [++]between-site reliability.

1. Each subject evaluated with the same diagnostic interview by at least two independent interviewers at different times. Reliability represented by the kappa statistic, indicating chance-corrected agreement between independent assessments. Kappa values of 0.75 and higher indicate excellent reliability, values of 0.60–0.74 represent good reliability, values of 0.40–0.59 indicate fair reliability and values of 0.39 or lower indicate poor reliability (Fleiss 1981).
2. This study did not report lifetime rates; table includes kappas for "prior to last year" instead.
3. Only alcohol users are included in analysis.
4. This study was not clear whether the kappas were for lifetime or current rates.

TABLE 7–4B. ICD-10 test–retest reliability[1] of alcohol abuse and dependence diagnoses, Part 2

	NICOTINE		OPIATES		OPIATES (LICIT)		SEDATIVES		STIMULANTS	
Study	Current	Life	Current	Life	Current	Life	Current	Life	Current	Life
AUDADIS[+]										
Chatterji et al. 1997, n=495; general population and substance treatment patients: India, Romania, Australia										
Dependence			0.93	0.94			0.84	0.85	0.94	0.87
Abuse			—	—			0.62	0.58	0.30	0.38
AUDADIS[+2]										
Grant et al. 1995, n=664; urban community participants: USA										
Dependence										
Abuse										
Dependence or abuse										
AUDADIS-ADR[+3]										
Vrasti et al. 1998, n=149; substance and general care patients: Romania										
Dependence										
Abuse										
CIDI-Auto[+]										
Rubio-Stipec et al. 1999, n=286; treated alcohol drinkers: Australia and Puerto Rico										
Dependence			0.85	0.92			0.62	0.70	0.66	0.73
Abuse			—	—			—	—	0.80	0.66

TABLE 7–4B. ICD-10 test–retest reliability[1] of alcohol abuse and dependence diagnoses, Part 2 *(continued)*

Study	NICOTINE		OPIATES		OPIATES (LICIT)		SEDATIVES		STIMULANTS	
	Current	Life	Current	Life	Current	Life	Current	Life	Current	Life
CIDI[+]										
Üstün et al. 1997, $n=288$; general population and substance treatment patients: San Juan and Sydney										
Dependence			—	0.80			—	0.48	—	0.76
Abuse			—	—			—	—	—	0.62
SCAN[++]										
Easton et al. 1997, $n=287$; community residents, substance treatment and general care patients: USA, Turkey										
Dependence			0.97	0.98						
Abuse			—	—						
SDSS[+4]										
Miele et al. 2001, $n=137$ (alc), 68 (can), 92 (coc), 74 (her); treated substance users: USA										
Dependence										
Abuse										

[+]Test–retest reliability using different interviewers; [++]between-site reliability.

1. Each subject evaluated with the same diagnostic interview by at least two independent interviewers at different times. Reliability represented by the kappa statistic, indicating chance-corrected agreement between independent assessments. Kappa values of 0.75 and higher indicate excellent reliability, values of 0.60–0.74 represent good reliability, values of 0.40–0.59 indicate fair reliability and values of 0.39 or lower indicate poor reliability (Fleiss 1981).
2. This study did not report lifetime rates; table includes kappas for "prior to last year" instead.
3. Only alcohol users are included in analysis.
4. This study was not clear whether the kappas were for lifetime or current rates.

was diagnosed as an independent category. These results indicate that part of the reliability problem with alcohol abuse stems from the category's conditional relationship to dependence rather than intrinsically unreliable criteria.

Validation of Dependence and Abuse

PSYCHOMETRIC VALIDATION: MULTI-METHOD COMPARISONS

In practical terms, high concordance between DSM-IV and ICD-10 would suggest that, despite minor differences in criteria, rates and results can be compared across studies. In theoretical terms, high concordance would suggest that both nomenclatures tap the same underlying construct or condition, supporting its validity. Numerous studies have addressed DSM-IV/ICD-10 concordance (Table 7–5). Across substances, studies, and time frames, DSM-IV and ICD-10 diagnoses of dependence show excellent agreement. In contrast, more than three-quarters of the abuse/harmful use comparisons show poor agreement. Agreement was also poor for nonhierarchical abuse/harmful use diagnoses, indicating that the criteria themselves simply did not agree well. Concordance of DSM-IV and ICD-10 combined diagnoses (abuse/harmful use or dependence) was intermediate between dependence and abuse/harmful use.

Within age, sex and ethnic groups, ICD-10/DSM-IV concordance was addressed using National Longitudinal Alcohol Epidemiologic Study (NLAES) data (N=42,086). Grant[10] examined this for alcohol, cannabis and "any drug." We extended this for cocaine, stimulants, tranquilizers, hallucinogens, and sedatives (unpublished tables available from first author upon request). DSM-IV/ICD-10 concordance for dependence was very good to excellent across substances, time frames, and demographic groups. In contrast, abuse/harmful use diagnoses showed poor–fair concordance. For some substances (e.g., sedatives, hallucinogens, stimulants, tranquilizers) the *n* was too small to be informative. Curiously, for every substance and time frame, DSM-IV/ICD-10 agreement was higher for blacks than for nonblacks. DSM-IV/ICD-10 agreement for combined diagnoses (abuse and/or dependence) ranged from good to excellent.

Several studies[11,12] examined validity of DSM-IV and ICD-10 diagnoses by calculating between-measure agreement. Measures included the Composite Diagnostic Interview (CIDI), Schedule for Clinical Assessment in Neuropsychiatry (SCAN), Alcohol Use Disorders and Associated Disabilities Interview Schedule (AUDADIS), Psychiatric Research Interview for Substance and Mental Disorders (PRISM), Structured Clinical Interview for DSM-IV Disorders (SCID), and longitudinal, expert, all data (LEAD) procedure; studies included patients and nonpatients in the United States, Luxembourg, Athens, and Madrid, incorporating samples of 105–420 individuals. Between-measure agreement tended to be better for DSM-IV than ICD-10; for DSM-IV, 35% of kappas were good or excellent;

TABLE 7–5A. DSM-IV/ICD-10 agreement by substance (kappa values[1]), Part 1

	ALCOHOL		CANNABIS		COCAINE		NonA DRUG		HALLUCINOGENS		HEROIN	
Study	Current	Life	Current	Life	Current	Life	Current	Life	Current	Life	Current	Life
AUDADIS												
Grant 1996, n=42,862; representative general population: USA												
Dependence	0.80	0.72	0.85	0.91	0.92	0.97	0.88	0.93	0.86	0.92		
Abuse	0.06	0.13	0.14	0.23	0.25	0.48	0.15	0.32	0.01	0.23		
Dependence or abuse	0.62	0.73	0.43	0.61	0.77	0.82	0.53	0.70	0.55	0.69		
AUDADIS												
Hasin et al. 1996b, n=962; random community population: NJ, USA												
Dependence	0.69	0.81										
Abuse	–0.04	0.03										
Dependence or abuse	0.59	0.65										
Nonhierarchical	0.20	0.17										
AUDADIS												
Hasin et al. 1997, n=1,811; community, psychiatric and medical participants: 12 international sites												
Dependence	0.90	0.90	0.86	0.89	0.98	1.00						
Abuse	0.24	0.23	0.26	0.34	0.60	0.51						

TABLE 7–5A. DSM-IV/ICD-10 agreement by substance (kappa values[1]), Part 1 *(continued)*

	ALCOHOL		CANNABIS		COCAINE		NonA DRUG		HALLUCINOGENS		HEROIN	
Study	Current	Life	Current	Life	Current	Life	Current	Life	Current	Life	Current	Life
CIDI												
Hasin et al. 1997, n=1,811; community, psychiatric and medical participants: 12 international sites												
Dependence	0.90	0.87	0.84	0.90	0.96	0.96						
Abuse	0.40	0.31	0.22	0.28	0.01	0.09						
CIDI												
Howard et al. 2001, n=76; lifetime inhalant users: USA												
Dependence or abuse												
CIDI[2]												
Rounsaville et al. 1993, n=521; community and clinical participants: CT, USA												
Dependence	0.84	—	0.63	—	0.84	—						
Abuse	0.08	—	0.15	—	0.19	—						
Dependence or abuse	0.79	—	0.52	—	0.82	—						
SCAN												
Hasin et al. 1997, n=1,811, community, psychiatric and medical participants: 12 international sites												
Dependence	0.92	0.92	0.88	0.90	0.97	0.98						
Abuse	0.27	0.38	0.38	0.49	0.48	0.43						

TABLE 7–5A. DSM-IV/ICD-10 agreement by substance (kappa values[1]), Part 1 *(continued)*

	ALCOHOL		CANNABIS		COCAINE		NonA DRUG		HALLUCINOGENS		HEROIN	
Study	Current	Life	Current	Life	Current	Life	Current	Life	Current	Life	Current	Life
SCID												
Pollock et al. 2000, n=413; community and clinical adolescent participants: Pittsburgh												
Dependence	—	0.81										
Abuse	—	0.06										
Dependence or abuse	—	0.55										
Nonhier-archical	—	0.10										
SSAGA												
Schuckit et al. 1994, n=1,922; alcohol-dependent probands and relatives from random population, medical and dental clinics: COGA sample, USA												
Dependence	—	0.71	—	0.78	—	0.76						
Abuse	—	0.05	—	0.05	—	0.04						
Dependence or abuse	—	0.44	—	0.39	—	0.51						

1. Each subject evaluated with the same diagnostic interview by at least two independent interviewers at different times. Reliability represented by the kappa statistic, indicating chance-corrected agreement between independent assessments. Kappa values of 0.75 and higher indicate excellent reliability, values of 0.60–0.74 represent good reliability, values of 0.40–0.59 indicate fair reliability and values of 0.39 or lower indicate poor reliability (Fleiss 1981).

2. DSM-IV criteria were still under development at the time of this study; they are not exactly like the finalized criteria. This study appears to compare lifetime DSM-IV diagnosis to current ICD-10 diagnosis.

TABLE 7–5B. DSM-IV/ICD-10 agreement by substance (kappa values[1]), Part 2

	INHALANTS		LICIT DRUG		OPIATES		SEDATIVES		STIMULANTS	
Study	Current	Life	Current	Life	Current	Life	Current	Life	Current	Life
AUDADIS										
Grant 1996, n=42,862; representative general population: USA										
Dependence			0.82	0.95			1.00	0.93	0.80	0.95
Abuse			0.05	0.30			0.53	0.34	0.05	0.30
Dependence or abuse			0.54	0.72			0.95	0.74	0.54	0.70
AUDADIS										
Hasin et al. 1996b, n=962; random community population: NJ, USA										
Dependence										
Abuse										
Dependence or abuse										
Nonhierarchical										
AUDADIS										
Hasin et al. 1997, n=1,811; community, psychiatric and medical participants: 12 international sites										
Dependence					0.98	0.98	0.92	0.93	0.86	0.93
Abuse					0.42	0.54	0.45	0.44	0.46	0.37

TABLE 7–5B. DSM-IV/ICD-10 agreement by substance (kappa values[1]), Part 2 *(continued)*

	INHALANTS		LICIT DRUG		OPIATES		SEDATIVES		STIMULANTS	
Study	Current	Life	Current	Life	Current	Life	Current	Life	Current	Life
CIDI										
Hasin et al. 1997, n=1,811; community, psychiatric and medical participants: 12 international sites										
Dependence					0.96	0.98	0.98	0.46	1.00	0.92
Abuse					0.42	0.34	—	0.24	—	0.34
CIDI										
Howard et al. 2001, n=76; lifetime inhalant users: USA										
Dependence or abuse		0.76								
CIDI[2]										
Rounsaville et al. 1993, n=521; community and clinical participants: CT, USA										
Dependence					0.95	—	0.85	—	0.78	—
Abuse					0.11	—	0.35	—	0.27	—
Dependence or abuse					0.92	—	0.74	—	0.70	—
SCAN										
Hasin et al. 1997, n=1,811; community, psychiatric and medical participants: 12 international sites										
Dependence					0.98	0.98	0.89	0.91	0.93	0.95
Abuse					0.27	0.30	0.29	0.31	0.61	0.45

TABLE 7–5B. DSM-IV/ICD-10 agreement by substance (kappa values[1]), Part 2 *(continued)*

	INHALANTS		LICIT DRUG		OPIATES		SEDATIVES		STIMULANTS	
Study	**Current**	**Life**	**Current**	**Life**	**Current**	**Life**	**Current**	**Life**	**Current**	**Life**
SCID										
Pollock et al. 2000, n=413; community and clinical adolescent participants: Pittsburgh										
Dependence										
Abuse										
Dependence or abuse										
Nonhierarchical										
SSAGA										
Schuckit et al. 1994, n=1,922; alcohol-dependent probands and relatives from random population, medical and dental clinics: COGA sample, USA										
Dependence					—	0.75	—	0.76	—	0.83
Abuse					—	0.16	—	0.29	—	0.07
Dependence or abuse					—	0.59	—	0.57	—	0.44

1. Each subject evaluated with the same diagnostic interview by at least two independent interviewers at different times. Reliability represented by the kappa statistic, indicating chance-corrected agreement between independent assessments. Kappa values of 0.75 and higher indicate excellent reliability, values of 0.60–0.74 represent good reliability, values of 0.40–0.59 indicate fair reliability and values of 0.39 or lower indicate poor reliability (Fleiss 1981).
2. DSM-IV criteria were still under development at the time of this study; they are not exactly like the finalized criteria. This study appears to compare lifetime DSM-IV diagnosis to current ICD-10 diagnosis.

only 9% were good (none were excellent) for ICD-10. Dependence diagnoses showed fair to excellent between-measure concordance for alcohol (0.61–0.80), and cocaine (0.45–0.81). Cannabis and amphetamine dependence showed low to fair concordance across studies (cannabis, 0.35–0.67; amphetamine, 0.36–0.54). Concordance for abuse was very low, with 80% of kappas 0.00–0.20.

PSYCHOMETRIC VALIDATION: LONGITUDINAL STUDIES

Many clinicians assume that abuse is an early stage of dependence, in which case there is little reason for two separate diagnoses. However, if abuse and dependence have distinctive courses, then the validity of their separation is supported. This was first addressed prospectively in an analysis of national data.[13] Subjects who had been diagnosed with abuse at baseline were unlikely to have become dependent at 4 years follow-up. Instead, most cases of abuse remitted, while dependence cases tended to be chronic. These results were replicated in prospective studies of college men,[14] relatives of alcoholics,[15] a national survey of youth,[16] and a community sample of heavy drinkers.[17] The studies support the abuse/dependence distinction for alcohol; work of this type is needed for drug abuse and dependence.

PSYCHOMETRIC VALIDATION: FACTOR ANALYTICAL AND LATENT CLASS STUDIES

Factor and Latent Class Analyses of Alcohol Use Disorders

Early studies did not take account of methodological issues, such as the need for large samples when analyzing binary variables and problems arising when the sample is defined by characteristics included in the analysis.[18–20] Factor analyses of abuse and dependence in the general population avoid these problems. The first of these studies[21] found a single factor, although the data set was small and not designed initially to assess DSM-III-R or DSM-IV criteria. In a much larger national sample with items designed specifically for DSM-III-R and DSM-IV criteria, Muthén and colleagues[22] found two separate factors generally corresponding to dependence and abuse that showed stability in structure across drinkers, heavy drinkers, and problem drinkers. These two factors were correlated (approximately 0.74). Very similar results were found when data from the National Longitudinal Study of Youth[23] were used, with assessment in adulthood for the criteria. These results are consistent with the conceptualization of dependence described at the beginning of this chapter.

Two latent class analyses have been conducted with well-characterized, large samples. In a sample of male and female relatives of treated alcoholic individuals in a genetics study,[24] four classes were found, generally describing graded severity. While these results are not consistent with the DSM-IV division between abuse and dependence, it is not clear how the requirement for a relative with severe alcoholism may have affected generalizability. In male Australian twins, a five-class solution was selected: one class with no or very infrequent problems, one class characterized by hazardous use and drinking more than intended (closest to abuse), and three dependence-like classes with graded severity.[25] This model is more consistent with the DSM-IV abuse/dependence distinction.

Factor Analyses of Drug Use Disorders

Factor analyses of drug use disorders have been developed less extensively. A recent study by Teesson et al.[26] analyzed DSM-IV cannabis dependence and abuse criteria in 722 untreated cannabis users. They found two factors so highly correlated (0.99) that a one-factor model was preferred. While the analysis and interpretation were thoughtful in this study, the sample was small for binary variables. In larger samples, DSM-IV marijuana and cocaine dependence and abuse criteria were analyzed with 5,808 lifetime marijuana users and 1,593 cocaine users in the U.S. national survey NLAES (C. Blanco et al., under review).

Marijuana. Weighted exploratory factor analysis indicated a large factor accounting for approximately 60% of the variance, and a smaller factor accounting for approximately 7% of the variance. χ^2 tests of model fit indicated that the two-factor and one-factor solutions both fitted the data, with a smaller root mean square residual (RMSR) for the two-factor model (smaller values of RMSRs are preferred). The abuse factor had large loadings on three criteria: failing to fulfill role obligations, hazardous use and social problems. Other criteria loaded on dependence. The two factors were correlated (0.73), although not as highly as in Teesson et al.[26]

Cocaine. Weighted exploratory factor analysis indicated a large factor accounting for approximately 70% of the variance, and a smaller factor accounting for approximately 6% of the variance. Similar to the results for cannabis, both the one- and two-factor solutions fitted the data, and again, the RMSR was smaller for the two-factor solution. The abuse factor had large loadings on two criteria: failure to fulfill role obligations and hazardous use. Other criteria loaded on dependence. The two factors were correlated (0.77).

Conclusion. Both marijuana and cocaine dependence criteria describe valid dependence syndromes that are graded in severity rather than categorical. While parsimony might suggest combining the abuse and dependence factors because of their correlations, the significance tests of model fit and RMSRs suggest that abuse criteria describe a related yet somewhat distinct phenomenon from dependence.

PSYCHOMETRIC VALIDATION: CONSTRUCT VALIDATION STUDIES

Studies of this type compare individuals with abuse or dependence to nondiagnosed drinkers or drug users on hypothesized correlates of a serious substance use disorder.[13]

In an all-male sample, alcohol abuse and dependence had similar correlates, although associations were weaker for abuse.[15] Two gender-balanced studies included a community sample of 962 heavy drinkers[27] and a national sample of current drinkers.[28] In both, alcohol dependence had strong, significant associations with family history of alcoholism, suicidal ideation, blackouts, and drinking volume, all of which are correlates of a serious disorder. Associations with alcohol abuse were weaker and less often significant. Also, in former drinkers in a national sample, past DSM-IV alcohol dependence but not abuse predicted current major depressive disorder.[29] These findings show equivocal evidence for alcohol abuse but consistent support for the validity of alcohol dependence as a serious alcohol use disorder. More evidence of this type is needed for drug use disorders.

VALIDATION: ETIOLOGICAL FINDINGS FROM GENETIC STUDIES

Twin studies have indicated a genetic component to alcohol dependence[30,31] and to dependence on other drugs.[32,33] With regard to specific genes, however, when DSM-IV and ICD-10 were in preparation, little was known aside from Asian studies on alcohol-metabolizing polymorphisms (*ADH1B* and *ALDH2*). Since then, with the explosion of knowledge and methods in genetics, this picture has changed. The Collaborative Study on the Genetics of Alcoholism (COGA) family genetics study is now a major source of information on the genetics of alcohol dependence and related conditions. Via the National Institute on Drug Abuse (NIDA) Genetics Consortium, knowledge should catch up on specific genetic contributions with drug use disorders.

Strong validation of the disorder comes from changes in dependence risk due to genetic variation affecting proteins implicated in the dependence process. Variations in single nucleotide polymorphisms in the γ-aminobutyric acid ($GABA_A$) receptor gene *(GABRA2)* have shown strong relationships to alcohol dependence in three genotyping studies in U.S.[34,35] and Russian[36] populations. Covault et al.[35] also suggested that results were specific to alcohol dependence, as elimination of subjects with comorbid cocaine dependence from the analysis strengthened the results. Numerous other findings are emerging on GABA receptor genes.[37] These findings support the validity of the clinical alcohol dependence phenotype, although biologically based endophenotypes may eventually offer more or complementary information.

VALIDATION: ANIMAL MODELS

Animal models for excess consumption have existed for some time, including high- and low-alcohol-preferring rat lines from Indiana University, heavy-drinking primates (e.g., the work of Grant and Johanson[38]) and high- and low-cocaine self-administering rats (i.e., the work of Koob[39]). These animal models play an important role in medication development. However, animal models of a dependence syndrome of symptoms were developed further in two papers. Deroche-Gamonet and colleagues[40] demonstrated three cocaine dependence–like behaviors in rats. One was sustained persistence of drug-seeking after nonavailability was signaled (difficulty stopping or limiting use). The second was quantitatively increasing efforts to get the drug without giving up as the drug became harder to obtain (a lot of time spent obtaining the drug). The third was continued use despite harmful consequences (in this case, use despite knowledge that foot-shock was paired with use). Not all the rats evidenced these behaviors. Instead, they arose mainly among a susceptible subset, with susceptibility defined by rapid reinstatement of use patterns after acclimation to use, withdrawal of drug availability, and renewed access. Importantly, none of the rats evidenced dependence behaviors after brief exposure to drug access, but only after prolonged access. The fact that nonsusceptible rats reduced their drug use greatly when paired with foot-shock while susceptible rats showed little reduction in their drug use suggests that despite awkwardness in question wording within human studies, the concept of continued use despite knowledge of problems is valid across species. If this is the case, it is reasonable to assume that the concept is also valid cross-culturally among humans. Vanderschuren and Everitt[41] also demonstrated dependence-like behaviors in rats, again only after prolonged access to self-administration.

Animal models of substance use have contributed much to the study of etiology/treatment of substance dependence, and they may contribute further by suggesting refinements of the diagnostic criteria. Of course, foot-shock is neither a medical, psychological, social, or legal consequence of use, but rapid-reinstating rats who learn that foot-shock accompanies drug use but continue use anyway provide compelling evidence of dependence. Perhaps DSM-V/ICD-11 could be improved by taking the two existing criteria, "continued use despite physical or psychological problems" (dependence) and "continued use despite social or interpersonal problems" (abuse), and combining them into a single criterion, "continued use despite serious negative consequences" for dependence, with future research addressing whether this could be considered a defining characteristic of alcohol or drug dependence in humans.

Substance-Induced Disorders in DSM-IV and ICD-10

Substance-induced disorders are an important area that is approached differently in DSM-IV and ICD-10. For Axis I psychotic, affective, and anxiety disorders, DSM-IV requires a) a prominent symptom of the disorder group (e.g., hallucinations or delusions, depressed or elevated mood, anxiety, panic attacks, or obsessions or compulsions); b) evidence from the history, physical exam, or lab findings either that the symptoms developed during or within a month of substance intoxication or withdrawal or that the "disturbance" was etiologically related to the "medication" use; c) that the "disturbance" be not better accounted for by a disorder that is not substance induced; and d) that the symptoms cause clinically significant distress or impairment in social, occupational, or other important areas of functioning. DSM-IV therefore does not require that all other criteria for the disorder be met. DSM-IV does not include substance-induced personality disorders.

ICD-10 is similar in some ways, requiring that a substance-induced disorder be clearly related to substance use. In cases where onset of the disorder occurs after use of psychoactive substances, strong evidence is required to demonstrate a link. In contrast to DSM-IV, ICD-10 requires that the full criteria for the disorder be met in terms of numbers of symptoms and duration. ICD-10 also differs from DSM-IV in that it allows for substance-induced personality disorders. Finally, in ICD-10, for a substance-induced psychotic disorder, the criteria are quite specific: a) onset of psychotic symptoms during or within 2 weeks of use; b) duration of symptoms for longer than 48 hours; and c) duration of the disorder for less than 6 months. Given the level of clinical interest in improved methods of assessment and treatment for psychiatric disorders comorbid with substance use disorders, surprisingly little attention has been given to the reliability or validity of the substance-induced disorder definitions provided in DSM-IV or ICD-10. To our knowledge, only one study[42] has tested the reliability of these disorders. In this study, the PRISM was used, as it was structured specifically to operationalize DSM-IV substance-induced as well as primary diagnostic criteria. To ensure adequate reliability, the PRISM differs from DSM-IV but shares with ICD-10 the requirement that for substance-induced disorders to be diagnosed, full diagnostic criteria for the base disorder must also be met. In a test–retest study of 285 substance abuse and psychiatric patients, many substance-induced diagnoses (e.g., disorders such as major depression and psychosis) were nearly as reliable as primary diagnoses, which were highly reliable in the PRISM. Further, a LEAD validity study in Spain comparing the PRISM to the less-structured SCID approach to substance-induced disorders[12] showed better reliability for the PRISM in substance-abusing psychiatric patients.

Remission Criteria

ICD-10 gives undefined remission categories (early, partial, or full remission). DSM-IV details early (less than 12 months) versus sustained (12 months or longer) and full (no abuse or dependence criteria) versus partial (one or more abuse or dependence criteria) remission. Thus, according to DSM-IV, dependence can be in early full remission, early partial remission, sustained full remission, or sustained partial remission. DSM-IV and ICD-10 also offer categories for those in a controlled environment such as a prison or a hospital. Little is known about the adequacy of these categories, and they are seldom used. Given the need for adequate measures for treatment studies, definitions of remission warrant further study in both nomenclatures.

Users of DSM-IV, ICD-10, and Alternative Systems

Here we consider the relevance of DSM-IV or ICD-10 definitions of substance use disorders and supporting evidence to users of the nomenclatures, including clinicians, insurance companies, neuroscientists, geneticists, treatment researchers, epidemiologists, and policy makers. We also consider other assessment approaches and their relevance.

CLINICIANS

Informal input from U.S. clinicians working in nonresearch alcohol and/or drug treatment settings (including those affiliated with NIDA's Clinical Trials Network) indicates that many see DSM-IV and ICD-10 definitions as irrelevant to their work. Learning the definitions is part of professional training, but the assessments themselves are part of "paperwork," and patients seen in these settings are all assumed to be dependent. Diagnoses for "secondary" substances are often not made systematically, and the main diagnosis does not play a role in treatment planning. An exception is withdrawal, which is assessed to determine if specific treatment is warranted. Many clinicians in generalist settings where often alcohol- and drug-abusing patients are treated (e.g., emergency rooms, primary care) also do not assess substance use or substance use disorders carefully for a variety of reasons.[43,44]

INSURANCE COMPANIES

These require diagnoses to reimburse for treatment; a mild-sounding diagnosis is less reimbursable. Altering or removing diagnoses may affect treatment availability.

SCIENTISTS

Neuroscientists and geneticists need a valid common definition of the condition they study in order to define groups as homogeneously as possible; heterogeneity complicates their work. In the absence of biological endophenotypes that can be used across studies, these investigators regularly use the DSM-IV dependence diagnosis, assessed in a structured manner. They rarely use the abuse category by itself, and because the distinctions between abuse and dependence are increasingly recognized, neuroscientists and geneticists now seldom combine abuse and dependence as a single phenotype. (Because the seven dependence criteria can theoretically yield a diagnosis from 99 criteria combinations,[45] many consider dependence heterogeneous. However, in a U.S. national sample, six combinations of the DSM-IV alcohol dependence criteria accounted for the large majority of dependence cases, all including physiological and impaired control criteria).

TREATMENT RESEARCHERS

The attitude of such researchers toward DSM-IV or ICD-10 diagnoses varies widely. Some use diagnoses only because they are a common requirement for research. Others feel that the dependence diagnosis is useful in designing a sample with a known, important defining clinical characteristic. Even medication-oriented clinical investigators may believe that a fully assessed diagnosis of dependence is not necessary in a clinical trial, assuming that all patients in treatment are dependent. Recent National Epidemiologic Survey on Alcohol and Related Conditions findings suggest that this is not the case for drug patients.[46] Instead, many patients have past but not current diagnoses; others are in treatment due to external circumstances regarding drug use but do not actually meet criteria for dependence.

EPIDEMIOLOGISTS

Epidemiologists need a reliable, valid nomenclature in order to provide accurate rates, time trends, subgroup differences in populations, the need for and use of health services and (among genetic epidemiologists) phenotypes useful for genetic studies.

POLICY MAKERS

Although not a unitary group, policy makers can be generally defined as those allocating funds and other resources to prevention and treatment. It has been suggested that this group is especially interested not in dependence per se but rather in whether treatment reduces the social and legal consequences of substance use disorders. As such, many policy makers are interested in the Addiction Severity Index (ASI), a standard intake assessment form in most treatment facilities in the United States.

The Addiction Severity Index[47,48] includes simple measures of use frequency and five problem areas (consequences) commonly affected by addiction: physical health, psychiatric status (distress), family/social environment, employment/financial support, and legal issues. It is the most widely used instrument in U.S. substance abuse clinics[49] and is used increasingly in other countries. In particular, the EuropASI, a somewhat modified version, is used by many treatment facilities for clinical assessment, registration, research and management.[50] The ASI has been translated into numerous languages, with generally good reliability and validity across modified versions (e.g., Dutch: Hendriks et al.[51]; German: Scheurich et al.[52]; and French: Krenz et al.[53]). Lower reliability/validity is more likely in special populations such as dual-diagnosis patients or the homeless. Most ASI sections were reliable in Dutch alcoholic individuals,[54] and while some areas of the ASI had cross-cultural problems in Kuwaiti substance abusers, much of the instrument's validity was excellent.[55] Despite nonspecific concerns about cultural insensitivity,[56,57] the ASI is now used in studies in Taiwan,[58] Iran,[59] Pakistan,[60] Amsterdam,[61] Italy,[62] Spain,[63] and Israel.[64] NIDA is funding work by McLellan and Alterman to study and enhance ASI validity in Mexico and South America.[65] Given the widespread use of the ASI, it may be useful to determine if anything can be learned from it that can be applied to the DSM-V/ICD-11 development process, especially for the nondependence category. Possible ideas include assessment of consequences of substance use regardless of whether dependence is present or not, and differentiation of consequences into the five areas covered by the ASI.

Recommendations

As we consider the extensive work that has already been conducted to understand the diagnostic profiles of substance use disorders, the following serve as recommendations:

1. Retain substance dependence as a category. Standardize the criteria across DSM-V and ICD-11.
2. Consider a severity measure based on a count of DSM-V/ICD-11 criteria, to ensure continued standardization of the severity measure and a close link to the binary diagnostic categories (e.g., Helzer et al.[66] and Hasin et al.[67,68]). Although more complex severity rating schemes can doubtless be devised, these may be more applicable to specialized uses, while a simple severity indicator is likely to be more widely used.
3. Conduct further reliability and validity studies of cannabis withdrawal and, if supported, add the diagnosis to DSM-V and ICD-11, using the same criteria in both nomenclatures.
4. Investigate whether the briefer symptom set of withdrawal symptoms for each substance in ICD-10 is as informative as the longer symptom set of withdrawal symptoms in DSM-IV, and use a standard set that is most parsimonious in DSM-V and ICD-11.
5. Conduct further reliability and validity studies of the substance-induced psychiatric categories. Consider making DSM consistent with the ICD in requiring that full criteria for the primary disorder (e.g., duration, symptom count) be met to make a substance-induced diagnosis, in addition to chronologically plausible substance involvement.
6. Carry out theoretical work leading to empirical studies of remission criteria to provide improved measures of this aspect of course in DSM-V and ICD-11.
7. Plan and carry out clinician education programs on the value of careful assessment of current and past dependence and abuse for all substances so that evidence-based treatments can be applied to patients with evidence-based diagnoses. Design such programs to be suitable for specialist as well as generalist settings.

8. Measure consequences of heavy substance use (medical, psychological, social, occupational, legal) independently of dependence, either with the existing DSM-IV abuse criteria or with an instrument such as the ASI.
9. Consider a name change for substance abuse to "substance dysfunction disorder" to avoid the confusion of substance "abuse" with other types of abuse.
10. Conduct future research addressing whether "continued use despite serious negative consequences" could be considered a defining characteristic of alcohol or drug dependence in humans.

References

1. Edwards G, Gross M: Alcohol dependence: provisional description of a clinical syndrome. Br Med J 1:1058–1061, 1976.
2. Edwards G: The alcohol dependence syndrome: a concept as stimulus to enquiry. Br J Addict 81:171–183, 1986.
3. World Health Organization: Nomenclature and classification of drug- and alcohol-related problems: WHO memorandum. Bull World Health Organ 99:225–242, 1981.
4. Rounsaville BJ: Experience with ICD-10/DSM-IV substance use disorders. Psychopathology 35:82–88, 2002.
5. Rounsaville BJ, Spitzer RL, Williams J: Proposed changes in DSM-III substance use disorders: description and rationale. Am J Psychiatry 143:463–468, 1986.
6. World Health Organization: Lexicon of Alcohol and Drug Terms. Geneva, World Health Organization, 1994. Available online at http://www.who.int/substance_abuse/terminology/who_lexicon/en/index.html. Accessed April 20, 2006.
7. Budney AJ, Hughes JR, Moore BA, et al: Review of the validity and significance of cannabis withdrawal syndrome. Am J Psychiatry 161:1967–1977, 2004.
8. Canino GJ, Bravo M, Ramírez R, et al: The Spanish Alcohol Use Disorder and Associated Disabilities Interview Schedule (AUDADIS): reliability and concordance with clinical diagnoses in a Hispanic population. J Stud Alcohol 60:790–799, 1999.
9. Horton J, Compton W, Cottler LB: Reliability of substance use disorder diagnoses among African-Americans and Caucasians. Drug Alcohol Depend 57:203–209, 2000.
10. Grant BF: DSM-III-R and ICD-10 alcohol and drug abuse/harmful use and dependence, United States, 1992: a nosological comparison. Alcohol Clin Exp Res 21:79–84, 1996.
11. Cottler LB, Grant BF, Blaine J, et al: Concordance of DSM-IV alcohol and drug use disorder criteria and diagnoses as measured by AUDADIS-ADR, CIDI and SCAN. Drug Alcohol Depend 47:195–205, 1997.
12. Torrens M, Serrano D, Astals M, et al: Diagnosing comorbid psychiatric disorders in substance abusers: validity of the Spanish versions of the Psychiatric Research Interview for Substance and Mental Disorders and the Structured Clinical Interview for DSM-IV. Am J Psychiatry 161:1231–1237, 2004.
13. Hasin D, Grant BF, Endicott J: The natural history of alcohol abuse: implications for definitions of alcohol use disorders. Am J Psychiatry 147:1537–1541, 1990.
14. Schuckit MA, Smith TL, Landi NA: The 5-year clinical course of high-functioning men with DSM-IV alcohol abuse or dependence. Am J Psychiatry 157:2028–2035, 2000.

15. Schuckit MA, Smith TL: A comparison of correlates of DSM-IV alcohol abuse or dependence among more than 400 sons of alcoholics and controls. Alcohol Clin Exp Res 25:1–8, 2001.
16. Grant BF, Stinson FS, Harford TC: Age at onset of alcohol use and DSM-IV alcohol abuse and dependence: a 12-year follow-up. J Subst Abuse 13:493–504, 2001.
17. Hasin D, Van Rossem R, McCloud S, et al: Differentiating DSM-IV alcohol dependence and abuse by course: community heavy drinkers. J Subst Abuse 9:127–135, 1997.
18. Hasin DS, Grant BF, Endicott J, et al: Cocaine and heroin dependence compared in poly-drug abusers. Am J Public Health 78:567–569, 1988.
19. Bryant KJ, Rounsaville BJ, Babor TF: Coherence of the dependence syndrome in cocaine users. Br J Addict 86:1299–1310, 1991.
20. Feingold A, Rounsaville BJ: Construct validity of the dependence syndrome as measured by DSM-IV for different psychoactive substances. Addiction 90:1661–1669, 1995.
21. Hasin D, Muthén B, Wisnicki K, et al: Validity of the bi-axial dependence concept: a test in the US general population. Addiction 89:573–579, 1994.
22. Muthén B, Grant B, Hasin D: The dimensionality of alcohol abuse and dependence: factor analysis of DSM-III-R and proposed DSM-IV criteria in the 1988 National Health Interview Survey. Addiction 88:1079–1090, 1993.
23. Harford TC, Muthén B: The dimensionality of alcohol abuse and dependence: a multivariate analysis of DSM-IV symptom items in the National Longitudinal Survey of Youth. J Stud Alcohol 62:150–157, 2001.
24. Bucholz KK, Heath AC, Reich T, et al: Can we subtype alcoholism? A latent class analysis of data from relatives of alcoholics in a multicenter family study of alcoholism. Alcohol Clin Exp Res 20:1462–1471, 1996.
25. Heath AC, Bucholz KK, Slutske WS, et al: The assessment of alcoholism in surveys of the general community: what are we measuring? Some insights from the Australian twin panel interview survey. Int Rev Psychiatry 6:295–307, 1994.
26. Teesson M, Lynskey MT, Manor B, et al: The structure of cannabis dependence in the community. Drug Alcohol Depend 68:255–262, 2002.
27. Hasin D, Paykin A: DSM-IV alcohol abuse: investigation in a sample of at-risk drinkers in the community. J Stud Alcohol 60:180–187, 1999.
28. Hasin DS, Grant BF: The co-occurrence of DSM-IV alcohol abuse in DSM-IV alcohol dependence: results of the National Epidemiologic Survey on Alcohol and Related Conditions on heterogeneity that differ by population subgroup. Arch Gen Psychiatry 61:891–896, 2004.
29. Hasin DS, Grant BF: Major depression in 6,050 former drinkers: association with past alcohol dependence. Arch Gen Psychiatry 59:794–800, 2002.
30. Prescott CA, Kendler KS: Genetic and environmental contributions to alcohol abuse and dependence in population-based sample of male twins. Am J Psychiatry 156:34–40, 1999.
31. Heath AC, Whitfield JB, Madden PAF, et al: Towards a molecular epidemiology of alcohol dependence: analysing the interplay of genetic and environmental risk factors. Br J Psychiatry Suppl 40:s33–s40, 2001.
32. Kendler KS, Jacobson KC, Prescott CA, et al: Specificity of genetic and environmental risk factors for use and abuse/dependence of cannabis, cocaine, hallucinogens, sedatives, stimulants, and opiates in male twins. Am J Psychiatry 160:687–695, 2003.

33. Tsuang MT, Lyons MJ, Eisen SA, et al: Genetic influences on DSM-III-R drug abuse and dependence: a study of 3,372 twin pairs. Am J Med Genet 67:473–477, 1996.
34. Edenberg HJ, Dick DM, Xuei X, et al: Variations in GABRA2, encoding the alpha 2 subunit of the GABA(A) receptor, are associated with alcohol dependence and with brain oscillations. Am J Hum Genet 74:705–714, 2004.
35. Covault J, Gelernter J, Hesselbrock V, et al: Allelic and haplotypic association of GABRA2 with alcohol dependence. Am J Med Genet B Neuropsychiatr Genet 129: 104–109, 2004.
36. Lappalainen J, Krupitsky E, Remizov M, et al: Association between alcoholism and gamma-amino butyric acid alpha2 receptor subtype in a Russian population. Alcohol Clin Exp Res 29:493–498, 2005.
37. Radel M, Vallejo RL, Iwata N, et al: Haplotype-based localization of an alcohol dependence gene to the 5q34 γ-aminobutyric acid type A gene cluster. Arch Gen Psychiatry 62:47–55, 2005.
38. Grant KA, Johanson CE: Oral ethanol self-administration in free-feeding rhesus monkeys. Alcohol Clin Exp Res 12:780–784, 1988.
39. Koob GF: Neural mechanisms of drug reinforcement. Ann NY Acad Sci 654:171–191, 1992.
40. Deroche-Gamonet V, Belin D, Piazza VP: Evidence for addiction-like behavior in the rat. Science 305:1014–1017, 2004.
41. Vanderschuren LJ, Everitt BJ: Drug seeking becomes compulsive after prolonged cocaine self-administration. Science 305:1017–1019, 2004.
42. Hasin D, Samet S, Nunes E, et al: Diagnosis of comorbid disorders in substance users: Psychiatric Research Interview for Substance and Mental Disorders (PRISM-IV). Am J Psychiatry 163:689–696, 2006.
43. Caton CL, Drake RE, Hasin D, et al: Differences between early-phase primary psychotic disorders with concurrent substance use and substance-induced psychoses. Arch Gen Psychiatry 62:137–145, 2005.
44. Friedmann PD, McCullough D, Chin MH, et al: Screening and intervention for alcohol problems: a national survey of primary care physicians and psychiatrists. J Gen Intern Med 15:84–91, 2000.
45. Grant BF: Theoretical and observed subtypes of DSM-IV alcohol abuse and dependence in a general population sample. Drug Alcohol Depend 60:287–293, 2000.
46. Hasin DS, Hatzenbuehler M, Smith S, et al: Co-occurring DSM-IV drug abuse in DSM-IV drug dependence: results from the National Epidemiologic Survey on Alcohol and Related Conditions. Drug Alcohol Depend 80:117–123, 2005.
47. McLellan AT, Luborsky L, O'Brien CP, et al: An improved diagnostic instrument for substance abuse patients: the Addiction Severity Index. J Nerv Ment Dis 168:26–33, 1980.
48. McLellan AT, Kusher H, Metzger D, et al: The fifth edition of the Addiction Severity Index. J Subst Abuse Treat 9:199–213, 1992.
49. Leonhard C, Mulvey K, Gastfriend DR, et al: The Addiction Severity Index: a field study of internal consistency and validity. J Subst Abuse Treat 18:129–135, 2000.
50. Raes V, Lombaert G: EuropASI: a standard in de Sleutel, Belgium. J Subst Use 9:196–204, 2004.

51. Hendriks VM, Kaplan CD, van Limbeek J, et al: The Addiction Severity Index: reliability and validity in a Dutch addict population. J Subst Abuse Treat 6:133–141, 1989.
52. Scheurich A, Muller MJ, Wetzel H, et al: Reliability and validity of the German version of the European Addiction Severity Index (EuropASI). J Stud Alcohol 61:916–919, 2000.
53. Krenz S, Dieckmann S, Favrat B, et al: French version of the Addiction Severity Index (5th edition): validity and reliability among Swiss opiate-dependent patients. French validation of the Addiction Severity Index. Eur Addict Res 10:173–179, 2004.
54. DeJong CA, Willems JC, Schippers GM, et al: The Addiction Severity Index: reliability and validity in a Dutch alcoholic population. Int J Addict 30:605–616, 1995.
55. Bilal AM: Correlates of addiction-related problems in Kuwait: a cross-cultural view. Acta Psychiatr Scand 78:414–416, 1988.
56. Mäkelä K: Studies of the reliability and validity of the Addiction Severity Index. Addiction 99:398–410, 2004.
57. Schippers GM, Broekman TG, Koeter MWJ, et al: The Addiction Severity Index as a first-generation instrument: commentary on "Studies of the reliability and validity of the ASI" by K. Mäkelä. Addiction 99:416–417, 2004.
58. Horng FF, Chueh KH: Effectiveness of telephone follow-up and counseling in aftercare for alcoholism. J Nurs Res 12:11–20, 2004.
59. Ahmadi J, Fakoor A, Pezeshkian P, et al: Substance use among Iranian psychiatric inpatients. Psychol Rep 89:363–365, 2001.
60. Mufti KA, Said S, Farooq S, et al: Five year follow up of 100 heroin addicts in Peshawar. J Ayub Med Coll Abbottabad 16:5–9, 2004.
61. Langeland W, Draijer N, van den Brink W: Psychiatric comorbidity in treatment-seeking alcoholics: the role of childhood trauma and perceived parental dysfunction. Alcohol Clin Exp Res 28:441–447, 2004.
62. Pozzi G, Tacchini G, Di Giannantonia M, et al: Mental disorders of drug addicts in treatment: a study of prevalence with retrospective evaluation by means of structured diagnostic interviews [in Italian]. Minerva Psichiatr 36:139–154, 1995.
63. Ponce G, Jimenez-Arriero MA, Rubio G, et al: The A1 allele of the DRD2 gene (TaqI A polymorphisms) is associated with antisocial personality in a sample of alcohol-dependent patients. Eur Psychiatry 18:356–360, 2003.
64. Isralowitz RE: Cultural identification and substance use: immigrant and native heroin addicts in Israel. J Soc Psychol 144:222–224, 2004.
65. National Institute on Drug Abuse: International activities, in Director's Report to the National Advisory Council on Drug Abuse, May 2001. Rockville, MD, National Institute on Drug Abuse, 2001. Available online at http://www.nida.nih.gov/dirreports/dirrep501/DirectorReport11.html. Accessed April 22, 2006.
66. Helzer JE, Bucholz KK, Bierut LJ, et al: Should DSM-V include dimensional diagnostic criteria for alcohol use disorders? Alcohol Clin Exp Res 30:303–310, 2006.
67. Hasin D, Aharonovich E, Liu X, et al: Alcohol dependence symptoms and alcohol dehydrogenase 2 polymorphism: Israeli Ashkenazis, Sephardics and recent Russian immigrants. Alcohol Clin Exp Res 26:1315–1321, 2002.
68. Hasin D, Schuckit MA, Martin CS, et al: The validity of DSM-IV alcohol dependence: what do we know, what do we need to know? Alcohol Clin Exp Res 27:244–252, 2003.

8

COMORBIDITY OF SUBSTANCE USE DISORDERS WITH PSYCHIATRIC CONDITIONS

Marc A. Schuckit, M.D.

Most diagnoses in medicine are based on a combination of symptoms, their time course and a threshold beyond which the syndrome is felt to be clinically relevant.[1] No single indicator is likely to be sufficient to establish a diagnosis, because such indicators are rarely unique to one syndrome. For example, in medicine, chest pain could reflect a broken rib, an invasive tumor, a consequence of pneumonia, or a myocardial infarction. Diagnosis and treatment cannot rest with the pain itself, but this symptom is used as an entrée into a differential diagnosis that considers additional problems over time, along with biological tests, before appropriate treatment can be instituted. Similarly, in psychiatry, sadness could reflect grief, thyroid disease, adrenal abnormalities or a reaction to chronic pain, in addition to serving as the central signal for a potential major depressive episode, the depressive phase of manic-depressive,

---

This work was supported by the Veterans Affairs Research Service; by funds provided by the state of California for medical research on alcohol and substance abuse through the University of California, San Francisco; and by a grant from the CompassPoint Addiction Foundation.

Reprinted from Schuckit MA: "Comorbidity Between Substance Use Disorders and Psychiatric Conditions." *Addiction* 101 (suppl 1):76–88, 2006. Used with permission of the Society for the Study of Addiction.

disease, or a consequence of repeated intake of high doses of depressant drugs such as alcohol. Psychiatry is especially vulnerable to the nonspecificity of symptoms, as there are few (if any) biological tests that are sensitive and specific enough to establish a diagnosis.

Potential problems with the diagnostic process increase almost exponentially when substance use disorders (SUDs) and psychiatric syndromes occur together, as a reflection of at least four broad issues.[2–4] First, combinations of SUDs and psychiatric disorders may represent two or more independent conditions, each of which is likely to run the distinct clinical course relatively unique to that disorder. Here, both conditions must be treated comprehensively. This combination could occur through chance alone (roughly the prevalence of one disorder multiplied by the prevalence of the other) or be a consequence of the actions of the same predisposing factors (e.g., stress, personality, additional psychiatric disorders, childhood environment, and genetic influences) affecting the risk for multiple conditions.[5] Second, the first disorder could influence the development of the second condition in such a manner that the additional disorder then runs an independent course. For example, the frequent use of high doses of substance could unmask a latent predisposition toward a psychiatric disorder or cause permanent physiological changes in the brain that result in long-term or permanent psychoses, depression, and so on.[5–7] Again, both conditions must be treated for as long as necessary. Similarly, a psychiatric disorder (e.g., mania) could increase the risk for heavy and repetitive use of substances, an SUD that might continue even when the preexisting psychiatric condition is appropriately treated or remits. A third relationship could be seen if the second condition developed through an effort of the patient to diminish problems associated with the first syndrome. For example, a person might escalate the use of substances and develop an SUD in an attempt to alleviate feelings of depression, or to decrease side effects of psychiatric medications. Here, while the SUDs might become a long-term problem, the excessive use of alcohol or an illicit drug might disappear when the preexisting clinical syndrome is addressed appropriately.

This review focuses on a fourth category of contributors to the high prevalence of psychiatric comorbidities seen in individuals with SUDs. Some syndromes may be temporary psychiatric pictures (e.g., psychosis with features resembling schizophrenia) seen as a consequence of intoxication with specific types of substances (e.g., stimulants, such as amphetamines and cocaine) or withdrawal conditions (e.g., depressive syndromes with cessation of stimulants). These substance-induced syndromes represent an important challenge to both researchers and clinicians attempting to understand more about the complex relationship between psychiatric and substance-related disorders.

The distinction between the types of comorbidities, each of which is likely to operate in some patients, has important implications.[8,9] The etiologies may be different[10] (a factor of importance for research), and several categories, including substance-induced disorders, are likely to have distinct clinical courses and responses to treatment.[11] The following sections discuss comorbidity, with an emphasis on substance-induced disorders, by addressing the impact of methodology on research results; evidence that substance-induced disorders exist; the clinical and research relevance of these conditions; and some suggestions for research questions that might be addressed in the process of preparing for the *Diagnostic and Statistical Manual of Mental Disorders,* 5th edition (DSM-V).

Methodological Issues That Affect Results

DIFFERENT DEFINITIONS OF COMORBIDITY

Comorbidity has been defined in a variety of ways. Some studies emphasize "pure psychiatric diagnoses," defined as a psychiatric condition observed in the absence of any other major diagnosis during the same year.[12] More classically, multiple diagnoses have been placed into a primary versus secondary approach,[13] in which the first condition to develop is labeled as "primary," a notation that depends on chronology, not necessarily cause and effect. Other authors have labeled as primary the major reason for clinical care.

The independent versus substance-induced distinction is an extension of the primary/secondary approach. It was developed in recognition that a psychiatric syndrome (e.g., a major depressive episode) might also be identified during periods of abstinence and that labels should not be based solely on initial chronology.[9,14] Therefore, the ability to spot independent disorders should be enhanced.

Most data on comorbidities were developed regarding SUDs and Axis I conditions such as depressive syndromes, and these will be emphasized here. Of course, comorbidity of SUDs with each other and with Axis II personality conditions is also relevant[15] but is beyond the scope of the current review.

OPERATIONALIZATION AND EVALUATION OF THE DIAGNOSTIC CRITERIA

A number of questions arise regarding how the labels are used within a research protocol. For example, does the project require that the specific type of drug be relevant to the specific comorbid diagnosis? This is important because some drugs (e.g., intoxication with alcohol and sedative-hypnotics) can cause some temporary conditions (e.g., depression) but are less likely to cause others (e.g., mania).[16] A second issue is whether the diagnosis is required to be associated with great distress or impairment, or whether a simple endorsement of the symptoms by a respondent is enough to make a diagnosis.[17] Obviously, without this requirement the inclusion of many minor symptoms and life problems could markedly expand the number of people diagnosed. Third, a similar problem can occur if the criteria did not include the need for some problems to have occurred repeatedly (an issue relevant to many of the criterion items for SUDs), or did not determine if the items clustered together during the relevant period. Studies also vary regarding their emphasis on syndromes occurring in the last year versus during the lifetime, with the combination of time frames important for the primary versus secondary or induced versus independent approaches. It is also important to note whether the full diagnostic syndrome is required for establishing the ages at onset and for remission, or whether a diagnosis is considered valid if only some symptoms are present. In the absence of a full syndrome, the age at onset is likely to be much younger, but the process might be like determining the onset of major depression as the first time a person was ever sad. Differences across studies on any one of these items are likely to have a large impact on the results regarding the incidence, time course, and optimal treatment of comorbidities.

An additional and very important research issue relates to the types of interviewers employed and their level of supervision. The problem here is that different studies can have different, but complementary, assets and liabilities. Large-scale epidemiological investigations, such as the National Epidemiologic Survey on Alcohol and Related Conditions (NESARC), gather data on thousands of subjects over a very short time and can be excellent measures of patterns of problems in a wide range of people in the general population. However, such studies require large numbers of nonclinician interviewers, who can have difficulty interpreting the relevance of some complaints (e.g., mania) and determining whether the symptoms were relatively mild and transitory (e.g., for some simple phobias) versus those relevant to a diagnosis. The need for so many interviewers also means that the problems reported by subjects are less likely to be reviewed by clinicians, a time-consuming but useful process used in the Collaborative Study on the Genetics of Alcoholism. The clinician reviewer can then encourage interviewers to gather additional information about the clinical condition, rather than having them adhere rigidly to a fully structured interview. On the other hand, the high level of structure in the research instruments used by NESARC minimizes differences between interviewers. However, the approach that is necessary for large-scale studies may make it difficult to gather more detailed information required for the more subtle distinctions, such as those between induced and independent depressions.

Other problems reflect the approach used to deal with what appear to be multiple diagnoses in the same person. This occurs, for example, when a subject endorses depressive symptoms, reports panic attacks, and describes discomfort in social situations. In some studies these are listed as three separate diagnoses, but others establish a hierarchy, searching for one overarching diagnosis (e.g., major depression) that might explain the other complaints (e.g., temporary panic attacks and feelings of social discomfort).

THE INTERVIEW USED IN THE PROTOCOL

Some interviews were developed to gather information quickly on substance-related issues from a large number of diverse subjects, with administration carried out by hundreds of interviewers (e.g., the Alcohol Use Disorder and Associated Disabilities Interview Schedule for DSM-IV (AUDADIS–DSM-IV).[18] Others were constructed for large populations but with an emphasis on non-substance-related conditions, such as the Diagnostic Interview Schedule (DIS), the Composite International Diagnostic Interview (CIDI) and the Structured Clinical Interview for DSM-IV Axis I Disorders (SCID-IV).[19,20] With any of these measures, unless closely supervised, lay interviewers may have difficulties distinguishing periods of situational excitement or substance-related irritability from mania, or determining whether driving while impaired with alcohol occurred (i.e., what amount of alcohol was consumed over what period of time followed by driving how many hours later?). Thus, such epidemiological interview-based instruments are ideal for large epidemiological studies but might exaggerate the rates of psychiatric disorders and SUDs by reporting conditions that might not meet a full and clinically relevant syndrome. These interviews might not be optimal for exploring more complex questions such as comorbid conditions, especially with regard to substance-induced disorders.

Several instruments have been developed to overcome some of these problems, but are less efficient and can be too expensive for use in large epidemiological surveys. The Semi-Structured Assessment for the Genetics of Alcoholism (SSAGA) interview was created to help distinguish primary versus secondary or substance-induced versus independent conditions and to gather detailed information about substance-related issues.[21,22] Interviewers are trained to use a timeline approach to establish the age at onset of dependence, periods of abstinence, and ages at onset of Axis I syndromes. The SSAGA has a semistructured format to facilitate such determinations, using lay interviewers who probe for additional information along with close review by editors and a final diagnosis established through a clinician-based evaluation of all data sources. The semistructured nature encourages interviewers to gather additional information relevant to the clinical intensity, duration, and clustering of symptoms, with editors often asking the interviewer to return to the research subject to gather more information.

The Psychiatric Research Interview for Substance and Mental Disorders (PRISM)[23,24] can also help evaluate independent and induced psychiatric conditions. This instrument places sections dealing with drugs and alcohol early in the interview, and an effort is made to establish the age at onset of substance-related and psychiatric syndromes based on the age at which the full disorder was present. The interview is structured to optimize interpretation of substance-induced versus independent conditions, but gathering of additional information and clinician review are not always used.

ADDITIONAL RESEARCH ATTRIBUTES LIKELY TO HAVE AN IMPACT ON RESULTS

The population selected for study (patients, their relatives, general populations, and respondents to an advertisement) can influence results. However, no one study or single group of subjects can give the "true answer" regarding the prevalence and patterns of psychiatric and SUDs. Rather, it is important to evaluate patterns across different populations.

The timing of the evaluation is also important. For example, rates of comorbid psychiatric syndromes are likely to be temporarily elevated if substance-dependent subjects are interviewed during intoxication, withdrawal or the first several weeks of abstinence.[25] These are times of highest prevalence of substance-induced disorders.

It is also important to gather additional sources of data about subjects whenever possible. These include clinician reviews of all available information on a patient,[26] using additional informants (e.g., a spouse) regarding the subject and urine toxicology screens or state markers of heavy drinking. These can be key in determining whether, for example, depressive symptoms reported in a follow-up were truly independent of substance use. In addition, evaluations of risk factors for comorbidity require consideration of assortative mating in the families, a factor that increases comorbidity in the offspring, and such data often require interviewing relatives as well as the subject.[27]

Do Substance-Induced Disorders Exist?

Psychiatric nosologies have traditionally emphasized the importance of recognizing temporary psychiatric conditions observed in the context of biological influences. These include auditory hallucinations during Cushing's disease or hypothyroidism that may not be schizophrenia, and intense sadness in someone taking beta-blockers that may not be a typical major depressive episode. Similarly, psychiatric symptoms seen only in the context of substance intoxication and withdrawal can have distinct prognoses and treatments.[9,23] The goal of this section is to emphasize that there is enough support for the existence of substance-induced disorders for them to be included in DSM, not to provide a meta-analysis or a detailed contrast and comparison of all pro and con research.

DATA SUPPORTING STIMULANT-INDUCED PSYCHOSES

Temporary schizophrenia-like conditions of hallucinations (predominantly auditory) and/or delusions (usually paranoid) developing without insight and observed in a clear sensorium can be induced by stimulants. They should be distinguished from the lifelong schizophrenic disorders, as the former are likely to require only short-term antipsychotic medications, whereas schizophrenia often necessitates use of such drugs for many years.[28]

Schizophrenic-like psychoses can be induced in the laboratory with stimulants.[29] Angrist and colleagues[30,31] administered up to 50 mg of amphetamine per hour in nine healthy subjects, who became psychotic within 7–45 hours, usually following 200–300 mg of amphetamine. All recovered within 6 days of abstinence. Bell[32] gave doses of amphetamines necessary to increase blood pressure by 50% to 16 subjects, reporting psychoses in 12, with all psychoses disappearing with abstinence. Griffith[33] used a similar protocol in 4 males with no prior psychiatric or substance use history, demonstrating psychotic syndromes in all, usually with 120–250 mg of the drug, and reporting full recovery with abstinence.

Additional support for temporary stimulant-induced psychoses resembling schizophrenia comes from descriptions of clinical samples and surveys of populations. Following the first known report of temporary psychoses with stimulants,[34] "epidemics" of these syndromes were recorded after the Second World War in Japan and Germany, with subsequent case descriptions published from Europe, Asia, and the United States.[35–38] Psychotic symptoms are estimated to occur at some time in about 40% of amphetamine-dependent patients, especially with higher doses.[16,23] Stimulant-induced psychoses have been reported with a wide range of stimulants and may be a good model for evaluating evanescent neurochemical changes likely to be similar to more permanent changes observed in schizophrenia.[35,36,38,39] Stimulant-induced psychoses are *very likely to clear* within several days to about a month of abstinence.[31–33,37] Only 1%–15% of patients with stimulant-induced psychoses maintain some psychotic symptoms after a month. As described in the introduction to this chapter, these could reflect the fact that 1% or so of people in any group will develop schizophrenia, or could be the consequence of the precipitation of longer-term psychotic disorders in predisposed individuals. Thus, a person with schizophrenic relatives or someone in the early phases of this disorder is likely to deteriorate when he or she takes stimulants, a process that underscores the heterogeneity and complexity of the relationships between SUDs and schizophrenic symptoms.[6,29,37,40,41] This might contribute to reports that up to 60% of schizophrenic individuals in treatment have histories of abuse or dependence on illicit drugs such as amphetamines and cocaine.[4,6,42,43] It is also possible that heavy use of stimulants might cause more long-lasting, and hypothetically even permanent, neurochemical changes associated with long-term psychotic disorders in a small number of individuals, even if the individuals are not so predisposed. However, permanent psychoses caused solely by stimulants are likely to be fairly rare and, thus, difficult to study. In any event, if hallucinations and/or delusions without insight continue after a month to 6 weeks of abstinence, the symptoms may well represent an independent psychotic disorder that requires long-term antipsychotic medications.

The symptoms observed in stimulant psychoses closely resemble those seen in schizophrenia. Therefore, the best approach to initially establishing a working diagnosis might rest with a chronology-based time line.[32,36,37,39] Regarding specific symptoms, paranoid delusions have been reported in 25%–75% of stimulant-induced psychoses, auditory hallucinations in 50%–85%, ideas of reference in 15%–60%, and Schneiderian first-rank symptoms in 50% in some surveys.[29,36,37] Negative schizophrenia-like symptoms may be seen in approximately 30% of such subjects.[32,44]

DATA SUPPORTING A CANNABINOID-INDUCED PSYCHOSIS

Laboratory observations are limited to the documentation that intoxication with this drug can produce feelings of derealization, depersonalization and paranoia.[45] Therefore, most support for temporary cannabinoid-induced psychosis comes from clinical descriptions of temporary hallucinations and/or delusions without insight in cannabinoid users in India, Asia, the United Kingdom, South Africa, New Zealand, and the United States.[46–48] Of course, some cases may represent acute toxic drug effects associated with delirium, although most developed in a clear sensorium, and some might reflect precipitation of psychotic syndromes in predisposed individuals.[49] However, most studies indicate that the auditory hallucinations and paranoid delusions, including Schneiderian first-rank symptoms,[50] are very likely to disappear within several days to a month with abstinence.

Cannabinoids are also likely to enhance the risk for schizophrenia in people carrying a predisposition. A 15-year follow-up of approximately 50,000 Swedish military conscripts demonstrated a 2.4- to 6.0-fold increased risk for later hospitalization for schizophrenic-like disorders in individuals who used marijuana at baseline.[7,51] However, none of the heaviest users developed schizophrenia, and many who became psychotic were occasional users or lifelong abstainers. In addition, a 3-year follow-up of about 4,000 people in the Netherlands reported a 2.8-fold increased risk for subsequent schizophrenia in cannabinoid users,[52] with similar results in New Zealand.[53] Support for the conclusion that these figures represent precipitation of illness in predisposed people rather than cannabinoid-caused psychoses in the general population comes from observations that increased marijuana use across cohorts is not associated with a greater lifetime risk for schizophrenia across such cohorts or in countries with higher, compared to lower, marijuana use rates.[54] As described with stimulants, if true psychotic symptoms in a clear sensorium and without insight remain after 4–6 weeks of abstinence, the condition may represent a long-term and potentially permanent psychosis such as schizophrenia.

Before moving on to substance-induced depressive syndromes, it is important to emphasize that temporary substance-induced psychoses are also observed with some additional drugs, including alcohol and, perhaps, phencyclidine.[16,55,56] Rates of alcohol use disorders are also evaluated among schizophrenic individuals,[56] and there is a complex relationship between schizophrenia and nicotine dependence.[57,58] A review of these interesting and complex relationships must await additional papers.

EVIDENCE SUPPORTING SUBSTANCE-INDUCED MOOD DISORDERS

Temporary depressive symptoms have been reported in the context of intoxication or withdrawal for nicotine, cannabinoids, opioids, hallucinogens, and other drugs of abuse.[16,59] Because the question at hand is whether substance-induced disorders exist, this section focuses on the drug with the most available data, alcohol, but briefly mentions additional substances where appropriate.

Laboratory experiments have demonstrated that alcohol affects mood. One study of 10 subjects who consumed alcohol every 2 hours throughout the day (up to 25 standard drinks in 24 hours) reported that most developed depressive syndromes, including at least 4 with suicidal ideation who dropped out during the first week. All depressions cleared with abstinence.[60] In a second series of studies, 14 subjects paid to drink heavily for several weeks demonstrated increasing levels of depression, guilt, and feelings of anxiety, and all depressions disappeared with abstinence.[61,62] Another investigation, in which 12 volunteers were offered free access to alcohol over 7 days, reported temporary depression and anxiety in most subjects,[63] while a study of women reported that the consumption of two or more drinks during a session was associated with mild depressive symptoms both during the experiment and the next morning.[64]

SSAGA interviews with clinician review of diagnoses have documented that more than 40% of alcoholic persons have ever fulfilled criteria for major depressive-like syndromes, with almost 70% of these syndromes being substance-induced disorders. These include data from families in the six Collaborative Study on the Genetics of Alcoholism (COGA) centers, two Native American groups,[9,14,65,66] and alcoholic individuals entering treatment.[67] However, a large national epidemiological study using the AUDADIS and lay interviewers without clinical supervision reported high rates of depression in alcoholic persons but noted that few were substance induced.[18] These divergent results probably reflect different methods across studies as described in the section on methodological issues.

Additional support for the relevance of substance-induced mood disorders comes from prospective studies which suggest that heavy drinking at time 1 is likely to predict depressive symptoms at time 2. A 6-year follow-up of 176 subjects reported that drinking predicted an increased number of subsequent transitions from functioning well to periods of depression (perhaps reflecting substance-induced mood disorders), while individuals with prior (but not currently active) alcoholism had no increased number of transitions to depression over time.[68] Active alcoholism among depressed individuals made it less likely that they would demonstrate transitions to a euthymic mood. Another prospective study reported that heavier drinking during month 2 predicted depressive symptoms during month 3.[69] In addition, 3- and 12-month follow-ups of almost 200 alcoholic individuals revealed that only those who had returned to drinking were likely to demonstrate depressions,[67] while a longitudinal study of more than 700 adults reported that patterns of higher alcohol use during earlier follow-ups predicted a higher prevalence of depressive symptoms at subsequent contacts.[70] Finally, a follow-up of young subjects found no relationship between earlier heavy drinking and later alcohol use disorders (AUDs), unless the individuals continued heavy drinking.[71]

Prospective studies of populations at high risk for depression or alcoholism also generally support the existence of substance-induced mood disorders. First, despite evidence that some people may drink (not necessarily to the point of problems) in response to both positive and negative affect,[72,73] two follow-up studies of teenagers who had major depressive episodes reported no heightened risk for alcohol or drug dependence over the subsequent decades, despite a high prevalence of future depressions.[74,75] The results might also indicate that independent major depressions tend to run a true course and are not usually associated with later alcoholism, unless perhaps there are alcohol-dependent relatives as well.

Some studies of offspring of depressed subjects and those with early shyness or psychological symptoms report an increased subsequent risk for substance-related problems,[17,76,77] but others note no increased risk for AUDs in children of depressed individuals.[78–80] Relationships are complex and may differ across the sexes, and positive studies may include subjects with additional family histories of alcoholism or SUDs.[80,81] Similarly, several prospective studies of teenagers reported that young heavier drinkers or children of alcoholic parents may have increased depressive symptoms,[82,83] but others disagree and note these subjects were no more likely to develop mood problems or major depressive episodes than controls.[79,84,85] The negative studies include an evaluation of approximately 1,000 16- to 25-year-old subjects in New Zealand, where earlier drinking patterns were predictors of alcohol-related outcomes but not of depressive disorders.[86] A prospective evaluation of two generations of 453 families of alcoholic persons and controls noted that an alcoholic relative predicted higher rates of AUDs but not independent major depressive episodes.[16,80,87–89]

When substance-induced mood disorders are identified, they are likely to disappear soon after abstinence, a situation not seen with independent depressive episodes. Thus, overall continued abstinence in alcoholic individuals is likely to be associated with a decrease in depressive symptoms.[90–93] For example, follow-up of alcoholic individuals with substance-induced mood disorders reported that the proportion with marked depressive symptoms decreased from 42% to 6% with 1 month of abstinence.[67] A separate study of unmedicated male alcoholic individuals documented that for those with induced depressions, an average Hamilton Rating Scale for Depression score of 16 after 1 week of abstinence decreased to a score of 6 after 4 weeks dry, while similar decreases are not seen for subjects initially identified as having independent major mood disorders.[25,94] Similarly, in another investigation the proportion of alcoholic individuals with major depressive-like symptoms decreased from 67% to 13% over a month, without antidepressant treatment,[95] findings supported by several other clinical observations.[93,96–100] In addition, 85% of those with alcohol-induced mood disorders ran the course predicted regarding the temporary nature of the symptoms,[92] and an 18-month follow-up of inpatients dependent upon a variety of drugs or alcohol showed that the course of substance-induced depressions was different from independent mood disorders. A tendency toward diminution or disappearance of depressive symptoms with abstinence has also been reported for patients entering care for stimulant or opioid dependence.[101–108] At the same time, the diagnosis of induced depressive episodes cannot be based on cross-sectional symptom patterns, because depressive symptoms in the context of heavy drinking are almost identical to those seen during independent depression[9,109] and can include suicidal ideation.

There are several validators of the accuracy of timeline-based notations of substance-induced mood disorders. First, such substance-induced disturbances are more likely than independent disorders to diminish and disappear with time alone.[25,67,92] Second, an elevated risk for independent mood disorders in relatives may be only seen for those alcoholic persons who themselves had independent depressions.[9,81] Similarly, independent major depressive episodes may be most likely to be observed in alcoholic individuals who have relatives with such depressions.[110–113]

However, it is important to remember that not all studies agree and that groups of alcoholic individuals with depressive syndromes are heterogeneous. A national AUDADIS-based survey concluded that past alcoholism may be associated with an enhanced risk for major depressive disorders, even during apparent abstinence.[114] The relationship between alcoholism and depressive episodes in this study might reflect the presence of independent depressions among relatives of the alcoholic individuals or the possible impact of stresses or lower social supports associated with rebuilding one's life following abstinence.[13,80] This study did not gather data from additional informants or use blood or urine tests to corroborate the abstinence. On the other hand, a 1-year prospective follow-up of alcoholic persons, using a SSAGA-like interview along with data from additional informants and biological tests of abstinence, did not report higher rates of major depressive episodes, perhaps reflecting the smaller sample or the shorter time frame of follow-up.[116]

This discussion of the relationships between mood syndromes and SUDs would not be complete without a mention of two additional factors. While the acute phase of withdrawal from alcohol lasts 4 days or so, this is likely to be followed by a protracted abstinence syndrome that can last several months or more.[117] Here, while the alcoholic person is not depressed all day every day (i.e., does not fulfill criteria for a major depressive episode), he or she is likely to experience insomnia, problems concentrating, and irritability that improve with increasing time of abstinence. These mood-related conditions must be recognized by clinicians and treated, usually with education and cognitive-behavioral approaches.[16] These are not, however, independent major depressive episodes. The second proviso to emphasize is the importance of evaluating whether what appears to be a substance-induced mood disorder actually clears with abstinence. It is at least theoretically possible that some individuals predisposed toward major depressive episodes might develop their syndromes in the context of the stresses associated with SUDs. As many as 15% of any group of individuals (including those with alcoholism) are likely to show major depressive episodes as a reflection of the usual prevalence of these mood disorders. Therefore, when symptoms consistent with a DSM-IV major depressive episode continue to occur daily and almost all day following 4 or more weeks of abstinence, the clinician should consider carefully the possibility that a major independent depressive episode is present, and treat the patient accordingly.

In summary, there is no easy or perfect answer regarding the manner in which major depressive episodes and alcohol dependence are related. Multiple factors, including substance-induced disorders, are likely to contribute to this comorbidity. Nonetheless, the studies cited above document a high probability that substance-nduced mood disorders contribute to the comorbidity observed.

Clinical Relevance of Substance-Induced Disorders

There are three basic elements to this section: data indicating that substance-induced disorders 1) are prevalent enough to be worth recognizing; 2) have a relatively unique clinical course compared with independent disorders; and 3) have optimal treatments that may be different from those most appropriate for independent conditions.

SUBSTANCE-INDUCED DISORDERS ARE RELATIVELY COMMON

Estimates of the prevalence of substance-induced psychiatric syndromes range from about zero[18] to 65% or more of some psychiatric conditions seen in alcoholic individuals.[14] Lower estimates tend to come from large epidemiological studies, and higher rates are seen when the SSAGA is used with close clinical oversight of interviewers. Substance-induced conditions are also likely to vary across psychiatric diagnoses and categories of drugs.

The lifetime rate of temporary substance-induced psychoses in stimulant-dependent individuals may be at least 40%. The figures for cannabinoid-induced psychoses are more difficult to estimate, but the information presented earlier leaves little doubt that they exist.

Regarding the prevalence of other substance-induced conditions, it is helpful to review figures across studies using the same methods. I have chosen to emphasize data generated from the SSAGA or similar instruments with interviewer training and supervision similar to that used in the COGA. Here, while 40% or more of alcoholic individuals have histories of major depressive episodes, in as many as 70% of these cases the disorders are substance-induced.[9,25,65–67] Substance-induced conditions represented 20% of the panic disorders, 25% of social phobias, 40% of the obsessive-compulsive disorders, and 50% of agoraphobia conditions.[9,26] However, not all substances of abuse can induce all psychiatric pictures, and substance-induced conditions are observed less frequently in individuals dependent upon opioids and inhalants.[9,16,118] Therefore, in summary, most studies document substantial proportions of alcoholic individuals and stimulant-dependent subjects with substance-induced conditions.

SUBSTANCE-INDUCED DISORDERS OFFER USEFUL INFORMATION ABOUT PROGNOSIS

As reported in the previous subsection, the symptoms of most substance-induced conditions resemble closely those of the relevant independent psychiatric disorders.[9,36,37] However, 85% or more of substance-induced syndromes improve rapidly with abstinence, falling below the threshold for a diagnosis of an Axis I disorder within several days to a month. This clinical course is distinct from what would be expected with, for example, independent schizophrenia and major depressive episodes.

The required brevity of this review has not allowed for similar in-depth evaluations of anxiety conditions. However, stimulant intoxication is associated with temporary panic attacks and generalized anxiety–like and phobic-like conditions both in the laboratory and in clinical settings.[27,59,119,120] These anxiety conditions, too, are temporary and are very likely to clear with continued abstinence. Temporary substance-induced anxiety and mood syndromes have also been reported for hallucinogens and cannabinoids and can be observed for other Axis I disorders (e.g., sleep, sexual dysfunction).[16,118] Comorbidities of independent disorders also impact on outcomes. There is general agreement that comorbid substance dependence is associated with a more severe course of independent Axis I conditions, and that these long-term independent syndromes produce greater difficulty in treating the associated SUD.[6,52,121–123] The course of the second disorder (e.g., major depression) may improve if the first disorder (e.g., an AUD) is in remission, and visa versa.[124,125] However, while some studies report that independent depressions in the context of substance dependence have a worse prognosis,[105,106,126] others suggest a better than average outcome for the psychiatric condition.[127–129] It is likely that some of this diversity reflects the varying amounts of detail paid to separately evaluating substance-induced and independent disorders. Only carefully constructed studies will help to clarify the differences in the clinical course associated with comorbidities in substance-induced versus independent disorders, improve our level of knowledge about etiologies, and lead to more effective treatments. These steps will be facilitated by the continued use of clearly defined substance-induced disorders in DSM-V.

SUBSTANCE-INDUCED DISORDERS HAVE UNIQUE TREATMENTS

The differences in short- and long-term prognoses between substance-induced and independent psychiatric disorders have several implications. First, regarding psychoses, reflecting the beneficial effects of antipsychotic medications for all forms of hallucinations and delusions, these drugs are likely to help control such symptoms in substance-induced psychotic conditions. However, such medications should be limited to the several days to a month it takes for substance-induced psychotic symptoms to disappear. Patients with long-term psychoses (e.g., schizophrenia) exacerbated by stimulants or alcohol are, on the other hand, likely to require long-term antipsychotic medications.

The conclusions are a little more complex regarding the optimal use of antidepressant medications in substance-dependent individuals. Even in classical independent major depressive episodes, nonpharmacological treatments help,[130] and antidepressants often require 2–3 weeks to have an effect. In addition, there are few data to demonstrate whether antidepressants work equally well in depressive episodes induced by medications, medical disorders, or substances of abuse. However, one might hypothesize that these medications would be more effective than placebo in independent depressive episodes in substance-dependent patients and, reflecting the disappearance of depression with abstinence alone, not be much better than placebo for substance-induced disorders when patients abstain. Thus, the heterogeneity in clinical studies regarding steps used to identify substance-induced mood disorders may have contributed to differences in the reported usefulness of antidepressant drugs in patients with comorbid SUDs and depressive syndromes.

Studies from the 1980s indicated that alcoholic individuals with comorbid depressions were not likely to respond to tricyclic antidepressants.[131,132] However, in a recent review of 14 controlled antidepressant trials in depressed patients with SUDs, half the papers reported a significant antidepressant response.[103] Regarding specific positive studies, a 12-week trial of 51 alcoholic individuals with comorbid depression indicated that fluoxetine was associated with a greater improvement in depressive symptoms than placebo.[133] Perhaps these results reflect a several weeks' period of abstinence before patients began active medications, a step that might have diminished the proportion of participants with substance-induced depressions. Another study reported the use of desipramine in 12 alcoholic individuals who completed the trial and who had an onset of a depression following the development of alcoholism, comparing the results with 10 similar individuals treated with placebo.[134] Here, the medication was superior to placebo, but the group with active drug was small, subjects were abstinent between 1 and 12 weeks prior to entering the protocol, and depressive symptoms were required to have lasted for at least 3 weeks in this 24-week trial. Other studies have evaluated the use of antidepressants in treating depressive episodes observed in opioid- and stimulant-dependent individuals, with results not offering strong support for the use of medications.[104,135]

Regarding the impact of antidepressants on drinking behaviors among alcoholic individuals, a recent review indicated that three of nine controlled trials showed no difference between placebo and antidepressants, five reported a modest level of improvement with active treatment, and one study showed that the antidepressant was clearly superior to placebo.[103] Another review of selective serotonin reuptake inhibitors indicated that in only one of six such investigations was the active drug clearly superior to placebo regarding drinking outcomes.[136,137] At the same time, manic-depressive alcoholic individuals have been reported in one study to decrease drinking when treated with valproic acid.[138] Therefore, regarding antidepressant treatment of depressive episodes or drinking in individuals with alcoholism, the answer may depend on how the question is asked. The variation in results across studies might reflect approaches that resulted in differences across trials in the number of individuals with temporary, substance-induced depressive episodes, cases where placebo and the passage of time might have been as effective as the antidepressants.

Space constraints do not allow for a more detailed review of the use of medications in the treatment of comorbid anxiety disorders in individuals with substance dependence. It is likely that a clear answer regarding the usefulness of medications will require investigations that evaluate data separately for individuals with substance-induced versus independent anxiety disorders.

Some Conclusions

The analysis in this chapter has focused on several questions relevant to the considerations required for the development of DSM-V. The material presented herein indicates that substance-induced disorders exist, they are prevalent enough to contribute significantly to the rates of comorbidity between SUDs and psychiatric conditions, and these disorders have treatment implications. However, it is important to remember that substance induced conditions explain only a subgroup of patients with comorbid SUDs and major psychiatric conditions. The current literature review underscores the heterogeneous nature of comorbidity and raises the importance of identifying these subgroups of individuals with comorbid conditions in order to address both research and clinically based questions. This brief review has focused mainly on alcohol, cannabinoids, and stimulants regarding psychoses and mood disorders, with brief mention of anxiety conditions, but the same general conclusions are likely to apply to some other drugs and psychiatric conditions.

This chapter points toward several research priorities for comorbid conditions. There is a need to establish and standardize definitions and research methods relevant to studies of substance-induced disorders. Consensus is needed on a preferred definition of comorbidity along with clearer definitions of criterion items for SUDs (e.g., repeatedly), as well as greater consistency across studies on impairment or distress, clustering, and remission. Research groups need to agree on the optimal methods to study comorbidities, possibly through a national cooperative study focusing on comorbidity, including substance-induced disorders. Such a study could be patterned after national collaborations regarding depressive disorders and after COGA. In the absence of such approaches, the field is unlikely to be able to draw valid and generalizable conclusions regarding important aspects of comorbidity, including data regarding the expected clinical course, treatments, etiologies, and prevention of these syndromes.

In considering the definitions of comorbidity and substance-induced conditions for DSM-V, it is important to keep several issues in mind. The criteria should build on data available to date, and not turn to major alterations of existing approaches unless supported by robust studies. Recognizing that the editions of DSM are primarily clinical manuals, it is also important that the criteria be relatively straightforward to encourage use by clinicians, insurers, and administrators. Diagnoses must be flexible enough to be applicable across different categories of drugs, diverse psychiatric conditions, and different ethnic and demographic groups, because the development of separate criteria for each drug and psychiatric diagnosis would result in an approach of such complexity as to jeopardize general use.

In summary, this review has underscored the importance of comorbidity in SUDs, the heterogeneous and complex nature of these conditions, the relevance of substance-induced disorders, and the difficulties inherent in establishing cause and effect or more generalizable treatment approaches based on the current literature. However, questions of the optimal approaches (note the emphasis on the plural) to types of comorbidities between SUDs and psychiatric conditions are important topics for future research as our field prepares for the development of DSM-V.

References

1. Regier DA, Narrow WE, Rae DS: For DSM-V, it's the "disorder threshold," stupid (letter). Arch Gen Psychiatry 61:1051, 2004.
2. Helzer JE, Pryzbeck TR: The co-occurrence of alcoholism with other psychiatric disorders in the general population and its impact on treatment. J Stud Alcohol 49:219–224, 1988.
3. Kessler RC, Crum RM, Warner LA, et al: Lifetime co-occurrence of DSM-III-R alcohol abuse and dependence with other psychiatric disorders in the National Comorbidity Survey. Arch Gen Psychiatry 54:313–321, 1997.
4. Regier DA, Farmer ME, Rae DS, et al: Comorbidity of mental disorders with alcohol and other drug abuse: results from the Epidemiologic Catchment Area (ECA) Study. JAMA 264:2511–2518, 1990.
5. Volkow ND: The reality of comorbidity: depression and drug abuse. Biol Psychiatry 56:714–717, 2004.
6. Rabinowitz J, Bromet EJ, Lavelle J, et al: Prevalence and severity of substance use disorders and onset of psychosis in first admission psychotic patients. Psychol Med 28: 1411–1419, 1998.

7. Zammit S, Allebeck P, Andreasson S, et al: Self reported cannabis use as a risk factor for schizophrenia in Swedish conscripts of 1969: historical cohort study. BMJ 325: 1199–1201, 2002.
8. Hasin D, Liu X, Nunes E, et al: Effects of major depression on remission and relapse of substance dependence. Arch Gen Psychiatry 59:375–380, 2002.
9. Schuckit MA, Tipp JE, Bergman M, et al: Comparison of induced and independent major depressive disorders in 2,945 alcoholics. Am J Psychiatry 154:948–957, 1997.
10. Ries RK, Demirsoy A, Russo JE, et al: Reliability and clinical utility of DSM-IV substance-induced psychiatric disorders in acute psychiatric inpatients. Am J Addict 10:308–318, 2001.
11. O'Brien CP, Charney DS: Priority actions to improve care of persons with co-occurring substance abuse and other mental disorders: call to action. Biol Psychiatry 56:703–713, 2004.
12. de Graaf R, Bijl RV, Smit F, et al: Risk factors for 12-month comorbidity of mood, anxiety, and substance use disorders: findings from the Netherlands Mental Health Survey and Incidence Study. Am J Psychiatry 159:620–629, 2002.
13. Winokur G, Coryell W, Endicott J, et al: Familial alcoholism in manic-depressive (bipolar) disease. Am J Med Genet 67:197–201, 1996.
14. Schuckit MA, Tipp JE, Bucholz KK, et al: The life-time rates of three major mood disorders and four major anxiety disorders in alcoholics and controls. Addiction 92:1289–1304, 1997.
15. Grant BF, Hasin DS, Stinson FS, et al: Co-occurrence of 12-month mood and anxiety disorders and personality disorders in the US: results from the National Epidemiologic Survey on Alcohol and Related Conditions. J Psychiatric Res 39:1–9, 2005.
16. Schuckit MA: Drug and Alcohol Abuse: A Clinical Guide to Diagnosis and Treatment, 6th Edition. New York, Springer, 2006.
17. Weissman MM, Wickramaratne P, Nomura Y, et al: Families at high and low risk for depression: a 3-generation study. Arch Gen Psychiatry 62:29–36, 2005.
18. Grant BF, Stinson FS, Dawson DA, et al: Prevalence and co-occurrence of substance use disorders and independent mood and anxiety disorders: results from the National Epidemiologic Survey on Alcohol and Related Conditions. Arch Gen Psychiatry 61: 807–816, 2004.
19. First MB, Spitzer RL, Gibbon M, et al: Structured Clinical Interview for DSM-IV Axis I Disorders, Patient Edition. New York, New York State Psychiatric Institute, 1997.
20. Robins LN, Wing J, Wittchen HU, et al: The Composite International Diagnostic Interview: an epidemiologic instrument suitable for use in conjunction with different diagnostic systems and in different cultures. Arch Gen Psychiatry 45:1069–1077, 1988.
21. Bucholz KK, Cadoret R, Cloninger CR, et al: A new, semistructured psychiatric interview for use in genetic linkage studies: a report on the reliability of the SSAGA. J Stud Alcohol 55:149–158, 1994.
22. Schuckit MA, Smith TL, Danko GP, et al: Five-year clinical course associated with DSM-IV alcohol abuse or dependence in a large group of men and women. Am J Psychiatry 158:1084–1090, 2001.
23. Caton CLM, Drake RE, Hasin DS, et al: Differences between early-phase primary psychotic disorders with concurrent substance use and substance-induced psychoses. Arch Gen Psychiatry 62:137–145, 2005.

24. Hasin DS, Trautman KD, Miele GM, et al: Psychiatric Research Interview for Substance and Mental Disorder (PRISM): reliability for substance abusers. Am J Psychiatry 153:1195–1201, 1996.
25. Brown SA, Vik PW, Patterson TL, et al: Stress, vulnerability and adult alcohol relapse. J Stud Alcohol 56:538–545, 1995.
26. Torrens M, Serrano D, Astals M, et al: Diagnosing comorbid psychiatric disorders in substance abusers: validity of the Spanish versions of the Psychiatric Research Interview for Substance and Mental Disorders and the Structured Clinical Interview for DSM-IV. Am J Psychiatry 161:1231–1237, 2004.
27. Schuckit MA, Hesselbrock VM, Tipp J, et al: The prevalence of major anxiety disorders in relatives of alcohol dependent men and women. J Stud Alcohol 56:309–317, 1995.
28. Kane JM, Marder SR: Schizophrenia: somatic treatment, in Comprehensive Textbook of Psychiatry. Edited by Sadock BJ, Sadock VA. Philadelphia, PA, Lippincott Williams & Wilkins, 2004, pp 1467–1476.
29. Janowsky DS, Risch C: Amphetamine psychosis and psychotic symptoms. Psychopharmacology 65:73–77, 1979.
30. Angrist B: Amphetamine psychosis: clinical variations of the syndrome, in Amphetamine and Its Analogs. Edited by Cho AK, Segal DS. New York, Academic Press, 1995.
31. Angrist BM, Gershon S: The phenomenology of experimentally induced amphetamine psychosis: preliminary observations. Biol Psychiatry 2:95–107, 1970.
32. Bell DS: The experimental reproduction of amphetamine psychosis. Arch Gen Psychiatry 29:35–40, 1973.
33. Griffith JD: Experimental psychosis induced by the administration of D-amphetamine, in Amphetamine and Related Compounds. Edited by Costa E, Garattini S. New York, Raven, 1970, pp 876–904.
34. Young D, Serorille WB: Paranoid psychosis in narcolepsy and possible dangers of Benzedrine treatment. Med Clin North Am 22:637–643, 1938.
35. Calello DP, Osterhoudt KC: Acute psychosis associated with therapeutic use of dextroamphetamine (letter). Pediatrics 113:1466, 2004.
36. Chen C-K, Lin S-K, Sham PC, et al: Pre-morbid characteristics and co-morbidity of methamphetamine users with and without psychosis. Psychol Med 33:1407–1414, 2003.
37. Segal DS, Geyer MA, Schuckit MA: Stimulant-induced psychosis: an evaluation of animal models, in Essays in Neurochemistry and Neuropharmacology, Vol 5. Edited by Youdim MGH, Lovenberg W, Sharman DF, et al. London, England, Wiley, 1981, pp 95–129.
38. Surles LK, May HJ, Garry JP: Adderall-induced psychosis in an adolescent. J Am Board Fam Pract 15:498–500, 2002.
39. Yeh H-S, Lee Y-C, Sun H-J, et al: Six months follow-up of patients with methamphetamine psychosis. Zhonghua Yi Xue Za Zhi (Tapei) 64:388–394, 2001.
40. Hides L, Lubman DI, Dawe S: Models of co-occurring substance misuse and psychosis: are personality traits the missing link? Drug Alcohol Rev 23:425–432, 2004.
41. Miller P, Lawrie SM, Hodges A, et al: Genetic liability, illicit drug use, life stress and psychotic symptoms: preliminary findings from the Edinburgh study of people at high risk for schizophrenia. Soc Psychiatry Psychiatr Epidemiol 36:338–342, 2001.
42. Hambrecht M, Häfner H: Substance abuse and the onset of schizophrenia. Biol Psychiatry 40:1155–1163, 1996.

43. Kessler RC, McGonagle KA, Zhao S, et al: Lifetime and 12-month prevalence of DSM-III-R psychiatric disorders in the United States: results from the National Comorbidity Survey. Arch Gen Psychiatry 51:8–19, 1994.
44. Griffith JD, Cavanaugh J, Held J, et al: Dextroamphetamine: evaluation of psychotomimetic properties in man. Arch Gen Psychiatry 26:97–100, 1972.
45. Thomas H: A community survey of adverse effects of cannabis use. Drug Alcohol Depend 42:201–207, 1996.
46. Chaudry HR, Moss HB, Bashir A, et al: Cannabis psychosis following bhang ingestion. Br J Addict 86:1075–1081, 1991.
47. Solomons K, Neppe VM, Kuyl JM: Toxic cannabis psychosis is a valid entity. S Afr Med J 78:476–481, 1990.
48. Wylie AS, Scott RTA, Burnett SJ: Psychosis due to "skunk" (letter). BMJ 311:125, 1995
49. Hall W, Degenhardt L, Teesson M: Cannabis use and psychotic disorders: an update. Drug Alcohol Rev 23:433–443, 2004.
50. Basu D, Malhotra A, Bhagat A, et al: Cannabis psychosis and acute schizophrenia: a case control study from India. Eur Addict Res 5:71–73, 1999.
51. Andreason S, Allebeck P, Engstrom A, et al: Cannabis and schizophrenia: a longitudinal study of Swedish conscripts. Lancet 2:1483–1486, 1987.
52. van Os J, Bak M, Hanssen M, et al: Cannabis use and psychosis: a longitudinal population-based study. Am J Epidemiol 156:319–327, 2002.
53. Arseneault L, Cannon M, Poulton R, et al: Cannabis use in adolescence and risk for adult psychosis: longitudinal prospective study. BMJ 325:1195–1199, 2002.
54. Degenhardt L, Hall W, Lynskey M: Testing hypotheses about the relationship between cannabis use and psychosis. Drug Alcohol Depend 71:37–48, 2003.
55. Tien AY, Anthony JC: Epidemiological analysis of alcohol and drug use as risk factors for psychotic experiences. J Nerv Ment Dis 178:473–480, 1990.
56. Tsuang JW, Lohr JB: Effects of alcohol on symptoms in alcoholic and nonalcoholic patients with schizophrenia. Hosp Community Psychiatry 45:1229–1230, 1994.
57. Grant BF, Hasin DS, Chou P, et al: Nicotine dependence and psychiatric disorders in the United States. Arch Gen Psychiatry 61:1107–1115, 2004.
58. Zammit S, Allebeck P, Dalman C, et al: Investigating the association between cigarette smoking and schizophrenia in a cohort study. Am J Psychiatry 160:2216–2221, 2003.
59. Gawin FH: Abstinence symptomatology and psychiatric diagnosis in cocaine abusers. Arch Gen Psychiatry 43:107–113, 1986.
60. Isbell H, Fraser HR, Wikler A, et al: An experimental study of the etiology of "rum fits" and delirium tremens. J Stud Alcohol 16:1–33, 1955.
61. Tamerin JS, Weiner S, Mendelson JH: Alcoholics' expectancies and recall of experiences during intoxication. Am J Psychiatry 126:1697–1704, 1970.
62. Tamerin JS, Mendelson JH: The psychodynamics of chronic deterioration: observation of alcoholics during the process of drinking in an experimental group setting. Am J Psychiatry 125:886–899, 1969.
63. McNamee HB, Mello NK, Mendelson JH: Experimental analysis of drinking patterns of alcoholics. Am J Psychiatry 124:1063–1069, 1968.
64. Birnbaum I, Taylor T, Parker E: Alcohol and sober mood state in female social drinkers. Alcohol Clin Exp Res 7:362–368, 1983.

65. Gilder DA, Wall TL, Ehlers CL: Comorbidity of select anxiety and affective disorders with alcohol dependence in Southwest California Indians. Alcohol Clin Exp Res 28:1805–1813, 2004.
66. Hesselbrock MN, Hesselbrock VM, Segal B, et al: Ethnicity and psychiatric comorbidity among alcohol-dependent persons who receive inpatient treatment: African Americans, Alaska Natives, Caucasians, and Hispanics. Alcohol Clin Exp Res 27:1368–1373, 2003.
67. Brown SA, Schuckit MA: Changes in depression among abstinent alcoholics. J Stud Alcohol 49:312–317, 1988.
68. Mueller TI, Lavori PW, Keller MB, et al: Prognostic effect of the variable course of alcoholism on the 10-year course of depression. Am J Psychiatry 151:701–706, 1994.
69. Conner KR, Sörensen S, Leonard KE: Initial depression and subsequent drinking during alcoholism treatment. J Stud Alcohol 66:401–406, 2005.
70. Brook DW, Brook JS, Zhang C, et al: Drug use and the risk of major depressive disorder, alcohol dependence, and substance use disorders. Arch Gen Psychiatry 59:1039–1044, 2002.
71. Jessor R, Donovan J, Costa P: Beyond Adolescence: Problem Behavior and Young Adult Development. Cambridge, United Kingdom, Cambridge University Press, 1991.
72. Cooper ML, Frone MR, Russell M, et al: Drinking to regulate positive and negative emotions: a motivational model of alcohol use. J Pers Soc Psychol 69:990–1005, 1995.
73. Labouvie E, Bates ME: Reasons for alcohol use in young adulthood: validation of a three-dimensional measure. J Stud Alcohol 63:145–155, 2002.
74. Harrington R, Fudge H, Rutter M, et al: Adult outcomes of childhood and adolescent depression, I: psychiatric status. Arch Gen Psychiatry 47:465–473, 1990.
75. Rao U, Ryan ND, Birmaher B, et al: Unipolar depression in adolescents: clinical outcome in adulthood. J Am Acad Child Adolesc Psychiatry 34:566–578, 1995.
76. Caspi A, Moffitt T, Newman D, et al: Behavioral observations at age 3 years predict adult psychiatric disorders. Arch Gen Psychiatry 53:1033–1039, 1996.
77. Chen Y-Y, Weitzman ER: Depressive symptoms, DSM-IV alcohol abuse and their comorbidity among children of problem drinkers in a national survey: effects of parent and child gender and parent recovery status. J Stud Alcohol 66:66–73, 2005.
78. Bennett ME, McCrady BS, Johnson V, et al: Problem drinking from young adulthood to adulthood: patterns, predictors and outcomes. J Stud Alcohol 60:605–614, 1999.
79. Jacob T, Windle M: Young adult children of alcoholic, depressed and nondistressed parents. J Stud Alcohol 61:836–844, 2000.
80. Schuckit MA, Smith TL, Chacko Y: Evaluation of a depression-related model of alcohol problems in 430 probands from the San Diego Prospective Study. Drug Alcohol Depend 82:194–203, 2006.
81. Ohannessian CM, Hesselbrock VM, Kramer J, et al: The relationship between parental alcoholism and adolescent psychopathology: a systematic examination of parental comorbid psychopathology. J Abnorm Child Psychol 32:519–533, 2004.
82. Colder CR, Chassin L: Affectivity and impulsivity: temperamental risk for adolescent alcohol involvement. Psychol Addict Behav 11:83–97, 1997.
83. West MO, Prinz RJ: Parental alcoholism and childhood psychopathology. Psychol Bull 102:204–218, 1987.

84. Chassin L, Pitts SC, LeLucia C, et al: A longitudinal study of children of alcoholics: predicting young adult substance use disorders, anxiety, and depression. J Abnorm Psychol 108:106–119, 1999.
85. Newcomb M, Bentler P: Consequences of Adolescent Drug Use: Impact on the Lives of Young Adults. Newbury Park, CA, Sage, 1988.
86. Wells JE, Horwood LJ, Fergusson DM: Drinking patterns in mid-adolescence and psychosocial outcomes in late adolescence and early adulthood. Addiction 99:1529–1541, 2004.
87. Preuss UW, Schuckit MA, Smith TL, et al: Mood and anxiety symptoms among 140 children from alcoholic and control families. Drug Alcohol Depend 67:235–242, 2002.
88. Schuckit MA, Smith TL, Radziminski S, et al: Behavioral symptoms and psychiatric diagnoses among 162 children in nonalcoholic or alcoholic families. Am J Psychiatry 157:1881–1883, 2000.
89. Schuckit MA, Smith TL, Danko GP, et al: Evaluation of a level of response to alcohol-based structural equation model in adolescents. J Stud Alcohol 66:174– 184, 2005.
90. Hatsukami D, Pickens RW: Posttreatment depression in an alcoholic and drug abuse population. Am J Psychiatry 139:1563–1566, 1982.
91. Kiefer F, Barocka A: Secondary depression in weaned alcoholics: implications of Lesch's typology of chronic alcoholism. Alcohol Alcohol 34:916–919, 1999.
92. Ramsey SE, Kahler CW, Read JP, et al: Discriminating between substance-induced and independent depressive episodes in alcohol dependent patients. J Stud Alcohol 65: 672–676, 2004.
93. Willenbring ML: Measurement of depression in alcoholics. J Stud Alcohol 47:367–372, 1986.
94. Brown SA, Inaba RK, Gillin JC, et al: Alcoholism and affective disorder: clinical course of depressive symptoms. Am J Psychiatry 152:45–52, 1997.
95. Davidson KM: Diagnosis of depression in alcohol dependence: changes in prevalence with drinking status. Br J Psychiatry 166:199–204, 1995.
96. Coryell W, Keller M, Endicott J, et al: Bipolar II illness: course and outcome over a five-year period. Psychol Med 19:129–141, 1989.
97. Dackis CA, Gold MS, Pottash ALC: Evaluating depression in alcoholics. Psychiatry Res 17:105–109, 1986.
98. Gibson S, Becker J: Changes in alcoholics' self-reported depression. Q J Stud Alcohol 34:829–836, 1973.
99. Penick EC, Powell BJ, Liskow BI, et al: The stability of coexisting psychiatric syndromes in alcoholic men after one year. J Stud Alcohol 49:395–405, 1988.
100. Pottenger M, McKernon J, Patrie LE, et al: The frequency of persistence of depressive symptoms in the alcohol abuser. J Nerv Ment Dis 166:562–570, 1978.
101. Kosten TR, Morgan CH, Kosten TA: Depressive symptoms during buprenorphine treatment of opioid abusers. J Subst Abuse Treat 7:51–54, 1990.
102. Kosten T, Oliveto A, Feingold A, et al: Desipramine and contingency management for cocaine and opiate dependence in buprenorphine maintained patients. Drug Alcohol Depend 70:315–325, 2003.
103. Nunes EV, Levin FR: Treatment of depression in patients with alcohol or other drug dependence: a meta-analysis. JAMA 291:1887–1896, 2004.

104. Nunes EV, Sullivan MA, Levin FR: Treatment of depression in patients with opiate dependence. Biol Psychiatry 56:793–802, 2004.
105. Rounsaville BJ: Treatment of cocaine dependence and depression. Biol Psychiatry 56:803–809, 2004.
106. Rounsaville BJ, Kosten TR, Weissman MM, et al: Prognostic significance of psychopathology in treated opiate addicts: a 2.5-year follow-up study. Arch Gen Psychiatry 43:739–745, 1986.
107. Rounsaville BJ, Anton SF, Carroll K, et al: Psychiatric diagnoses of treatment-seeking cocaine abusers. Arch Gen Psychiatry 48:43–51, 1991.
108. Strain EC, Stitzer ML, Bigelow GE: Early treatment time course of depressive symptoms in opiate addicts. J Nerv Ment Dis 179:215–221, 1991.
109. Preuss UW, Schuckit MA, Smith TL, et al: A comparison of alcohol-induced and independent depression in alcoholics with histories of suicide attempts. J Stud Alcohol 63:498–502, 2002.
110. Merikangas KR, Leckman JF, Prusoff BA, et al: Familial transmission of depression and alcoholism. Arch Gen Psychiatry 42:367–372, 1985.
111. Merikangas KR, Prusoff BA, Weissman MM: Parental concordance for affective disorders: psychopathology in offspring. J Affect Disord 15:279–290, 1988.
112. Weissman MM, Warner V, Wickramaratne P, et al: Offspring of depressed parents: 10 years later. Arch Gen Psychiatry 54:932–940, 1997.
113. Weissman MM, Wolk S, Goldstein RB, et al: Depressed adolescents grown up. JAMA 281:1707–1713, 1999.
114. Hasin DS, Grant BF: Major depression in 6050 former drinkers: association with past alcohol dependence. Arch Gen Psychiatry 59:794–800, 2002.
115. Schuckit MA, Smith TL: An evaluation of the level of response to alcohol, externalizing symptoms, and depressive symptoms as predictors of alcoholism. J Stud Alcohol 67:215–227, 2006.
116. Schuckit MA, Irwin M, Smith TL: One-year incidence rate of major depression and other psychiatric disorders in 239 alcoholic men. Addiction 89:441–445, 1994.
117. Satel SL, Kosten TR, Schuckit MA, et al: Should protracted withdrawal from drugs be included in DSM-IV? Am J Psychiatry 140:695–704, 1993.
118. American Psychiatric Association: Diagnostic and Statistical Manual of Mental Disorders, 4th Edition, Text Revision. Washington, DC, American Psychiatric Association, 2000.
119. Goodwin RD, Lieb R, Hoefler M, et al: Panic attack as a risk factor for severe psychopathology. Am J Psychiatry 161:2207–2214, 2004.
120. Schuckit MA, Hesselbrock V: Alcohol dependence and anxiety disorders: what is the relationship? Am J Psychiatry 151:1723–1734, 1994.
121. Caspari D: Cannabis and schizophrenia: results of a follow-up study. Eur Arch Psychiatry Clin Neurosci 249:45–49, 1999.
122. Castanada R, Galanter M, Lifschutz N, et al: Effect of drugs of abuse on psychiatric symptoms among hospitalized schizophrenics. Am J Drug Alcohol Abuse 17:313–320, 1991.
123. Weiser M, Reichenberg A, Rabinowitz J, et al: Self-reported drug abuse in male adolescents with behavioral disturbances, and follow-up for future schizophrenia. Biol Psychiatry 54:655–660, 2003.

124. Hasin DS, Tsai W-Y, Endicott J, et al: Five year course of major depression: effects of comorbid alcoholism. J Affect Disord 41:63–70, 1996.
125. Hasin DS, Tsai WY, Endicott J, et al: The effects of major depression on alcoholism. Am J Addict 5:144–155, 1996.
126. Gilman SE, Abraham HD: A longitudinal study of the order of onset of alcohol dependence and major depression. Drug Alcohol Depend 63:277–286, 2001.
127. Rounsaville BJ, Kleber H: Untreated opiate addicts: how do they differ from those seeking treatment? Arch Gen Psychiatry 42:1072–1077, 1985.
128. Rounsaville BJ, Dolinsky ZS, Babor TF, et al: Psychopathology as a predictor of treatment outcome in alcoholics. Arch Gen Psychiatry 44:505–513, 1987.
129. Schuckit MA, Winokur G: A short term follow-up of women alcoholics. Dis Nerv Syst 33:672–678, 1972.
130. McQuaid JR, Shuchter SR: Mood disorders: psychotherapy, in Comprehensive Textbook of Psychiatry. Edited by Sadock BJ, Sadock VA. Philadelphia, PA, Lippincott Williams & Wilkins, 2004, pp 1652–1660.
131. Ciraulo DA, Jaffe JH: Tricyclic antidepressants in the treatment of depression associated with alcoholism. J Clin Psychopharmacol 1:146–150, 1981.
132. Liskow BI, Goodwin DW: Pharmacological treatment of alcohol intoxication, withdrawal and dependence: a critical review. J Stud Alcohol 48:356–370, 1987.
133. Cornelius JR, Salloum IM, Ehler JG, et al: Fluoxetine in depressed alcoholics: a double blind, placebo-controlled trial. Arch Gen Psychiatry 54:700–705, 1997.
134. Mason BJ, Kocsis JH, Ritvo EC, et al: A double-blind placebo-controlled trial of desipramine in primary alcoholics stratified on the presence or absence of major depression. JAMA 275:1–7, 1996.
135. Carpenter KM, Brooks AC, Vosburg SK, et al: The effect of sertraline and environmental context on treating depression and illicit substance use among methadone maintained opiate dependent patients: a controlled clinical trial. Drug Alcohol Depend 74:123–134, 2004.
136. Hernandez-Avila CA, Modesto-Lowe V, Feinn R, et al: Nefazodone treatment of comorbid alcohol dependence and major depression. Alcohol Clin Exp Res 28:433–440, 2004.
137. Pettinati HM: Antidepressant treatment of co-occurring depression and alcohol dependence. Biol Psychiatry 56:785–792, 2004.
138. Salloum IM, Cornelius JR, Daley DC, et al: Efficacy of valproate maintenance in patients with bipolar disorder and alcoholism: a double-blind placebo-controlled study. Arch Gen Psychiatry 62:37–45, 2005.

9

COMORBIDITY OF SUBSTANCE USE WITH DEPRESSION AND OTHER MENTAL DISORDERS

From DSM-IV to DSM-V

Edward V. Nunes, M.D.
Bruce J. Rounsaville, M.D.

The *Diagnostic and Statistical Manual of Mental Disorders*, 4th Edition (DSM-IV), approach to co-occurring psychiatric and substance use disorders, based on the distinction between primary or independent and substance-induced disorders,[1] was unquestionably an important advance for the field. This provided clinicians with clear guidelines for determining when a mental disorder could be considered independently of substance use. Even more importantly, the "substance-induced"

This work was supported by grants K02 DA00288, P50DA09236, K05 DA00089 and P50 DA09241 from the National Institute on Drug Abuse, and the U.S. Veterans Administration Mental Illness Research, Education and Clinical Center. The authors are grateful to Marc Schuckit, M.D., for his suggestions, and to Carrie Davies for assistance with preparation of the manuscript.

Reprinted from Nunes EV, Rounsaville BJ: "Comorbidity of Substance Use With Depression and Other Mental Disorders." *Addiction* 101 (suppl 1):89–96, 2006. Used with permission of the Society for the Study of Addiction.

category reflected recognition that some psychiatric syndromes that occur only during substance use may have clinical implications for prognosis and treatment. These categories provided clarity and consensus in an area that previously had been a source of confusion and controversy, and allowed clinicians to think more freely and precisely about these difficult patients. At the same time, this approach has limitations and, despite its 10-year existence, has generated only a limited body of research. Following a discussion of the roots of the DSM-IV approach to comorbidity in prior diagnostic systems, we discuss limitations of DSM-IV and potential changes in the criteria, as well as developments that might be considered in moving toward DSM-V and beyond. The focus of the discussion is on depression, because this is where most of the evidence lies. It should be borne in mind, however, that virtually every psychiatric disorder is associated with increased prevalence of substance use disorders and vice versa and, if anything, the associations with substance use disorders are even stronger for other psychiatric disorders, including schizophrenia, bipolar illness, antisocial personality disorder, and some of the anxiety disorders.[2–4]

Research Versus Clinical Perspectives: A Caveat

A common theme that has emerged from the series of papers on which the chapters in this volume are based pertains to the important differences between the priorities of researchers and of clinicians, and the implications of this for nosology and for DSM-V. Researchers are interested in etiology and pathophysiology and in the multiple possible relationships between psychiatric syndromes and substance abuse and dependence. Although clinicians share an interest in these important issues, they have a more pragmatic, immediate focus—namely, to distinguish transient substance-induced psychiatric symptoms from disorders that are clinically significant (i.e., syndromes that persist, that are predictive of poor prognosis, and that potentially warrant specific treatment with psychotropic medications or specific behavioral and psychotherapeutic techniques). Arguably, with some fine-tuning, the current DSM-IV system approaches these clinical goals.

Further, there are costs to enacting major changes in nosology that suggest setting a relatively high threshold to change in moving from DSM-IV to DSM-V. These costs include the burden on clinicians, who must learn a new system; disruptions in research, particularly in longitudinal studies and in the ability to compare past and future studies; apparent changes in prevalence rates, which mainly reflect artifacts of syndrome definitions; the need to modify existing instruments or develop new instruments; and a negative public perception of vacillation or uncertainty.

Pre-DSM-IV Diagnostic Systems and Comorbidity

As the field entered the modern era of neo-Kraepelinian nosology based on observable symptoms, clinicians were sharply divided on the meaning of co-occurring psychiatric syndromes among substance-dependent patients. Some clinicians, particularly those involved in treatment of substance use disorders, tended to view psychiatric syndromes as manifestations of the substance use disorder and even suggested that focus on such psychiatric syndromes might represent a serious distraction and would interfere with the work of achieving and maintaining sobriety. Other clinicians, particularly those more involved in treating psychiatric disorders, tended to see substance use disorders as part of the psychopathology, at the risk of missing the need to provide primary treatment for the substance use disorder. Both points of view were perhaps the result of the poorly specified diagnostic syndromes of DSM-I and DSM-II, which tended to be based on inferences about internal states, rather than observable behavioral symptoms. This division was reflected in both the public and private treatment systems, in which, to the detriment of patients suffering from combinations of psychiatric and substance use problems, separate programs existed for treating these disorders, with little coordination between programs. These opposing points of view have spurred subsequent research.

FEIGHNER AND RESEARCH DIAGNOSTIC CRITERIA (RDC): THE CHRONOLOGICAL PRIMARY VERSUS SECONDARY DISTINCTION

The Feighner[5] and RDC[6] codified the classification of syndromes based on their order of age at first onset. As a result, psychiatric syndromes such as depression that occurred together with substance use disorders were classified as primary if the onset of the psychiatric syndrome during the lifetime occurred prior to onset of the substance use disorder; otherwise the syndrome was classified as secondary. This led to useful research, including findings from Schuckit and Brown[7,8] among primarily male veteran populations, that suggested that most depression among alcoholic individuals is chronologically secondary and tends to resolve with enforced abstinence on an inpatient unit, whereas primary depression in such patients is less prevalent but tends to persist despite abstinence. This suggests a useful distinction with clear prognostic and treatment implications. However, one problem is that primary disorders are relatively rare due to the typical early onset of substance use disorders,[9] raising the concern that many meaningful co-occurring psychiatric syndromes may be missed or ignored by the simple application of this system.

DSM-III AND DSM-III-R: THE ORGANIC SKIP-OUT

RDC and DSM-III introduced the notion that diagnosis of a psychiatric syndrome should include a review of concurrent substance use and that if the syndrome appeared possibly or probably caused by the substance use, then an organic disorder should be diagnosed.[6,10] This criterion was vaguely defined, having been based almost entirely on clinical judgment, and it ultimately generated little research. On the other hand, it represented recognition that the chronological primary versus secondary distinction might be too narrow.

EXPANSIONS OF THE PRIMARY/SECONDARY DISTINCTION

The pre-DSM-IV era saw a variety of efforts to expand the definition of primary and secondary disorders to render them more clinically useful. At Yale, the Schedule for Affective Disorders and Schizophrenia (SADS) was modified in such a way that co-occurring syndromes, such as depression, could be diagnosed if the psychiatric symptoms emerged during a stable period of substance use. The rationale for this was that during stable periods of use, toxicity (which would be expected during accelerating use) or withdrawal (which would be expected during sharp reductions in use) would not apply as explanations. A series of studies showed that psychiatric disorders, including depression, diagnosed in this way were predictive of poor outcome among opiate-dependent patients, as well as alcohol-dependent and cocaine-dependent patients.[11–14] Not surprisingly, the prevalence of depression and other psychiatric disorders, diagnosed in this way, was much higher than with the simple chronological primary distinction (in the range of 30%–50% for lifetime disorders and 20%–30% for current depression). These rates were comparable to rates typically less than 10% for the chronological primary.[9]

During the same period, groups engaged in clinical trials of antidepressant medications among substance-dependent patients expanded the definition of *primary* to include disorders not only that were chronologically primary but that had also persisted during past abstinent periods during the history. Disorders that were not primary by this definition were considered secondary if the full criteria for a depressive syndrome (major depression or dysthymia) were met and a stringent chronicity criterion was also met—namely, a requirement for 3–6 months' duration in the current episode. A series of clinical trials suggested that both primary and secondary depressions defined in this way were responsive to antidepressant medication treatment, although sample sizes in individual studies were too small to examine differences in effect size between the primary and secondary subgroups.[15–18] A version of the Structured Clinical Interview for DSM-IV Axis I Disorders (SCID) was also developed to capture these expanded chronological criteria for primary and secondary.[19] A related effort[20] showed that chronologically secondary depression among alcoholic individuals responded to antidepressant medication in a placebo-controlled trial as long as there was a brief period of abstinence of at least a week during which depression persisted prior to the initiation of treatment, whereas antidepressant medication was not helpful in the portion of the sample without such persistent depression.

Common elements of these efforts, which were reflected in the DSM-IV criteria, include the expanded notion of primary disorders as those with prior onset and those with persistence during abstinent periods. For secondary syndromes, these efforts suggest the notion that full criteria for the syndrome (e.g., major depression) should be met and that some effort should be made, perhaps by documenting chronicity or persistence during at least a brief period of abstinence, to establish that the psychiatric symptoms, such as depression, exceed what would be expected from the toxic or withdrawal effects of substances.

DSM-IV: Strengths and Limitations

DSM-IV defined primary or independent depression as a depression that can be shown to be temporally independent of substance use during the lifetime history (i.e., it either precedes the onset or has persisted during an abstinent period of at least 1 month). Ideally, the abstinence would be current and directly observed, although the criteria are not specific about this. Substance-induced depression was defined as a depression that could not be established as temporally independent based on the criteria for primary, but the depression symptoms exceed what would be expected from the usual toxic or withdrawal effects of substances and warrant clinical attention. By inference, a third category consists of the usual effects of substances, for which one can refer to the DSM criteria for intoxication and syndromes for the various commonly abused substances. In summary, DSM-IV posited two types of disorders: primary and substance-induced, and three types of symptoms, including primary, substance-induced and usual effects of substances.

STRENGTHS

The strengths of the DSM-IV system include a fairly clear definition of primary or independent disorders that has a good empirical basis in longitudinal and treatment studies and has probable prognostic and treatment implications. Further, in the "substance-induced" category, there is the recognition that some psychiatric syndromes that have occurred only in the setting of substance use may be clinically significant, warranting attention and specific treatment.

THE TERMINOLOGY PROBLEM

The terms *primary* and *substance-induced* seem to imply causality. "Substance-induced" suggests that the substances have caused the psychiatric symptoms. However, the DSM-IV criteria state that symptoms of a substance-induced disorder should "exceed the usual effects" of substances, implying something more. From a theoretical standpoint, questions of causality between co-occurring disorders are complicated and are probably best considered in the realm of future research rather than nosology at this point. Further, clinicians may tend to lump "substance-induced" with "usual effects of substances" and, thereby, dismiss the substance-induced syndrome, which seems contrary to the spirit of the category as representing something "more than usual effects" and warranting clinical attention. Thus, one recommendation might be that DSM-V consider terms that are more neutral with respect to the direction of causality. The use of "independent" as opposed to "primary" is already occurring in the literature and seems appropriate. Rather than "substance-induced," a term such as "substance-related" or "substance-associated" might be considered.

PROBLEMS WITH THE CRITERIA: CONCEPT VERSUS OPERATIONALIZATION

The DSM-IV criteria are vague in some respects, and this imprecision may work against reliability and validity. The definition of a primary or independent disorder leaves unclear under what conditions a current disorder may qualify as primary (i.e., must it occur during a current period of at least 1 month of abstinence, or can the co-occurring disorder qualify for an independent diagnosis if it occurred during a past period of abstinence, or if a past episode occurred during abstinence?). The criteria also do not specify whether a full syndrome is required versus a syndrome that is partially remitted.

The definition of "substance-induced" specifies only that some symptoms of a disorder, such as depression or anxiety, be present. Thus, it is not clear whether a full syndrome, such as the syndrome of major depression, is required. The latter requirement is part of the ICD-10 criteria. At the symptom level, it is not clear how to determine whether symptoms "exceed the usual effects" of substances. Relatedly, for usual effects of substances, the DSM-IV symptoms listed for the intoxication and withdrawal syndromes for the various substances are, arguably, not always complete.

MEASUREMENT AND THE SUBSTANCE-INDUCED SYNDROME

Systems for the diagnosis or measurement of the substance-induced syndromes have varied considerably. Ries and colleagues developed a simple Likert scale item for use by clinicians to indicate the extent to which a particular syndrome is substance-induced. They were able to show in a large clinical sample of inpatients that this rating was reliable and had some evidence of concurrent and predictive validity, in that it was associated with a more rapid resolution of psychiatric symptoms while, at the same time, being associated with a history of suicidal behavior.[21,22]

Hasin and colleagues developed the Psychiatric Research Interview for Substance and Mental Disorders (PRISM) on the basis of an analysis of sources of the poor reliability of the SCID in diagnosing co-occurring disorders.[23,24] The PRISM operationalizes a rigorous definition of substance-induced depression. This requires that the full major depression syndrome be met (i.e., a total of at least five symptoms) and that each of these symptoms exceed the usual effects of the particular substances that the patient is abusing. In a clinical sample of patients who were hospitalized on a dual-diagnosis inpatient unit, approximately 50% of major depressive syndromes were classified by the PRISM as substance-induced. In a 1-year follow-up on this sample, substance-induced depression was found to predict failure to remit and suicidal behavior in patients with a substance use disorder.[25,26] "Usual effects" of substances were not coded, essentially being discarded. Relatedly, a study that modified the SCID to incorporate some of the features of the PRISM showed that approximately one-third of cases of major depression diagnosed at baseline in a clinical sample converted to independent depression over a subsequent 1-year follow-up—that is, during the follow-up interval, the depression was shown to persist during periods of at least 1 month of abstinence.[27] Taken together, these data suggest that a more rigorous definition of substance-induced depression (requiring the full syndrome and some effort to operationalize the notion of exceeding usual effects) results in a syndrome with relatively clear prognostic and treatment implications, as well as a syndrome that may convert over time to primary or independent depression.

Other instruments that have operationalized the independent versus "substance-induced" distinction for depression include the Alcohol Use Disorder and Associated Disabilities Interview Schedule (AUDADIS),[28] which was developed for use by lay interviewers in two large community-based studies (the National Longitudinal Alcohol Epidemiologic Study [NLAES] and the more recent National Epidemiologic Survey on Alcohol and Related Conditions [NESARC]), and the Semi-Structured Assessment for the Genetics of Alcoholism (SSAGA), which was developed for use in the Collaborative Study on the Genetics of Alcoholism (COGA).[29] Interestingly, the NESARC yielded a very low prevalence of substance-induced depression, such that almost all major depression that was diagnosed was classified as independent or primary.[2] A cross-sectional study based on the COGA data set showed that, compared with substance-induced depression, independent depression was associated with a number of features that suggested greater vulnerability to true affective disease, such as past history of suicide attempts and a family history of depression.[30] A related study showed independent depression to be more associated with a depressive cognitive style.[31]

Clearly, data sets such as these have strong potential to be mined for analyses that can shed light on how to construct meaningful specific criteria for independent and substance-induced disorders.[32]

Recommendations and Potential Changes for DSM-V

Considering the rationale and background for the DSM-IV system for handling co-occurring psychiatric and substance use disorders, and the evidence accumulated to date as reviewed briefly above, our assessment is that DSM-V should preserve the basic distinction elaborated in DSM-IV between independent and substance-induced disorders, and symptoms that are usual effects of substances. Research leading up to DSM-V should focus on fine-tuning the criteria. Considerations should include adding greater precision to the criteria regarding 1) the timing of psychiatric and substance use symptoms; 2) the requisite severity of symptoms; 3) specifying whether full criteria for a co-occurring psychiatric syndrome need to be met in order to qualify for a "substance-induced" diagnosis; and 4) greater specificity regarding the definition of symptoms that exceed the usual effects of substances. This effort should lead ultimately to improved reliability, predictive validity, and, one hopes, clinical utility.

This work has already been initiated in the form of newly developed structured interviews, such as the PRISM, which have erected more specific rules for operationalizing the basic concepts of independent and substance-induced disorders elaborated in DSM-IV.[23,24] A variety of high-quality existing data sets could be brought to bear for fine-tuning the criteria. In addition to the NLAES,[33] NESARC,[2] and COGA[30] studies mentioned above, long-term follow-ups on the Epidemiologic Catchment Area (ECA) study,[34] the National Comorbidity Survey (NCS) study,[35] Breslau's Detroit study,[36] Kendler's twin studies,[37] Gelernter's genomewide scan sample,[38] and clinical studies employing the PRISM[25] and other structured instruments could be brought to bear. The broad strokes of a recommendation based on the current evidence would look something like the following:

1. For independent disorders, specify whether a past independent episode counts toward an overall independent diagnosis if the current episode would otherwise be considered substance-induced, or whether a past independent episode should be noted separately but not influence the diagnosis of the current episode; the latter preserves more information and encourages a careful lifetime history, and is thus perhaps preferable.
2. For substance-induced disorders, a) require that the full criteria for a syndrome, such as major depression, to be met; b) require that each of the component symptoms entering into a diagnosis be shown to exceed the usual effects of the substances involved; and c) suggest guidelines for making those distinctions.
3. Consider a more neutral terminology, such as "substance-associated" or "substance-related," that does not carry the causal implication of "substance-induced."

More rigorous criteria for substance-induced disorders, as in (2) above, would probably identify substance-induced syndromes that behave more like primary syndromes and that are perhaps likely to manifest ultimately as such if followed over time.[25,27] However, an important caveat would be that this would also produce more diagnostic orphans in the form of subthreshold psychiatric symptoms in the setting of substance use that might have important prognostic or treatment implications, and thus should still warrant clinical attention and should not be ignored in research efforts. A simple recommendation might be as follows:

4. Identify both substance-induced syndromes otherwise meeting full syndromal criteria (e.g., "substance-induced major depression"), and subsyndromal disorders (e.g., "substance-induced subsyndromal depression").
5. Consider features of substance-induced syndrome criteria that may be specific to particular substances or syndromes, particularly the more common depressive or anxiety syndromes as opposed to psychosis.

As already reflected in DSM-IV criteria, different substances produce different symptoms as part of intoxication or withdrawal. This specificity is built into the PRISM[24] and is implicit in recommendation (2) above. The duration of these symptoms may also differ by substance and is less clearly specified in DSM-IV. Cocaine, alcohol, and opioid withdrawal symptoms usually clear quickly, within a week or two,[39] but alcohol and opioid withdrawal may be subacute and last longer,[40] especially in the case of opioid withdrawal, if a long-acting agonist such as methadone is involved. Finally, different psychiatric syndromes may have different implications in defining what is independent, versus substance-induced, versus usual effects of substances. The more common substance-related symptoms fall on the depression-anxiety spectrum. Psychosis as a toxic effect of substances (mainly stimulants) is more rare and less systematically studied, and the stakes are higher in making the distinction with schizophrenia or schizoaffective disorder, which are chronic lifelong conditions generally requiring chronic treatment with neuroleptics.

An important goal for DSM-V and beyond is for the criteria to have clear prognostic and treatment implications. As noted above, in the short term a number of currently existing data sets could be mined to address predictive validity. However, more research will be needed, especially clinical trials to establish treatment implications of independent versus substance-induced syndromes, variously defined. Determining appropriate types of treatment and levels of care for patients with combinations of substance and psychiatric disorders has been an ongoing problem for service providers in the field. An effort is afoot to adapt the widely used American Society of Addiction Medicine Patient Placement Criteria,[41] which focus currently on substance use disorders, to evaluate the appropriate treatment for patients with co-occurring psychiatric and substance use disorders.[42] This would address such issues as whether the treatment plan should emphasize primarily substance use disorder treatment with some level of psychiatric consultation (as might be the case for a severe chronic substance use disorder with mild to moderate psychiatric symptoms), primarily psychiatric treatment (as for someone with a severe independent mood or psychotic disorder plus mild to moderate substance use disorder), or some intermediate plan. Coordination with this effort, so that the DSM-V criteria provide meaningful input into the Patient Placement Criteria, would seem highly desirable.

A fundamental theme of the conference series on which the chapters in this book are based has been that the ultimate goal for psychiatric nomenclature is to approach a model in which diagnosis is based on an understanding of etiology and pathophysiology. As reviewed in the companion chapter by Schuckit (see Chapter 8, this volume), there are several broad types of potential etiological relationships between co-occurring psychiatric and substance use disorders. Within these, multiple specific relationships are possible based on the unique pharmacology and pathophysiology of various drug–psychiatric disorder combinations, examples including nicotine and depression[43] and nicotine, cannabis, alcohol or stimulants and schizophrenia,[44] or the "reward deficiency syndrome" hypothesized to contribute to attention-deficit/hyperactivity disorder and other disorders of impulsivity.[45] The alcoholism typologies considered by Hesselbrock and Hesselbrock in this volume (see Chapter 10) have generally included a subtype with early onset of alcohol and substance abuse and dependence and frequent psychiatric comorbidity, particularly traits in the antisocial spectrum,[46,47] and some have added a subtype with prominent affective and anxiety symptoms.[48,49] While a nomenclature based on etiology would seem premature in the time frame of DSM-V, this clearly presents a rich opportunity for research and suggests that comorbidity is likely to play a part in any etiology-based nosology of the substance use disorders.

Another theme has been the potential for dimensional approaches to psychopathology, as covered in other chapters in this book. Advantages of a dimensional approach might include reducing a large number of categories to a smaller number of dimensions or spectra, facilitating research on shared pathophysiological mechanisms, and heightening attention to the possible clinical significance of subsyndromal or orphan disorders.[50,51] The typologies just discussed are reminiscent of the dimensional model of externalizing and internalizing psychopathology. As discussed earlier, attention to subsyndromal disorders would become particularly important if more rigorous criteria are adopted for substance-induced syndromes (e.g., substance-induced major depressive disorder).

In any case, it would seem clear that the substance use disorder diagnoses themselves should be preserved, even in the face of comorbidity due to their clear irreducible elements at the clinical and pathophysiological levels. These disorders have a unique precursor, namely substance use, and neuroadaptations in response to addictive substances, reflected in tolerance and withdrawal phenomena. Separate substance use disorder diagnoses, in all likelihood, would also retain utility regardless of advances in knowledge about shared causes or pathophysiology with other mental disorders.

Ultimately, research on etiological relationships between psychiatric and substance use disorders and common and shared aspects of pathophysiology will be important for advancing the entire field beyond clinical syndromes toward a more basic understanding of psychopathology. Such work would define phenotypes for family and genetic studies, neuroimaging studies, and other sorts of biological studies. In the end, however, the use of nonhierarchical, phenomenological diagnoses, such as those elaborated in DSM-IV, and fine-tuned criteria that we anticipate for DSM-V would seem the best approach to maintain at this point. Such nosology, along with comprehensive psychiatric diagnostic assessment, should be an ongoing part of the research agenda in fields such as genetics and neuroimaging that are at the cutting edge of biological psychiatry.

References

1. American Psychiatric Association: Diagnostic and Statistical Manual of Mental Disorders, 4th Edition. Washington, DC, American Psychiatric Association, 1994.
2. Grant BF, Stinson FS, Dawson DA, et al: Prevalence and co-occurrence of substance use disorders and independent mood and anxiety disorders: results from the National Epidemiologic Survey on Alcohol and Related Conditions. Arch Gen Psychiatry 61: 807–816, 2004.
3. Kessler RC, Crum RM, Warner LA, et al: Lifetime co-occurrence of DSM-III-R alcohol abuse and dependence with other psychiatric disorders in the National Comorbidity Survey. Arch Gen Psychiatry 54:313–321, 1997.
4. Regier DA, Farmer ME, Rae DS, et al: Comorbidity of mental disorders with alcohol and other drug abuse: results from the Epidemiologic Catchment Area (ECA) Study. JAMA 264:2511–2518, 1990.
5. Feighner JP, Robins E, Guze SB, et al: Diagnostic criteria for use in psychiatric research. Arch Gen Psychiatry 26:57–63, 1972.
6. Spitzer RL, Endicott J, Robins E: Research Diagnostic Criteria: rationale and reliability. Arch Gen Psychiatry 35:773–782, 1978.
7. Brown SA, Inaba RK, Gillin JC, et al: Alcoholism and affective disorder: clinical course of depressive symptoms. Am J Psychiatry 152:45–52, 1995.
8. Brown SA, Schuckit MA: Changes in depression among abstinent alcoholics. J Stud Alcohol 49:412–417, 1988.
9. Hasin D, Nunes E, Meydan J: Comorbidity of alcohol, drug and psychiatric disorders: epidemiology, in Dual Diagnosis and Treatment: Substance Abuse and Comorbid Disorders, 2nd Edition. Edited by Kranzler HR, Tinsley JA. New York, Marcel Dekker, 2004, pp 1–30.
10. American Psychiatric Association: Diagnostic and Statistical Manual of Mental Disorders, 3rd Edition. Washington, DC, American Psychiatric Association, 1980.
11. Carroll KM, Power ME, Bryant K, et al: One-year follow-up status of treatment-seeking cocaine abusers: psychopathology and dependence severity as predictors of outcome. J Nerv Ment Dis 181:71–79, 1993.
12. Rounsaville BJ, Dolinsky ZS, Babor TF, et al: Psychopathology as a predictor of treatment outcome in alcoholics. Arch Gen Psychiatry 44:505–513, 1987.

13. Rounsaville BJ, Kosten TR, Weissman MM, et al: Prognostic significance of psychopathology in treated opiate addicts: a 2.5-year follow-up study. Arch Gen Psychiatry 43:739–745, 1986.
14. Rounsaville BJ, Weissman MM, Crits-Christoph K, et al: Diagnosis and symptoms of depression in opiate addicts: course and relationship to treatment outcome. Arch Gen Psychiatry 39:151–156, 1982.
15. Nunes EV, McGrath PJ, Quitkin FM, et al: Imipramine treatment of alcoholism with comorbid depression. Am J Psychiatry 150:963–965, 1993.
16. Nunes EV, McGrath PJ, Quitkin FM, et al: Imipramine treatment of cocaine abuse: possible boundaries of efficacy. Drug Alcohol Depend 39:185–195, 1995.
17. McGrath PJ, Nunes EV, Stewart JW, et al: Imipramine treatment of alcoholics with primary depression: a placebo-controlled clinical trial. Arch Gen Psychiatry 53:232–240, 1996.
18. Nunes EV, Quitkin FM, Donovan SJ, et al: Imipramine treatment of opiate-dependent patients with depressive disorders: a placebo-controlled trial. Arch Gen Psychiatry 55:153–160, 1998.
19. Nunes EV, Goehl L, Seracini A, et al: A modification of the Structured Clinical Interview for DSM-III-R to evaluate methadone patients: test–retest reliability. Am J Addict 5:241–248, 1996.
20. Mason BJ, Kocsis JH, Ritvo EC, et al: A double-blind, placebo-controlled trial of desipramine for primary alcohol dependence stratified on the presence or absence of major depression. JAMA 275:761–767, 1996.
21. Ries RK, Demirsoy A, Russo JE, et al: Reliability and clinical utility of DSM-IV substance-induced psychiatric disorders in acute psychiatric inpatients. Am J Addict 10:308–318, 2001.
22. Comtois KA, Russo JE, Roy-Byrne P, et al: Clinicians' assessments of bipolar disorder and substance abuse as predictors of suicidal behavior in acutely hospitalized psychiatric inpatients. Biol Psychiatry 56:757–763, 2004.
23. Hasin DS, Trautman KD, Miele GM, et al: Psychiatric Research Interview for Substance and Mental Disorders (PRISM): reliability for substance abusers. Am J Psychiatry 153:1195–1201, 1996.
24. Hasin D, Samet S, Nunes E, et al: Diagnosis of comorbid psychiatric disorders in substance users assessed with the Psychiatric Research Interview for Substance and Mental Disorders for DSM-IV. Am J Psychiatry 163:689–696, 2006.
25. Hasin D, Liu X, Nunes E, et al: Effects of major depression on remission and relapse of substance dependence. Arch Gen Psychiatry 59:375–380, 2002.
26. Aharonovich E, Liu X, Nunes E, et al: Suicide attempts in substance abusers: effects of major depression in relation to substance use disorders. Am J Psychiatry 159:1600–1602, 2002.
27. Ramsey SE, Kahler CW, Read JP, et al: Discriminating between substance-induced and independent depressive episodes in alcohol dependent patients. J Stud Alcohol 65:672–676, 2004.
28. Grant BF, Hasin DS: The Alcohol Use Disorder and Associated Disabilities Interview Schedule. Rockville, MD, National Institute of Alcohol Abuse and Alcoholism, 1992.

29. Bucholz K, Cadoret R, Cloninger R, et al: A new semi-structured psychiatric interview for use in genetic linkage studies: a report on the reliability of the SSAGA. J Stud Alcohol 55:149–158, 1994.
30. Schuckit MA, Tipp JE, Bergman M, et al: Comparison of induced and independent major depressive disorders in 2,945 alcoholics. Am J Psychiatry 154:948–957, 1997.
31. Kahler CW, Ramsey SE, Read JP, et al: Substance-induced and independent major depressive disorder in treatment-seeking alcoholics: associations with dysfunctional attitudes and coping. J Stud Alcohol 63:363–371, 2002.
32. Robins LN: Using survey results to improve the validity of the standard psychiatric nomenclature. Arch Gen Psychiatry 61:1188–1194, 2004.
33. Grant BF, Harford TC: Comorbidity between DSM-IV alcohol use disorders and major depression: results of a national survey. Drug Alcohol Depend 39:197–206, 1995.
34. Swartz KL, Pratt LA, Armenian HK, et al: Mental disorders and the incidence of migraine headaches in a community sample: results from the Baltimore Epidemiologic Catchment Area follow-up study. Arch Gen Psychiatry 57:945–950, 2000.
35. Kessler RC, Berglund P, Demler O, et al: The epidemiology of major depressive disorder: results from the National Comorbidity Survey Replication (NCS-R). JAMA 289:3095–3105, 2003.
36. Breslau N, Peterson EL, Schultz LR, et al: Major depression and stages of smoking: a longitudinal investigation. Arch Gen Psychiatry 55:161–166, 1998.
37. Kendler KS, Prescott CA, Myers J, et al: The structure of genetic and environmental risk factors for common psychiatric and substance use disorders in men and women. Arch Gen Psychiatry 60:929–937, 2003.
38. Gelernter J, Panhuysen C, Weiss R, et al: Genome-wide linkage scan for cocaine dependence and related traits: significant linkages for a cocaine-related trait and cocaine-induced paranoia. Am J Med Genet B Neuropsychiatr Genet 136:45–52, 2005.
39. Nunes EV, Raby WN: Comorbidity of depression and substance abuse, in Biology of Depression, Vol 2. Edited by Licinio J, Wong M-L. Weinheim, Germany, Wiley-VCH-Verlag GmbH KGaA, 2005, pp 341–364.
40. Satel SL, Kosten TR, Schuckit MA, et al: Should protracted withdrawal from drugs be included in DSM-IV? Am J Psychiatry 150:695–704, 1993.
41. Gastfriend DR, Mee-Lee D: The ASAM patient placement criteria: context, concepts and continuing development. J Addict Dis 22(suppl 1):1–8, 2003.
42. Minkoff K, Zweben J, Rosenthal R, et al: Development of service intensity criteria and program categories for individuals with co-occurring disorders. J Addict Dis 22:113–129, 2003.
43. Glassman AH: Cigarette smoking: implications for psychiatric illness. Am J Psychiatry 150:546–553, 1993.
44. Ziedonis D, Steinberg ML, D'Avanzo K, et al: Co-occurring schizophrenia and addiction, in Dual Diagnosis and Psychiatric Treatment: Substance Abuse and Comorbid Disorders, 2nd Edition. Edited by Kranzler HR, Tinsley JA. New York, Marcel Dekker, 2004, pp 387–435.
45. Blum K, Noble E Reward deficiency syndrome (RDS): a biogenic model for the diagnosis and treatment of impulsive, addictive, and compulsive behaviors. Mol Psychiatry 6:S1, 2001.

46. Babor TF, Hofmann M, Del Boca FK, et al: Types of alcoholics, I: evidence for an empirically derived typology based on indicators of vulnerability and severity. Arch Gen Psychiatry 49:599–608, 1992.
47. Cloninger CR: Neurogenetic adaptive mechanisms in alcoholism. Science 236:410–416, 1987.
48. Del Boca FK, Hesselbrock M: Gender and alcoholic subtypes. Alcohol Health Res World 20:56–62, 1996.
49. Lesch OM, Ades J, Badawy A, et al: Alcohol dependence—classificatory considerations. Alcohol Alcohol Suppl 2:127–131, 1993.
50. Sarr M, Bucholz KK, Phelps DL: Using cluster analysis of alcohol use disorders to investigate "diagnostic orphans": subjects with alcohol dependence symptoms but no diagnosis. Drug Alcohol Depend 60:295–302, 2000.
51. Judd LL, Akiskal HS, Zeller PJ, et al: Psychosocial disability during the long-term course of unipolar major depressive disorder. Arch Gen Psychiatry 57:375–380, 2000.

10

ARE THERE EMPIRICALLY SUPPORTED AND CLINICALLY USEFUL SUBTYPES OF ALCOHOL DEPENDENCE?

Victor M. Hesselbrock, Ph.D.
Michie N. Hesselbrock, Ph.D., M.S.W.

Drinking, as an example of drug use behavior in the general population, varies considerably from severe alcohol dependence through simple abuse, to low-risk drinking patterns, to abstinence. Further, alcohol abuse and dependence often co-occur with other Axis I and Axis II disorders. These additional phenomena create problems in defining the nature of alcoholism, separating it from normal drinking, and identifying distinct boundaries between alcohol use disorders and other psychiatric disorders. These problems are common when examining most substances of abuse and illustrate the critical role and importance of properly defined criteria in clinical assessment.

Although many drug dependencies are often defined in clinical studies as a single diagnostic entity, their clinical expression is likely to be heterogeneous. Indeed, people with alcohol or other drug dependencies are heterogeneous in terms of their history and patterns of substance use, demography, and other co-occurring

---

This work was supported, in part, by NIH grants P50 AA-03510 and U10-AA08403.

Reprinted from Hesselbrock VM, Hesselbrock MN: "Are There Empirically Supported and Clinically Useful Subtypes of Alcohol Dependence?" *Addiction* 101 (suppl 1):97–103, 2006. Used with permission of the Society for the Study of Addiction.

psychiatric conditions. Further, different family backgrounds and rearing patterns and a variety of biological, social, and psychiatric problems have been associated with chronic drug use. These factors may influence treatment-seeking behavior, treatment outcomes, and the life course of substance abuse or dependence by moderating or mediating its clinical expression.[1] Because most of the published efforts in identifying "subtypes" of substance abuse or dependence have focused on *alcoholism,* a term that often encompasses both alcohol dependence and alcohol abuse, this review will focus on that literature.

Multivariate Typologies of Alcoholism

A variety of multivariate, multidimensional typologies of alcoholism have been proposed[2,3] but have seldom been developed and examined in well-characterized samples. A well-known example of a multidimensional classification of alcoholism was proposed by Cloninger and colleagues,[4] who identified two separate forms of alcoholism based on differences in alcohol-related symptoms, patterns of transmission, and personality characteristics using data derived from a cross-fostering study of Swedish adoptees. Type 1 is characterized by either mild or severe alcohol abuse in the probands and no criminality in the fathers. Individuals with type 1 alcoholism came from relatively high socioeconomic backgrounds, and alcohol abuse in the biological mothers was frequent. Persons with type 1 alcoholism are hypothesized to be responsive to environmental influence, to have relatively mild alcohol-related problems with few hospitalizations, and to have onset of alcoholism after age 25 years. These individuals are thought to be dependent on social approval (high reward dependence), be cautious (high harm avoidance), and prefer non-risk-taking situations (low novelty-seeking). On the other hand, type 2 alcoholism is characterized as being associated with familial alcoholism, having severe and violence-related alcohol problems, other drug use, and having an onset of alcohol problems before 25 years of age. Low reward dependence, low harm avoidance, and high novelty-seeking characterize these individuals. Although multivariate statistical methods were used to identify subtypes, Cloninger's types of alcoholism have been criticized due to the small sample size of both males ($n=151$) and females ($n=31$), sample selection methods, indirect assessment of family variables, and other methodological limitations.[5]

The heritability of the type 1/type 2 forms of alcoholism has been examined in twins[6] and among the family members of alcohol-dependent patients.[7] In both cases the more severe, type 2 form was found to have a higher heritability than the type 1 form.

Type A and Type B Subtypes of Alcoholism

A second multidimensional classification of alcoholism was proposed by Babor et al.[8] on the basis of a sample of 321 male and female alcoholic inpatients. Seventeen defining characteristics covering the areas of premorbid risk factors, the pathological use of alcohol and other substances, and the chronicity and consequences of drinking were used to identify homogeneous groups of alcoholics. Type A, resembling Cloninger's type 1, was characterized by a later onset of the disorder, fewer childhood behavior problems, and less psychopathology. Type B resembled type 2 alcoholism and was defined by a high prevalence of childhood behavior problems, familial alcoholism, early onset of alcohol problems, a more chronic treatment history, more psychopathology, and more life stress. While Cloninger et al.'s type 2 male-limited alcohol abuse was associated with moderate alcohol abuse, Babor et al.'s type B was associated with severe alcoholism and its more chronic consequences. Further, the Babor et al. subtypes of alcoholism were found in both male and female patients.

The Babor et al.[8] alcoholism subtypes have been examined by different authors, who used either the original data set[9–11] or similar defining characteristics and statistical methods (see references 12–13, among others). Schuckit et al.,[12] using a clustering algorithm approximating that described by Babor et al., found two similar groups as Babor et al. Type A individuals were characterized by a later onset of alcohol symptoms, fewer childhood behavior problems, somewhat fewer alcohol-related symptoms, and fewer other psychological/psychiatric problems (e.g., anxiety and depressive symptoms). Type B individuals reported more childhood problems (mainly conduct problems), an earlier onset of alcohol problems, greater severity of alcohol dependence, more physical problems, more polydrug use, and greater psychological dysfunction.

Type A/B clusters do occur within different ethnic groups. When methods similar to those of Babor et al.[8] and Schuckit et al.[12] were used, a two-cluster solution similar to type A/B was found in separate analyses of Hispanic ($n = 106$), African American ($n = 351$), and Alaska Native ($n = 442$) alcohol-dependent samples.[14]

More Than Two Subtypes?

Most cluster analytical studies of alcoholism indicate that the majority of cases can be classified into one of two clusters. The remaining cases are dropped from further analyses or cluster solution parameters are changed to include the maximum amount of cases. However, two-group solutions do not fully capture the clinical or general population samples. Further, most data reduction techniques (e.g., cluster analysis, factor analysis) are not governed by prescribed rules, so the final solution may be influenced by a variety of factors, including sample characteristics and sample size, the clinical information available and the theory underlying the original analysis. The indeterminate nature of cluster-derived typologies is exemplified by a reanalysis of the Babor et al.[8] data by Del Boca and Hesselbrock.[11] With lifetime alcoholism risk and severity variables as defining characteristics, the resulting four-cluster solution revealed important sex differences, as well as distinctions within the broader types that have etiological and clinical significance. The high-risk/high-severity (HRHS) cluster contained equal proportions of males and females (22% from each group) and included those cases highest in family history of alcoholism loading and the earliest age at onset of alcoholism. HRHS subjects were, on average, the youngest and were characterized by moderate alcohol involvement; a high frequency of other psychiatric symptoms, including conduct problems; and other drug use. The low-risk/low-severity cluster (LRLS) contained 31% of the cases (28% of males, 39% of females) and was characterized by relatively low alcohol involvement, low drug use, low levels of alcohol-related consequences and low rates of other psychiatric symptoms. The "internalizers" cluster contained 32% of females and only 11% of males in the sample who were characterized by high levels of depressive and anxiety symptoms. The "externalizers" cluster was characterized by a high prevalence of childhood behavior problems; this group had the highest rates of alcohol use for self-medication, benzodiazepine use, alcohol dependence, and medical/physical consequences. Fewer externalizing subjects had a family history of alcoholism, but subjects had high rates of alcohol use and alcohol-related social consequences and high rates of antisocial personality disorder. This cluster contained 38% of the males and 7% of females in the sample.

Unlike for most other multivariate substance dependence subtypes, longitudinal follow-up data are available for the subtypes of alcohol dependence proposed by Del Boca and Hesselbrock.[11] They compared the four clusters described above in relation to their 1- and 3-year posttreatment outcome data. In general, the differences between the four clusters were in the expected direction. At the 1-year follow-up, the HRHS and the externalizing groups reported the most drinking days during the year prior to follow-up. The HRHS group also reported the most total drinking at the 3-year follow-up assessment. The internalizing group reported the fewest total drinking days at both follow-up assessments. Consistent with this finding, the internalizing group and the LRLS group also reported the most days abstinent/occasional drinking at 1 and 3 years posttreatment, whereas the externalizing group reported the fewest abstinent days at both intervals. The majority of the sample received additional treatment for alcoholism after the index hospitalization, but the highest rate (85%–90%) was found among the externalizer subtype at both follow-up assessments. This is consistent with the group's increased level of alcohol-related consequences at intake. However, the HRHS subtype spent the largest number of weeks in treatment, reporting an average of 5 weeks at the 1-year interval and about 7.5 weeks in the year prior to the 3-year follow-up. Internalizers had spent the fewest weeks in treatment at both follow-up assessments, with less than 2 weeks at each.

A 2-year posttreatment follow-up of this sample was made through a search of Social Security Death Index records and death certificates. Crude death rates and average age at death varied among the four types of alcoholism. The rate of death was 21.4% among HRHS subjects, 34% among internalizers, 37.2% among externalizers, and 46.9% among the LRLS subjects. The youngest age at death was found among the HRHS (39.9 years), followed by the internalizers (51.1 years), the externalizers (54.6 years), and the LRLS (59.1 years).[13]

Windle and Scheidt[15] studied 481 male and 321 female alcohol-dependent inpatients, using defining characteristics similar to those of Babor et al. They identified four subtypes of alcohol dependence: mild course, polydrug, negative affect, and chronic/antisocial personality disorder (ASPD). The mild course subtype had a later onset of alcohol dependence, had fewer years of drinking, tended to drink less than the other groups, and reported impairment and withdrawal symptoms and few childhood conduct symptoms. The polydrug users subtype had the highest level of drug use, including benzodiazepines. The negative affect cluster reported the highest number of symptoms of affective and anxiety symptoms, along with the greatest number of characteristics. The chronic/ASPD cluster had the highest levels of alcohol consumption and alcohol impairment, and the most years drinking at high levels of consumption. The four types differed by gender but not by ethnicity. A higher percentage of the women than the men were found in the mild course, the polydrug, and the negative affect clusters. Males were overrepresented in the chronic alcohol use/ASPD cluster. The clusters did not vary in relation to socioeconomic status, including educational level. In general, these clusters are consistent with those identified by Zucker and Gomberg,[16] Schuckit et al.,[12] Del Boca and Hesselbrock,[11] and Hesselbrock.[17]

Latent Class–Derived Subtypes of Alcohol Dependence

Bucholz et al.[18] used latent class analysis to fit 37 lifetime symptoms of alcohol dependence with data from 1,360 female and 1,191 male relatives of alcoholic probands. Separate solutions were identified for males and females. A four-class solution was selected as the best fitting among those examined; individuals were assigned to their most probable class. The four classes included nonproblem drinkers (37.8% males, 50% females); mild alcoholics (persistent desire to stop, tolerance and blackouts) (31.1% males, 28.8% females); moderate alcoholics (social health, and emotional problems) (19.9% males, 14.6% females); and severely affected alcoholics (withdrawal, inability to stop drinking, craving, health and emotional problems) (11.2% males, 6.7% females). There was little evidence for the construct of alcohol abuse. Endorsement probabilities for abuse symptoms (e.g., arrests, driving while intoxicated [DWI]) were very low for all classes, while hazardous use was common among non–problem drinking men. In this high risk for alcohol dependence sample, latent classes did not differ qualitatively with distinct symptom profiles. Rather, they appeared to lie, for the most part, on a continuum of severity. One exception was "withdrawal," which characterized only severely affected individuals.

Genetic Analysis of Latent Classes of Alcohol Dependence

Foroud et al.,[19] on the basis of a sample of male and female alcoholic probands (N=830), used the following defining characteristics: persistent desire/being unable to quit or cut down on drinking, morning drinking, craving for alcohol, one or more episodes of binge drinking (defined as drinking for 2 or more days without sobering up), spending a great deal of time drinking or recovering from the effects of alcohol, narrowing of the drinking repertoire, giving up activities in order to drink, having 12 or more blackouts with 5 or more co-occurring withdrawal symptoms, having any health problems from drinking and having any psychological problems from drinking. A four-class solution was selected: an unaffected group with very low symptom endorsement probabilities for most items and containing 47% of the individuals in the sample, a mildly problematic group accounting for 23% of the sample; a moderately affected group, including 17% of individuals; and a severely affected group containing 13% of the sample. Post hoc analyses indicated that classes 3 and 4 defined an affected group of individuals with more severe alcohol dependence, and these two classes were combined to conduct an exploratory series of affected sib-pair analyses. Evidence for a locus on chromosome 16, near the marker D16D675, for classes reflecting alcohol dependence was found, with a maximum multipoint lod score of 4.0.

Subtypes of Alcohol Dependence Based on Co-occurring Psychopathology

A number of studies have demonstrated that the majority of male and female people with alcohol dependence (both treated and untreated) have associated comorbid psychiatric symptoms/conditions (cf. Hesselbrock et al.[20]; Helzer and Pryzbeck[21]). Some of these symptoms may represent preexisting psychiatric disorders, while others may be related to the chronic use of alcohol. For alcoholic males, the most common preexisting disorder observed is ASPD, with estimated prevalence rates ranging from 16% to 49%. Alcoholic females are also found to have significant rates of ASPD, possibly approaching 20%. The importance of comorbid ASPD for the course, consequences, and treatment outcome of alcoholism among both males and females with alcohol dependence has been shown in a number of studies (e.g., Hesselbrock et al.[22,23]). Alcoholic probands with comorbid ASPD have been characterized by an earlier onset of regular drinking, regular drinking to intoxication and problem drinking compared with non-ASPD alcoholic individuals. Further, both alcohol-dependent males and females with ASPD have a more severe course of the disorder and are more likely to relapse sooner and at a higher rate following treatment than non-ASPD alcoholic individuals.

Childhood Conduct and Adult Antisocial Personality Disorder Symptoms

As mentioned in the previous section, the association of ASPD with alcohol dependence has been established in both clinical and general population samples. Further, features of ASPD and conduct disorder have been implicated as important differentiators of subtypes of alcoholics in two well-known alcoholism typologies (Cloninger et al.[4]; Babor et al.[8]). Because ASPD is a diverse collection of symptoms reflecting patterns of irresponsible and antisocial behaviors that begin in childhood and persist into adulthood, the question arises as to whether certain ASPD symptom patterns might be associated more closely with certain phenotypes of alcohol dependence. To address this question, Bucholz et al.,[24] using latent class analysis, examined childhood and adult symptoms reflecting lifetime DSM-III-R criteria of ASPD reported by 2,834 female and 3,504 male relatives of probands and controls. A four-class (A–D) solution for females and a five-class (A–E) solution for males were selected. The classes ranged from unaffected to severely affected in both men and women for both child and adult misbehaviors. There was no evidence for a class expressing only childhood conduct problems. Rather, high endorsement of childhood symptoms was associated with high endorsement of adult symptoms as well.

Among women, both childhood conduct disorder and ASPD were found almost exclusively in the most severely affected class. Strong evidence for a linear trend was found for alcohol dependence severity, with each successive ASPD class manifesting a higher prevalence of alcohol dependence than the previous class. Milestones of drinking showed a strong association with class severity, with more severe ASPD classes having an earlier age at first intoxication and at regular drinking, and also a higher maximum of drinks consumed on one occasion. For women, comorbidity with other substance dependence and with panic disorder also increased with ASPD class severity, but neither depression nor social phobia increased with ASPD class severity. Among men, the majority of Class E (74.6%) but only a small percentage of Class D (19.8%) met the criteria for ASPD. Class D men had a milder spectrum of childhood misbehaviors, but an adult ASPD profile with other psychiatric comorbidity comparable to their Class E counterparts. Both classes were virtually indistinguishable in terms of lifetime prevalence of alcohol dependence. However, an increased prevalence of dependence on other substances was observed with each successive class. Findings from both men and women did not support the existence of distinct subtypes of ASPD, but rather indicated a disorder distributed on a severity spectrum.[24]

Are Multivariate Typologies of Alcohol Dependence Clinically Useful?

While all the published typologies have demonstrated an ability to identify relatively homogeneous groups of people with alcohol dependence based on aspects of their clinical features, few of the typological classifications have received rigorous testing to examine their diagnostic validity. Robins and Guze[25] proposed five research activities necessary for establishing a clinically relevant psychiatric diagnosis that are probably still appropriate here: 1) clinical description; 2) laboratory studies; 3) delimitation from other disorders; 4) follow-up studies, and 5) family studies. Many of the multivariate typologies of alcohol dependence found in the literature meet the "clinical description" criterion very well, as Robins and Guze indicated that not only should clinical features be used to form a diagnosis but demographic features, precipitating factors, age at onset, and so forth, should also be included to define the clinical picture more precisely. The types of alcoholism/alcohol dependence proposed by Knight,[26] Jellinek,[27] Cloninger et al.,[4] Babor et al.,[8] Zucker and Gomberg,[16] DelBoca and Hesselbrock,[11] Lesch and Walter,[28] Windle and Scheidt,[15] and others all tend to meet this criterion. The primary limitation of multivariate typologies in the clinical setting is that most typologies contain too many defining characteristics, thus requiring a lengthy clinical assessment. Few treatment facilities are willing to devote additional time or personnel to obtaining the information necessary to permit reliable typological categorization of patients. Consequently, in order to increase their clinical utility, most typologies need to identify a limited number of critical indicators that can be readily identified, even if other features may have some theoretical importance.

Further, few subtypes of alcohol or other substance dependence have been subjected to either clinical or basic laboratory investigation, certainly not to the extent proposed by Robins and Guze. In part, this is due to the lack of reliable biological indicators of alcohol or other substance dependence. Some studies have identified differences in monoamine oxidase–A (MAO-A) levels, aspects of the serotonin system, ethanol metabolism rates, and brain electrophysiological features in different subtypes of alcohol dependence. However, these biological variables have been examined in other psychiatric conditions as well, and the differences found between affected and non-affected individuals are not unique to any specific diagnosis. In the near future, as susceptibility genes are identified for different substances of abuse or dependence, typologies may be identified based on genotypic differences. While the familial nature and heritability of some of the typologies have been examined using biometric analyses (cf. van den Bree et al.[6]; Gilligan et al.[7]; Hesselbrock[5]), only Foroud et al.[19] have looked for genotypic differences in their latent class–derived subtypes of alcohol dependence.

For the statistically derived typologies of alcohol dependence, the Robins and Guze criterion of "delimitation from other disorders" is a problem in at least two respects. First, some of the samples upon which the subtypes were based were heterogeneous in terms of their abuse or dependence upon drugs other than alcohol. Further, many subjects in these samples also had a history of other psychiatric disorders. While these two issues reflect the natural occurrence of alcohol dependence in clinical and general populations, none of the typologies in the literature provide any "control" for these other comorbid conditions. In fact, several typologies include features of other psychiatric conditions such as conduct disorder, depressive symptoms or other drug use/abuse as defining characteristics. While the presence of symptoms, alone does not indicate the presence of another disorder, many typologies of alcohol dependence are not clearly delimited from depressive disorder, ASPD, or other substance dependencies.

Few subtypes of alcohol dependence have been followed up posttreatment or studied longitudinally to determine the clinical relevance of the subtypes. Follow-up studies are important to determine the stability of the subtype over time, to characterize the subtype's course of illness and to determine the subtype's response to treatment. The lone exception in the current literature is the work of Hesselbrock et al.,[13] who reevaluated the four-cluster typology suggested by Del Boca and Hesselbrock[11] at several different points in time. At follow-up, differences were found between the four alcohol dependence clusters in relation to drinking behavior, relapse rates, and treatment utilization. At 20 years posttreatment, the subtypes differed in terms of their mortality rates.[13]

The final criterion suggested by Robins and Guze is the use of family studies to examine more carefully hereditary and environmental causes of an illness leading to a diagnosis. Again, few statistically derived subtypes of alcohol dependence meet this criterion. The heritability of Cloninger's type 1/type 2 (particularly type 2) has been established by Gilligan et al.[7] and van den Bree et al.,[6] while Hesselbrock[17] found moderate heritability for several of his five clusters of alcohol dependence. In the near future other investigators may follow the lead of Foroud et al.[19] and begin to examine the genotypic bases of alcohol/substance dependence typologies. Further, none of the typologies examined (other than Cloninger et al.'s) included contextual factors as defining characteristics. Nor has the etiology of the alcohol dependence typologies been examined in relation to environmental factors such as parental home environment, marital home environment, level of perceived stress, neighborhood variables or treatment history.

In spite of the different theoretical backgrounds of the investigators, the samples examined and the methods used to form the typologies, there is a remarkable similarity across many of the multivariate typologies of alcohol dependence proposed in the literature. Several authors have suggested a chronic/severe type, a depressed/anxious type, a mildly affected type, and an antisocial type, although using their own labels. These four types of alcohol dependence are found within both genders and across several different ethnic groups. It is also likely these typologies vary in their heritability, although their biological and genotypic bases remain unknown. Also, each multivariate typology in the literature provides a clinical description that identifies homogeneous subgroups. Unfortunately, few have examined outcomes longitudinally to determine their clinical utility in predicting variations in illness course and response to treatment occurring across different subtypes. Thus, typologies still remain a viable and potentially valuable tool for the investigation of etiological pathways into alcohol use disorders, the investigation of both psychological[29,30] and pharmacological[28,31] therapies, and studies of the long-term course of alcohol use disorders.

References

1. Hesselbrock V, Hesselbrock M: Social and behavioral factors which may affect the genetic expression of alcoholism, in Genetics and Biology of Alcoholism. Edited by Cloninger CR, Begleiter H. Cold Spring Harbor, NY, Cold Spring Harbor Laboratory Press, 1990, pp 75–88.
2. Morey LC, Blashfield RK: Empirical classifications of alcoholics. J Stud Alcohol 42:925–937, 1981.
3. Skinner HA: Statistical approaches to the classification of alcohol and drug addiction. Br J Addict 77:259–273, 1982.
4. Cloninger CR, Bohman M, Sigvardsson S: Inheritance of alcohol abuse: cross-fostering analyses of adopted men. Arch Gen Psychiatry 38:861–868, 1981.
5. Hesselbrock M: Genetic determinants of alcoholic subtypes, in The Genetics of Alcoholism. Edited by Begleiter H, Kissen B. New York, Oxford University Press, 1995, pp 40–69.
6. van den Bree MBM, Svikis DS, Pickens RW: Genetic influences in antisocial personality and drug use disorders. Drug Alcohol Depend 49:177–181, 1998.
7. Gilligan SB, Reich T, Cloninger CR: Etiologic heterogeneity in alcoholism. Gen Epidemiol 4:395–414, 1987.
8. Babor T, Hofmann M, Del Boca FK, et al: Types of alcoholics, I: evidence for an empirically derived typology based on indicators of vulnerability and severity. Arch Gen Psychiatry 49:599–608, 1992.
9. Brown J, Babor TF, Litt M, et al: The type A/type B distinction: subtyping alcoholics according to indicators of vulnerability and severity. Ann NY Acad Sci 708:23–33, 1994.
10. Del Boca FK: Sex, gender and alcoholic typologies. Ann NY Acad Sci 708:34–48, 1994.
11. Del Boca FK, Hesselbrock MN: Gender and alcoholic subtypes. Alcohol Health Res World 20:56–66, 1996.
12. Schuckit MA, Tipp J, Smith TL, et al: An evaluation of type A and type B alcoholics. Addiction 90:1189–1204, 1995.
13. Hesselbrock M, Hesselbrock V, Del Boca F: Typology of alcoholism, gender and 20-year mortality. Alcohol Clin Exp Res 25:151A, 2001.
14. Hesselbrock V, Hesselbrock M, Segal B: Multivariate phenotypes of alcohol dependence among Alaskan Natives: type A/type B. Alcohol Clin Exp Res 24(suppl):107A, 2000.

15. Windle M, Scheidt DM: Alcoholic subtypes: are two sufficient? Addiction 99:1508–1519, 2004.
16. Zucker RA, Gomberg E: Etiology of alcoholism reconsidered: the case for a biopsychosocial process. Am Psychol 41:783–793, 1986.
17. Hesselbrock V: A five cluster phenotype of alcohol dependence. Paper presented at the Annual Meeting of the Research Society on Alcoholism, Hilton Head, SC, June 1998.
18. Bucholz KK, Heath A, Reich T, et al: Can we subtype alcoholism? A latent class analysis of data from relatives of alcoholics in a multi-center study. Alcohol Clin Exp Res 20:1462–1471, 1996.
19. Foroud T, Neuman R, Goate A, et al: Evidence for linkage of an alcohol-related phenotype to chromosome 16. Alcohol Clin Exp Res 22:2035–2042, 1998.
20. Hesselbrock MN, Meyer RE, Keener JJ: Psychopathology in hospitalized alcoholics. Arch Gen Psychiatry 42:1050–1055, 1985.
21. Helzer JE, Pryzbeck TR: The co-occurrence of alcoholism with other psychiatric disorders in the general population and its impact on treatment. J Stud Alcohol 49:219–224, 1988.
22. Hesselbrock M, Hesselbrock V, Babor T, et al: Antisocial behavior, psychopathology, and problem drinking in the natural history of alcoholism, in Longitudinal Research in Alcoholism. Edited by Goodwin D, Van Dusen K, Mednick SA. Boston, MA, Kluwer-Nijhoff Publishing, 1984, pp 197–214.
23. Hesselbrock V, Hesselbrock M, Stabenau J: Subtyping of alcoholism in male patients by family history and antisocial personality. J Stud Alcohol 49:89–98, 1985.
24. Bucholz KK, Hesselbrock VM, Heath AC, et al: A latent class analysis of antisocial personality disorder symptom data from a multi-centre family study of alcoholism. Addiction 95:553–567, 2000.
25. Robins E, Guze SB: Establishment of diagnostic validity in psychiatric illness: its application to schizophrenia. Am J Psychiatry 126:983–988, 1970.
26. Knight RP: Psychoanalytic treatment in a sanatorium of chronic addiction to alcohol. JAMA 111:1443–1448, 1938.
27. Jellinek EM: Alcoholism: a genus and some of its species. Can Med Assoc J 83:1341–1345, 1960.
28. Lesch OM, Walter H: Subtypes of alcoholism and their role in therapy. Alcohol Alcohol Suppl 1:63–67, 1996.
29. Kadden RM, Litt MD, Cooney NL, et al: Prospective matching of alcoholic clients to cognitive-behavioral or interactional group therapy. J Stud Alcohol 62:359–364, 2001.
30. Basu D, Ball SA, Feinn R, et al: Typologies of drug dependence: comparative validity of a multivariate and four univariate models. Drug Alcohol Depend 73:289–300, 2004.
31. Kranzler HR, Burleson J, Brown J, et al: Fluoxetine treatment seems to reduce the beneficial effects of cognitive-behavioral therapy in type B alcoholics. Alcohol Clin Exp Res 20:1534–1541, 1997.

11

SUBTYPES OF SUBSTANCE DEPENDENCE AND ABUSE

Implications for Diagnostic Classification and Empirical Research

Thomas F. Babor, Ph.D., M.P.H.
Raul Caetano, M.D., Ph.D.

Despite the general conviction that dependence on alcohol and other psychoactive substances is a unitary phenomenon, there is ample evidence that people with substance use disorders differ with respect to a variety of demographic, personal, and clinical characteristics.[1,2] Recognition of this heterogeneity has led to attempts to identify subgroups of persons with substance-related problems (herein referred to as *subtypes*) according to a variety of defining indicators, such as onset age, chronicity of problems, patterns of substance abuse, antecedent psychopathology, and childhood vulnerability factors[2,3] (see also Chapter 10, "Are There Empirically Supported and Clinically Useful Subtypes of Alcohol Dependence?," in this volume).

The writing of the paper reproduced in this chapter was supported in part by a Distinguished International Scientist Collaboration Award from the U.S. National Institute on Drug Abuse.

Reprinted from Babor TF, Caetano R: "Subtypes of Substance Dependence and Abuse: Implications for Diagnostic Classification and Empirical Research" *Addiction* 101 (suppl 1): 104–110, 2006. Used with permission of the Society for the Study of Addiction.

The goal of this chapter is to review practical, theoretical, and conceptual issues relevant to subtype descriptors for the classification of substance-related disorders in forthcoming editions of the American Psychiatric Association's *Diagnostic and Statistical Manual of Mental Disorders* (DSM) and the World Health Organization's *International Classification of Diseases* (ICD). We examine the definition and functions of typologies, the empirical evidence supporting substance-related subtypes, and the possible need for an adolescent subtype that takes into account recent epidemiological findings about the manifestation of dependence symptoms in young adults. The ultimate goal of this chapter is to improve diagnostic classification, facilitate clinical decision-making, and improve the allocation of patients to different modalities and intensities of treatment services.

Background Issues

For the purposes of this chapter, a typology is a classification system and a set of decision rules used to differentiate relatively homogeneous groups, called *subtypes.* A subtype is an abstract category organized according to some conceptual, theoretical, or clinical principle. According to one student of clinical subtyping,[4] subtypes of complex clinical phenomena are "splendid fictions" that are created in part by the human need for simplicity and order. This realization should not discourage us from attempting to make sense of complex clinical phenomena and heterogeneous groups, if we keep in mind that our primary purpose is to improve diagnostic classification and to make the most efficient use of our clinical services.

To that end, it is important to consider the potential benefits of typological classification in regard to substance-related disorders. Several theoretical, clinical, and practical functions suggest themselves. Theoretical functions deal with fundamental questions about the mechanisms through which individuals develop alcohol and drug dependence. If there is evidence for different etiologies of dependence (e.g., genetic predisposition or environmental risk factors), then it may be valuable to subtype on these dimensions, to the extent that such information may provide a guide to further research or a valuable resource for the planning of treatment measures.

A second function of typological formulations is to facilitate client–service matching. Here we are concerned with the most efficient and effective use of scarce clinical resources. The idea of treatment matching is guided by the assumption that treatment outcomes can be improved by matching patients to the most appropriate levels, modalities, and intensities of care.[5] Service matching is a broader perspective that includes not only clinical interventions but other services such as housing, case management, and employment counseling.[6] Ideally, the typology should be relevant to the types of services that are appropriate, feasible, and available to people with substance-related problems.

Typological formulations are also used to summarize important diagnostic, prognostic, and descriptive information in a simple, understandable classification scheme. Not only should they provide an empirical basis for client–service matching, they should also improve the specificity of prediction of short-term as well as long-term outcomes in relation to services received. Another function of subtyping is to inform and motivate the patient about the nature of the disorder he or she is experiencing. Finally, typologies could have the potential to prevent further development of substance dependence by suggesting candidates for secondary prevention efforts.

There is a long tradition of typological research in psychiatry that may be useful in the development of typological approaches to DSM classification of substance-related disorders. For example, the fourth edition of DSM[7] describes subtypes for schizophrenia, schizoaffective disorder, anxiety disorders, affective disorder, delusional disorder, and substance-induced psychotic disorder. These subtyping schemes are derived primarily from clinical experience rather than from empirical research, and each one relies on a different organizing principle. The subtypes of schizophrenia (paranoid, catatonic, disorganized, undifferentiated, and residual) are organized on the basis of "the clinical picture," which presumably refers to presenting symptoms. The subtypes of schizoaffective disorder (bipolar type, depressive type) are organized according to affect disturbance. The subtypes of delusional disorder (erotomanic, grandiose, jealous, persecutory, somatic, mixed) are organized according to the predominant delusion. What these subtyping schemes have in common is their apparent ability to facilitate the classification of psychiatric patients who share the same general condition into more meaningful or clinically useful subgroups.

Overview of Recent Typology Research

In the field of alcoholism, two general approaches to subtyping can be distinguished: single-domain typologies based on key defining characteristics (e.g., sex, age at onset) and multidimensional classification schemes based on combinations of defining characteristics. The tradition of clinical subtyping according to single domains extends back to the nineteenth century[3] and includes subtypes such as childhood learning disorders, conduct problems, familial alcohol dependence, early age at onset and comorbid psychopathology. Over the past century there has been an evolution of typological theory from these single-domain subtypes to multidimensional typologies based on a variety of defining characteristics, such as etiological elements, personality characteristics, drinking patterns, and course of illness.[3] This evolution in typological thinking has been influenced in part by the development of multivariate statistical techniques as well as reliable and valid measurement procedures that make it possible to search for homogeneous subgroups within a population of alcoholic individuals.

Because the literature on typology research has been reviewed periodically (see, e.g., reference 3 and Chapter 10 in this volume), we provide here only a brief update of recent research in three areas relevant to the future of diagnostic classification: developmental studies focusing on new typologies; validation studies of earlier typologies; and treatment-matching studies.

DEVELOPMENTAL STUDIES OF NEW TYPOLOGIES

Several new typological theories have been added to the international literature, which is dominated by American research and theory, and attempts have been made to expand alcoholism typologies to people with drug dependence. Driessen et al.[8] developed and validated a clinical typology of alcohol withdrawal in a sample of German detoxification patients. They found five clusters representing increasing severity of alcohol withdrawal, based on a combination of vegetative and psychopathological symptoms. The authors suggested that the typology may be useful to predict the course of alcohol withdrawal at the first day of treatment.

Cardoso et al.[9] used multivariate statistical techniques to identify five types of alcoholism in a sample of patients at Santa Maria's General Hospital, Lisbon, Portugal: anxiopathic (anxious functioning); heredopathic (family and genetic influences); thimopathic (affective symptomatology); sociopathic (disruptive behaviors under alcohol); and adictopathic (polysubstance use at younger age). The authors conclude that the resulting "NETER" typology represents a continuum of increasingly polymorphic subtypes that contain both genetic/family and psychosocial factors.

Windle and Scheidt[1] conducted an extensive investigation to determine whether two subtypes are sufficient for understanding the heterogeneity of alcoholism. Using cluster analytical techniques, they identified four subtypes: mild course, polydrug, negative affect, and chronic/antisocial. Their study replicates the consistent finding of a core group of highly dependent individuals who score toward the extreme end on dimensions of risk and problem severity and who tend to evidence antisocial personality.

Ball et al.[10] investigated the construct, concurrent, and predictive validity of Babor et al.'s[11] type A/type B distinction in cocaine abusers. In contrast to cocaine users classified as type A, type B cocaine abusers exhibited higher rates of premorbid risk factors (family history, childhood behavior problems, personality disorder, early age at onset) as well as more severe psychopathology and multiple substance use. The results suggest that the type A/type B approach to classification could be applied to drug users as well as alcoholic individuals.

VALIDATION STUDIES

Validation research has focused on the evaluation of existing typological theories in terms of their construct, concurrent, and predictive validity. With advances in genetic markers and pharmacological treatments, new methodologies have been applied to typological research. Johnson and Pickens[12] studied whether a typology defined by mild, severe, and dyssocial characteristics distinguished cases of alcohol dependence with high familial liability from those with low familial liability to alcoholism. The results suggest construct validity for the alcoholism typology in distinguishing subtypes with differing degrees of familial liability to alcoholism. Hillemacher et al.[13] used craving and number of previous detoxifications as a way of validating differences among subtypes. Anthenelli et al.[14] investigated platelet monoamine oxidase (MAO) activity in subgroups of alcoholic individuals. The results indicated that phenotypes of alcoholic individuals (e.g., Cloninger et al.'s[15] type 1 vs. type 2; type A vs. type B; primary vs. secondary) did not differ in platelet MAO activity. They concluded that decreased platelet MAO activity is not a trait marker of alcoholism or one of its subtypes. Johann et al.,[16] in a study of 5-HTT/ 5-HT_{2C} genotype characteristics in 314 German alcoholic individuals, found that comorbidity of alcoholism and attention-deficit/hyperactivity disorder forms a distinct phenotype that shows an increased severity of the substance disorder. This phenotype contributes substantially to type 2 alcoholism according to Cloninger et al.[15]

In validation research on the fourfold typology developed by Windle and Scheidt,[1] the polydrug subtype had the highest rate of family criminality, high-risk sexual behavior, and intravenous drug use, whereas the negative affect subtype had the highest rate of childhood sexual abuse, attempted suicide, and childhood homelessness. In addition, the chronic/antisocial personality (ASP) subtype had the most severe pattern of drinking and antisocial behavior.

Epstein et al.[2] conducted a construct validation study of four common alcoholism typologies in a sample of 342 alcoholic individuals recruited into five treatment outcome studies. Cloninger's type 1/type 2 had poor construct validity and was redundant with age-at-onset subtypes. The clinical utility of the ASP/non-ASP typology was limited due to low prevalence. The type A/type B schema was found to be relatively inclusive, and the groups were distinct. However, the authors suggest that dichotomous typologies may not be complex enough to be clinically useful descriptors of alcoholic samples. Aside from ASP and type B, there appears to be heterogeneity within groups typically considered homogeneous, such as "early versus late onset" alcoholic individuals.

TREATMENT-MATCHING STUDIES

Patient–treatment-matching studies can be considered as a special form of validation research, to the extent that they are designed to demonstrate the predictive validity of subtype differentiation in relation to a particular mechanism of action derived from typology theory. For example, Litt et al.[17] found that type B alcoholic individuals had better treatment outcomes when they were assigned to cognitive-behavioral therapy, whereas type A alcoholic individuals fared better with interactional group therapy. In a subsequent and much larger study of treatment matching in alcoholism,[5] the type A/type B classification was not found to be useful in identifying matching effects with different forms of individual psychotherapy.

Several studies have evaluated subtype differences in relation to pharmacotherapy for alcohol dependence. Kranzler and colleagues[18] reported that type B alcoholic individuals had less favorable drinking outcomes in response to treatment with fluoxetine, a selective serotonin reuptake inhibitor, than with placebo. This medication effect was not seen in type A alcoholic individuals. In a subsequent study,[19] a significant interaction between alcoholic subtype and medication condition was also found. However, contrary to the earlier findings, type A subjects had more favorable outcomes when treated with sertraline, a serotonin reuptake inhibitor, compared to placebo. Dundon et al.[20] found that type A alcoholic individuals had better treatment response to 14 weeks of sertraline than placebo, and this was not found for type B alcoholic individuals. The good outcomes were maintained for at least 6 months after pharmacotherapy. In contrast, heavy drinking in type B alcoholic individuals increased over the 6 months after pharmacotherapy in those initially treated with sertraline. Brady et al.[21] investigated the use of sertraline in treating co-occurring symptoms of alcohol dependence and posttraumatic stress disorder (PTSD). Participants with more severe alcohol dependence and later-onset PTSD had better drinking outcomes if they were in the placebo group, leading the authors to conclude that there may be subtypes of alcohol-dependent individuals who respond differently to serotonin reuptake inhibitor treatment.

SUMMARY

Del Boca[22] has summarized current methodological issues in relation to developmental and validation research in the following terms. First, clustering-derived typologies vary in the number of subtypes identified and the features defining the types, depending on sample size and attributes, contextual (cultural and historical) factors, method of analysis, and the predilections of investigators. Thus, in addition to the question of how many subtypes, there are important conceptual, theoretical, and analytical issues that need to be addressed before a convincing validation can be conducted.

Second, Del Boca argues that investigators need to confront the limitations of conventional clustering techniques and expand their use of alternative approaches for explicating data structure and examining process. Because subtypes can enhance our understanding of the etiology and course of alcoholism, researchers should make greater use of longitudinal data and methods of analysis, such as latent growth mixture modeling, which can identify multiple processes of change. In contrast to conventional clustering procedures, such methods have the further advantage of probabilistic assignment of individuals to classes.

Third, careful attention should be given to the domains chosen to serve as the basis of classification and to how independent evidence can be used for validation. As both personal and environmental factors influence the development of alcohol dependence, these should be included. Other candidate variables for validating subtypes might include factors studied by molecular geneticists, as well as measures of affect regulation and early family and peer experiences.

Fourth, most typology studies have used treatment samples recruited in the United States. Research should be conducted on nontreatment participants, and inclusion of samples from other cultures would undoubtedly improve understanding of the role that personal attributes and contextual factors play in producing differences among alcoholic individuals in etiology, course, and outcome.

Finally, it should be noted that treatment-matching research is ultimately one of the most important ways to validate typological classification systems. To date, the research suggests that treatment matching with neither pharmacotherapy nor psychotherapy has produced consistent results.

Conclusions and Recommendations: The Way Forward

With the advent of structured interview schedules, personality tests, and symptom inventories designed to collect descriptive clinical information, quantitative procedures have been used to identify homogeneous groups of patients with substance-related disorders. Subtype discrimination has been advanced by use of multivariate statistical techniques, including cluster analysis and latent class analysis, which can be used to identify homogeneous subgroups based on correlations among individuals sharing similar characteristics. From the experience gained in these other areas of clinical research, it is clear that classification theory can be grounded in objective clinical assessment. A fundamental question concerns the potential utility of subtyping schemes in DSM-V and ICD-11. To guide further work on this topic, it may be beneficial to evaluate the state of the existing literature in relation to a set of taxonomic standards suggested by Babor and Dolinsky.[23] Optimally, a typology of substance-related disorders should

- Be simple in its structure;
- Have practical utility (e.g., mediate judgments about clinical evidence);
- Allow matching to clinical and preventive services;
- Be easy to use and derive from available data;
- Permit inferences to underlying causes;
- Predict future behavior;
- Facilitate communication;
- Demonstrate empirical validity and reliability; and

- Identify subtypes that are homogeneous within categories, remain stable over time, and are comprehensive in their coverage of different substance-using populations.

By these standards, what can we conclude about the current state of typological research in relation to the improvement of diagnostic classification of substance use disorders? First, the research suggests that no consensus has emerged about the nature, much less the number, of subtypes that could be used to characterize the clinical heterogeneity assumed to be present in groups of people with substance use disorders. Although several relatively simple binary typologies have been developed (e.g., Cloninger's type 1 and type 2; Babor et al.'s type A and type B), validation research has produced mixed results in terms of the construct, concurrent, and predictive validity of these classifications. Moreover, the multidimensional nature of these typologies makes it difficult to achieve reliable classification based on simple assessments or clinical judgment. Although many typologies seem to have predictive validity, the treatment-matching literature suggests that subtyping schemes have limited clinical utility as a means of assigning patients to more effective interventions.

Nevertheless, research on subtypes of alcoholic individuals has consistently identified two basic groups defined by both vulnerability characteristics (e.g., a family history of alcohol problems; childhood conduct disorder) and severity indicators (e.g., a history of chronic drinking; severe dependence). These subtypes divide into a low-severity, low-vulnerability subgroup (similar to Babor's type A) and a high-vulnerability, high-severity subgroup (similar to Babor's type B).[3,11,24] The former is characterized by later onset of problem drinking, few childhood vulnerability factors, the relative absence of alcohol problems in the family history, a low level of antecedent psychopathology, and a drinking pattern characterized by less severe alcohol consumption, alcohol dependence and alcohol-related problems. The latter subtype is characterized by early onset of alcohol problems, a greater number of childhood vulnerability factors, a family history of alcohol problems, a variety of antecedent and concomitant psychopathology, and a drinking history characterized by excessive drinking, severe alcohol dependence, and serious alcohol-related problems. There is also evidence[1,25] (see also Chapter 10 in this volume) for further differentiation of some of these subgroups, particularly among the high-severity/high-vulnerability population. Such differentiation may be beneficial as a guide to more complex clinical decision-making, but may not be necessary if the typology is being used for more generic purposes, such as estimating clinical course, treatment response, and general prognosis. To a lesser extent, typological research has also been applied to the identification of drug abuse subtypes.[10,26] Consistent with the alcohol literature, this research has concluded that a relatively parsimonious binary classification fits the data for a variety of psychoactive substances, and the typology differentiates along dimensions of defining characteristics that are similar to those identified in the alcohol literature. Unfortunately, there have been few cross-national replications for alcohol typologies, and there is only limited evidence that the binary classification applies to other psychoactive substances. Under these circumstances, it would seem premature to recommend the adoption of a subtyping scheme in the DSM or ICD classification systems without further international research.

If there is general agreement that typological formulations at this time are not likely to contribute to the classification of substance use disorders, the following questions need to be addressed before continuing the search for clinically relevant subtypes:

- Should the typology be theory driven or directed by blind empiricism?
- Should the typology work within a single domain of variables, or should it be multidimensional?
- Should subtyping be approached in a cross-sectional way or situated in the larger context of developmental experience?
- Is one typology going to be sufficient, or should there be several?

Whether the typology should be theory driven or directed by blind empiricism depends to some extent on the current quality of addiction theory. Although there are many relevant theories about the etiology of substance-related disorders (e.g., neurobiological, genetic, psychological), there is no dominant theory (see reference 27). On the other hand, blind empiricism, especially that dictated by multivariate statistical procedures such as cluster analysis, also has serious limitations. Without some theoretical rationale for the selection of variables to include in a typological formulation, blind empiricism can result in the creation of categories that may have little intuitive appeal or clinical meaning. The answer to this question is therefore likely to be the recommendation to use a combination of approaches, borrowing basic assumptions from addiction theory and applying multivariate statistical techniques to determine whether the resulting subtypes are consistent with current theory.

Regarding the second question (single-domain or multidimensional typology), if a single domain is chosen (e.g., gender, age at onset, psychopathology, family history), it would certainly simplify the diagnostic and classification rules. The use of multiple domains, on the other hand, may be better suited to the clinical complexity of substance-related disorders but may limit the feasibility of using a typology classification in routine clinical practice.

Another issue is whether subtyping should be approached in a cross-sectional way or situated in the larger context of life-course development. Some types of substance-related disorders may be developmentally cumulative, becoming progressively worse over time, whereas others may be developmentally limited (e.g., manifested only during adolescence or early adulthood).[28] As suggested by Caetano and Babor in Chapter 12 ("Diagnosis of Alcohol Dependence in Epidemiological Surveys") in this volume, there may be a need to account for the kinds of substance use patterns that characterize adolescence or young adulthood. A typological formulation that captures this diversity would be desirable if it were not formulated at the expense of simplicity.

Other questions that arise are related to the differences among psychoactive substances and whether a classification scheme should apply equally well to all or most substances. Would it make sense, for example, to have the same classification for alcohol dependence as for cocaine or methamphetamine dependence? The same typology may not be optimal to capture the clinical profiles of all psychoactive substances, but a single typology would certainly be more efficient.

What would be the benefits of, for example, subtyping people with alcohol dependence in terms of severity and vulnerability indicators that take into account similarities and differences in family history, age at onset, psychopathology and problem severity? Based on the existing research, such a classification scheme would allow clinicians to differentiate among patients who require different levels and intensities of service, and perhaps allow "case mix" adjustments for comparisons across facilities where clinical profiles differ significantly. Similarly, there is a need to consider the criteria for substance abuse and dependence in terms of adolescent patterns of substance use that may not warrant a diagnosis of dependence in the classic sense of that term. From a very practical point of view, perhaps it would be best to start with an attempt to create a relatively simple typology using readily available measures of vulnerability (e.g., family history, antecedent psychopathology, early onset) and severity (e.g., substance-related consequences, dependence severity) that are particularly relevant to clinical concerns. This approach might provide a simple classification into the uncomplicated and complicated subtypes suggested in the literature.

Finally, observational and laboratory studies (e.g., genotyping, neuroimaging, electrophysiology, cue exposure) should be conducted as a reality check on phenomenological methods that may not be sufficient to provide an accurate classification of alcohol and drug dependence for the purposes of clinical management and prevalence estimation.

References

1. Windle M, Scheidt DM: Alcoholic subtypes: are two sufficient? Addiction 99:1508–1519, 2004.
2. Epstein EE, Labouvie E, McCrady BS, et al: Multi-site study of alcohol subtypes: classification and overlap of unidimensional and multi-dimensional typologies. Addiction 97:1041–1053, 2002.
3. Babor TF: The classification of alcoholics: typology theories from the 19th century to the present. Alcohol Health Res World 20:6–17, 1996.
4. Millon T: Classification in psychopathology: rationale, alternatives, and standards. J Abnorm Psychol 100:245–261, 1991.
5. Babor TF, Del Boca FK: Treatment Matching in Alcoholism. Cambridge, United Kingdom, Cambridge University Press, 2003.

6. McLellan AT, Grant GR, Zanis M, et al: Problem-service "matching" in addiction treatment. Arch Gen Psychiatry 54:730–735, 1997.
7. American Psychiatric Association: Diagnostic and Statistical Manual of Mental Disorders, 4th Edition. Washington, DC, American Psychiatric Association, 1994.
8. Driessen M, Lange W, Junghanns K, et al: Proposal of a comprehensive clinical typology of alcohol withdrawal: a cluster analysis approach. Alcohol Alcohol 40:308–313, 2005.
9. Cardoso JM, Barbosa A, Ismail F, et al: NETER alcoholic typology (NAT). Alcohol Alcohol 41:133–139, 2006.
10. Ball SA, Carroll KC, Babor TF, et al: Subtypes of cocaine abusers: support for a type A/type B distinction. J Consult Clin Psychol 63:115–124, 1995.
11. Babor TF, Hofmann M, DelBoca F, et al: Types of alcoholics, I: evidence for an empirically derived typology based on indicators of vulnerability and severity. Arch Gen Psychiatry 49:599–608, 1992.
12. Johnson EO, Pickens RW: Familial transmission of alcoholism among nonalcoholics and mild, severe, and dyssocial subtypes of alcoholism. Alcohol Clin Exp Res 25:661–666, 2001.
13. Hillemacher T, Bayerlein K, Wilhelm J, et al: Recurrent detoxifications are associated with craving in patients classified as type 1 according to Lesch's typology. Alcohol Alcohol 41:66–69, 2006.
14. Anthenelli RM, Tip J, Li TK, et al: Platelet monoamine oxidase activity in subgroups of alcoholics and controls: results from the Collaborative Study on the Genetics of Alcoholism. Alcohol Clin Exp Res 22:111–115, 1998.
15. Cloninger CR, Sigvardsson S, Bohman M: Type I and type II alcoholism: an update. Alcohol Health Res World 20:18–23, 1996.
16. Johann M, Bobbe G, Putzhammer A, et al: Comorbidity of alcohol dependence with attention-deficit hyperactivity disorder: differences in phenotype with increased severity of the substance disorder, but not in genotype (serotonin transporter and 5-hydroxytryptamine-2c receptor). Alcohol Clin Exp Res 27:1527–1534, 2003.
17. Litt MD, Kadden RM, Cooney NL, et al: Coping skills and treatment outcomes in cognitive-behavioral and interactional group therapy for alcoholism. J Consult Clin Psychol 71:118–128, 2003.
18. Kranzler H, Lappalainen J, Nellissery M, et al: Association study of alcoholism subtypes with a functional promoter polymorphism in the serotonin transporter protein gene. Alcohol Clin Exp Res 26:1330–1335, 2002.
19. Pettinati HM,Volpicelli JR, Kranzler HR, et al: Sertraline treatment for alcohol dependence: interactive effects of medication and alcoholic subtype. Alcohol Clin Exp Res 24:1041–1049, 2000.
20. Dundon W, Lynch KG, Pettinati HM, et al: Treatment outcomes in type A and B alcohol dependence 6 months after serotonergic pharmacotherapy. Alcohol Clin Exp Res 2:1065–1073, 2004.
21. Brady K, Sonne S, Anton R, et al: Sertraline in the treatment of co-occurring alcohol dependence and posttraumatic stress disorder. Alcohol Clin Exp Res 29:395–401, 2005.
22. Del Boca FK: Two subtypes or more, much work remains: a commentary on Windle and Scheidt (letter). Addiction 99:1609–1610, 2004.

23. Babor TF, Dolinsky ZS: Alcoholic typologies: historical evolution and empirical evaluation of some common classification schemes, in Alcoholism: Origins and Outcome. Edited by Rose RM, Barrett J. New York, Raven, 1988, pp 245–266.
24. Schuckit MA, Frances RJ, Talbott JA: Low level of response to alcohol as a predictor of future alcoholism. Year Book of Psychiatry & Applied Mental Health, 1995, pp 139–140.
25. Del Boca FK, Hesselbrock MH: Gender and subtypes of alcoholics. Alcohol Health Res World 20:56–62, 1996.
26. Basu D, Ball SA, Feinn R, et al: Typologies of drug dependence: comparative validity of a multivariate and four univariate models. Drug Alcohol Depend 73:289–300, 2004.
27. West R: Theory of Addiction. Oxford, England, Blackwell, 2006.
28. Zucker RA, Fitzgerald HE, Moses HD: Emergence of alcohol problems and the several alcoholisms: a developmental perspective on etiologic theory and life course trajectory, in Developmental Psychopathology, Vol 2: Risk, Disorder, and Adaptation. Edited by Cohen DJ. New York, Wiley, 1994, pp 677–711.

12

DIAGNOSIS OF ALCOHOL DEPENDENCE IN EPIDEMIOLOGICAL SURVEYS

An Epidemic of Youthful Alcohol Dependence or a Case of Measurement Error?

Raul Caetano, M.D., Ph.D.
Thomas F. Babor, Ph.D., M.P.H.

Epidemiological research on the distribution and determinants of alcohol dependence in the general population has important implications for the public health functions of psychiatric classification, including the estimation of prevalence rates, the use of classification to monitor mental health at the population level, and the assessment of predictors of psychiatric disease in the general population. This line of research has focused on the measurement and classification of alcohol use disorders into the most clinically popular diagnostic categories, alcohol abuse, and dependence. Several researchers[1–3] have noted that prevalence estimates for abuse and dependence diagnoses, derived from population surveys using structured di-

---

Reprinted from Caetano R, Babor TF: "Diagnosis of Alcohol Dependence in Epidemiological Surveys: an epidemic of youthful alcohol dependence or a case of measurement error?" *Addiction* 101 (suppl 1):111–114, 2006. Used with permission of the Society for the Study of Addiction.

agnostic instruments, have yielded higher rates for younger adults (e.g., 18- to 30-year age group) than for older adults (e.g., older than age 30). In this chapter, we review the literature on this phenomenon and present data illustrating the possibility that prevalence rates of alcohol dependence among young adults may be inflated because of measurement error. The literature being reviewed comes from general population epidemiological studies conducted in the United States in the past 20 years, all of which have used *Diagnostic and Statistical Manual of Mental Disorders,* 4th Edition (DSM-IV) criteria for identifying alcohol dependence. The age distribution of alcohol dependence in other countries may be different.

Survey Findings: Rates of Alcohol Dependence

Table 12–1 shows data from a review by Harford et al.,[2] who reported prevalence rates of alcohol dependence among younger and older age groups for current drinkers. The data for male current drinkers show that 4.6% of adolescents (aged 12–17) meet criteria for past-year dependence, and the rate increases to 8.5% in the 18–23 age group. Thereafter, prevalence declines for each succeeding age cohort. There are two potential explanations for these findings: 1) an emerging epidemic of alcohol dependence and 2) measurement error.

First, the findings could represent an emerging epidemic of alcohol dependence in the younger age cohorts, one that will be reflected eventually in an increasing demand for treatment with each successive age cohort. Alternatively, the findings could mean that alcohol dependence is not progressive in this early-onset group and that most early-onset alcoholic individuals "mature out" of their alcohol dependence as they become older. This latter hypothesis is, in fact, a distinct possibility given that the clustering of alcohol problems across time in general population samples is relatively low. Contrary to what happens in clinical samples, in the general population, having problems at a particular time is only a moderate predictor of having problems at another time.[4,5] In fact, correlations in longitudinal data are low even among alcohol dependence indicators, such as withdrawal symptoms, tolerance, and impaired control.[6] Taken at face value, the general population data are at variance with the assumption that alcohol dependence is cumulative and progressive and that early onset of alcohol dependence (as noted in the clinical typology literature; see Babor[7]) is associated with a more serious form of alcohol dependence characterized by multiple alcohol-related problems, poor treatment response, and a more severe course.

Caetano[8] suggested a number of ways to reconcile these differences between the presentation and course of alcohol dependence in general population and clinical samples. The first, which is directly relevant to subtyping efforts, is to view cases of alcohol dependence observed in the general population as a less severe form of the phenomenon seen in clinical samples. Data from clinical and general

TABLE 12–1. Dependence rates reported from the 2001 National Household Survey on Drug Abuse for current drinkers by age group and sex (n=16,600)

	Prevalence (%) by age group (years) and gender					
Gender	12–17	18–23	24–29	30–49	≥50	Total
Males	4.6	8.5	4.6	2.5	1.2	3.6
Females	4.5	5.2	1.7	2.4	0.9	2.4

Source. Harford et al.[2]

population samples support this contention. In general, most individuals identified as alcohol-dependent in general population surveys are classified on a minimum number of criteria (three or four). In clinical samples alcohol-dependent individuals usually report a larger number of symptoms.[9,10]

The concept of a continuum of alcohol dependence with various levels of severity is consistent with the original formulation of the alcohol dependence syndrome.[11] Unfortunately, as Caetano[8] has suggested, the identification of different levels of alcohol dependence is hindered by the characteristics of the DSM criteria, which do not set a threshold above which each criterion will be considered as present, and which do not require an assessment of the severity of each criterion diagnosed as present.

Difficulties in identifying thresholds for criteria or for rating severity of symptoms are also associated with the continuous nature of dependence-related behaviors. It has been argued, for example, that certain dependence criteria occur on a continuum of intensity that begins with "normal" behavior. For instance, Edwards[12] has proposed that withdrawal is a graded, rather than an "all-or-none," disturbance. Stockwell[13] has suggested that withdrawal may be arranged in a continuum of severity that begins with elements of hangover and proceeds to delirium tremens. Littleton and Little[14] suggested that early signs of withdrawal, such as anxiety, depression, dysphoria, headache, and tremors, are "familiar to some of us as a hangover."

The second explanation for the increased prevalence of alcohol dependence in younger age groups in the general population is measurement error. The dependence criteria now incorporated into DSM and the *International Classification of Diseases* (ICD)[15] for substance-related disorders were based on the World Health Organization's[11,16] formulation of the alcohol dependence syndrome, in which dependence was characterized as a biobehavioral disorder distinguished by impaired control over substance use; increased salience of the substance in the user's reward hierarchy,; narrowing of the substance-taking behavioral repertoire; the development of behavioral, metabolic, and physiological tolerance; and manifestation of a characteristic withdrawal syndrome following cessation of substance use. Although detailed symptom definitions were written to describe these criteria, the translation of the criteria into operational measures at the item level in highly structured interview schedules such as the Composite International Diagnostic Interview (CIDI) and the Alcohol Use Disorder and Associated Disabilities Interview Schedule (AUDADIS) is based on a rather literal interpretation of the criteria. As the criteria were being operationalized, little attention was paid to possible confounding of symptom reports with behaviors and consequences that were not implied or intended in the original formulation.

Evidence for the possible introduction of systematic error into the measurement of the dependence criteria comes from several lines of research. Two studies that evaluated symptom-level data in samples of adolescents found that tolerance and "drinking more or longer than intended" (i.e., impaired control) were the two most frequently endorsed symptoms.[3,17] In another study,[2] based on data from the 2001 U.S. National Household Survey on Drug Abuse, the alcohol dependence symptom with the highest prevalence in adolescents aged 12–17 was tolerance, which was reported by over 20% of current drinkers.

It has been suggested[18] that the high prevalence of reported tolerance in U.S. adolescent samples may represent a normal developmental phenomenon rather than a pathophysiological process. Thus, the rapid development of an ability to "hold one's liquor" during adolescence may not be the same process that allows a chronic heavy drinker to consume enormous amounts of alcohol for long periods of time without major behavioral or physical impairment. Although several researchers have reported that withdrawal symptoms have a lower prevalence in adolescents than adults (e.g., reference 18), other research[2] indicates that higher rates of withdrawal symptoms are reported by adolescent female drinkers (3.4%) than by any other age group. Among male current drinkers, the rates were 3.5% for adolescents (ages 12–17) and 4.2% for the 18- to 23-year age group, with less than 3% of the remaining age groups reporting this symptom in the past 12 months.

In DSM-IV, a characteristic withdrawal syndrome is described as two or more of the following symptoms: "autonomic hyperactivity (e.g., sweating or pulse rate greater than 100); increased hand tremor; insomnia; nausea or vomiting; transient visual, tactile, or auditory hallucinations or illusions; psychomotor agitation; anxiety; and grand mal seizures."[19] Given the apparent severity of withdrawal as a physiological dependence symptom, and its traditional centrality in clinical descriptions of alcoholism dating back to the nineteenth-century depiction of the "drunkard's progress," it is surprising to see even small percentages of American teenagers reporting withdrawal symptoms at the beginning of their drinking careers, and the rates of teenagers and young adults exceeding those of older age cohorts.

Consistent with the evidence from national surveys, a survey conducted in the state of Connecticut[20] found that the rates of dependence reported for young adults (ages 18–24) were almost twice as high (16%) as those for the next age group (9%, ages 25–34). Further examination of the symptom level prevalence estimates, shown in Table 12–2 for all respondents who met criteria for dependence (i.e., a total of three or more symptoms), indicates that contrary to what might be

TABLE 12–2. Rates of alcohol dependence symptoms observed in a statewide telephone survey of Connecticut adults using the Diagnostic Interview Schedule for DSM-IV

	Age group (years)	
Symptom	**18–24**	**25–34**
Tolerance	81%	75%
Withdrawal	95%	83%
More than intend	91%	91%
Persistent desire	45%	61%
Lots of time	40%	61%
Interfere—work	26%	45%
Continued use	22%	38%

predicted from dependence theory, the younger age group reports higher rates of tolerance and withdrawal symptoms than the older age group. These data suggest that young adults, whose drinking tends to be concentrated into episodes of heavy episodic drinking, may be reporting tolerance and withdrawal symptoms with a high frequency because of a tendency, attributable partly to the wording of structured interview schedules, to confuse binge drinking and its sequelae with more classic physical symptoms of alcohol dependence. This same phenomenon has been noted by Harford et al.,[2] who suggested that the explanation lies in the relative inexperience of younger drinkers with alcohol's effects and physiological reactions to excessive alcohol consumption rather than alcohol dependence per se. This explanation is more consistent with the likelihood that individuals with such a short duration of exposure to alcohol would experience dependence-like symptoms but not a classic dependence syndrome.

Other factors that can potentially contribute to measurement error in the diagnosis of alcohol dependence in the general population have been discussed by Caetano.[8] First, there are important differences between clinical interviews and interviews in epidemiological studies of the general population during which alcohol dependence indicators are assessed. Clinical interviews are conducted with individuals who have come to treatment because they have severe drinking problems. The severity of the problems makes identification of alcohol dependence indicators relatively easy, thus minimizing misdiagnosis. Second, many individuals presenting for treatment may have already had contact with alcohol treatment and may have been educated to recognize their symptoms. Third, clinical interviews are longer and allow for detailed probing of respondents' answers, which decreases the chance of misinterpretation of the reported information. In contrast, data collection in general population surveys is conducted with respondents who have a less severe spectrum of problems, who have had no prior involvement with treatment and who therefore cannot use previous treatment experiences to interpret their own behavior. Further, interview time is limited, and there is little opportunity for probing. In spite of being carefully trained to apply survey questionnaires in a standardized manner, interviewers in such surveys are not clinically trained. This, too, may increase the chances of misidentification of certain behavior as indicators of dependence.

Implications

If measurement error is the reason for the increased prevalence of alcohol dependence in younger age cohorts, there are several important implications for the development of improved diagnostic procedures and the possible inclusion of a dependence subtype for adolescents and young adults. First, there is a need to explore symptom-level data more thoroughly to determine whether young adults are confusing the sequelae of acute intoxication with alcohol withdrawal, and rapid initial tolerance with the alcoholic's ability to consume significant amounts of alcohol without apparent behavioral impairment. Second, epidemiologists and clinicians need to be more cautious, even skeptical, of the tendency of structured psychiatric interviews to classify young adults as being alcohol-dependent. Third, it may be useful to characterize individuals who meet alcohol dependence criteria at a young age (e.g., prior to age 25) without significant exposure to chronic alcohol consumption as manifesting a form of "adolescent alcohol dependence" that may represent a less severe form of alcohol use disorder than that observed in adults who develop these symptoms only after 15–20 years of regular heavy drinking. This may be similar to Jellinek's[21] classification of alpha and beta alcoholism, which represented drinking patterns that could be harmful in the absence of severe alcohol dependence.

References

1. Grant BF, Dawson DA, Stinson FS, et al: The 12-month prevalence and trends in DSM-IV alcohol abuse and dependence: United States, 1991–92 and 2001–02. Drug Alcohol Depend 74:223–234, 2004.
2. Harford TC, Grant BF, Yi H, et al: Patterns of DSM-IV alcohol abuse and dependence criteria among adolescents and adults: results from the 2001 National Household Survey on Drug Abuse. Alcohol Clin Exp Res 29:810–829, 2005.
3. Kessler RC, McGonagle KA, Zhao S, et al: Lifetime and 12-month prevalence of DSM-III-R psychiatric disorders in the United States: results from the National Comorbidity Survey. Arch Gen Psychiatry 51:8–19, 1994.
4. Caetano R: Prevalence, incidence and stability of drinking problems among whites, blacks and Hispanics—1984–92. J Stud Alcohol 58:565–572, 1997.
5. Hasin DS, Grant B, Endicott J: The natural history of alcohol abuse: implications for definitions of alcohol use disorders. Am J Psychiatry 147:1537–1541, 1990.

6. Cahalan D, Room R: Problem Drinking Among American Men. New Brunswick, NJ, Rutgers Center of Alcohol Studies, 1974.
7. Babor TF: The classification of alcoholics: typology theories from the 19th century to the present. Alcohol Health Res World 20:6–17, 1996.
8. Caetano R: The identification of alcohol dependence criteria in the general population. Addiction 94:255–267, 1999.
9. Caetano R: Correlates of DSM-III-R dependence in treatment and general populations. Drug Alcohol Depend 28:225–239, 1991.
10. Bucholz KK, Helzer JE, Shayka JJ, et al: Comparison of alcohol dependence in subjects from clinical, community, and family studies. Alcohol Clin Exp Res 18:1091–1099, 1994.
11. Edwards G, Arif A, Hodgson R: Nomenclature and classification of drug and alcohol related problems: a WHO memorandum. Bull World Health Organ 59:225–242, 1981.
12. Edwards G: Withdrawal symptoms and alcohol dependence: fruitful mysteries. Br J Addict 85:447–461, 1990.
13. Stockwell T: Alcohol withdrawal: an adaptation to heavy drinking of no practical significance? Addiction 89:1447–1453, 1994.
14. Littleton J, Little H: Current concepts of ethanol dependence. Addiction 89:1397–1412, 1994.
15. World Health Organization: The ICD-10 Classification of Mental and Behavioural Disorders: Clinical Descriptions and Diagnostic Guidelines. Geneva, Switzerland, World Health Organization, 1992.
16. Edwards G, Gross MM: Alcohol dependence: provisional description of a clinical syndrome. Br Med J 1:1058–1061, 1976.
17. Kilpatrick DG, Acierno R, Saunders B, et al: Risk factors for adolescent substance abuse and dependence: data from a national sample. J Consult Clin Psychol 68:19–30, 2000.
18. Martin CS, Winters KC: Diagnosis and assessment of alcohol use disorders among adolescents. Alcohol Health Res World 22:95–105, 1998.
19. American Psychiatric Association: Diagnostic and Statistical Manual of Mental Disorders, 4th Edition. Washington, DC, American Psychiatric Association, 1994.
20. Ungemack J, Babor TF, Bidiorini A: Connecticut Compendium on Substance Abuse Treatment Need. Hartford, Connecticut Department of Mental Health and Addiction Services, 2001.
21. Jellinek E: The disease concept of alcoholism. Q J Stud Alcohol 13:673–684, 1960.

13

ADOLESCENTS AND SUBSTANCE-RELATED DISORDERS

Research Agenda to Guide Decisions About DSM-V

Thomas J. Crowley, M.D.

Approximately 180,000 adolescents annually enter American substance treatment programs.[1] Although referred to loosely as "substance abusers," most meet full *Diagnostic and Statistical Manual of Mental Disorders,* 4th Edition (DSM-IV), diagnostic criteria for substance dependence (SD), and most of the others meet DSM-IV criteria for substance abuse (SA).[2–4] Among adolescents DSM-IV diagnoses of SA and SD show "discriminant validity"; the prevalence of these disorders is (as expected) very significantly greater among adolescent patients in substance treatment than among controls.[2] Further evidence of validity lies in the observation that in clinical samples of adolescents, there is the expected orderly progression in severity of prob-

---

The author consulted these colleagues in the preparation of this manuscript: Sandra Brown, Christian Hopfer, Paula Riggs, Joseph Sakai and Elizabeth Whitmore. The review was supported in part by grants DA 009842, 011015 and 012845 from the National Institute on Drug Abuse, a U.S. government agency.

Reprinted from Crowley TJ: "Adolescents and Substance-Related Disorders: Research Agenda to Guide Decisions on DSM-V." *Addiction* 101 (suppl 1):115–124, 2006. Used with permission of the Society for the Study of Addiction.

lems (e.g., frequency of drug use, adverse consequences) from those who have no diagnosis, to those who have the milder abuse diagnosis, to those who have the more serious dependence diagnosis.[5] These diagnoses also show good inter-rater reliability among adolescents, at least in the context of a single structured interview.[6]

Therefore, the DSM-IV substance use disorder (SUD) diagnoses "work" in adolescents, as they do in adults, showing good inter-rater reliability and validity. In this chapter, accordingly, I do not recommend studies of changes in overall criteria for SA and SD diagnoses to accommodate clinical issues with adolescents. I do, however, suggest six areas for adolescent-relevant studies, addressing how those criteria are applied, to improve their usefulness in diagnosing substance-related disorders in adolescents.

Cannabis Withdrawal

STATEMENT OF THE PROBLEM

Cannabis dependence is among the most frequent diagnoses of adolescents entering substance treatment. DSM-IV-TR states: "Symptoms of possible cannabis withdrawal (e.g., irritable or anxious mood accompanied by physiological changes such as tremor, perspiration, nausea, change in appetite, and sleep disturbances) have been described in association with the use of very high doses, but their clinical significance is uncertain. For these reasons, the diagnosis of cannabis withdrawal is not included in this manual." Given that statement, DSM-IV also is unclear as to whether reported withdrawal symptoms should be counted toward diagnoses of cannabis dependence. Research since 1994 may have helped to clarify the "clinical significance" of cannabis withdrawal.

REVIEW OF THE LITERATURE

A recent review[7] of cannabis withdrawal studies, conducted mainly in adults, concludes that strong evidence now supports a clinically significant withdrawal syndrome that apparently contributes to cannabis relapse among abstaining cannabis users. In this section, I review the four papers that extend those adult findings to adolescents.

In a 1998 report on a group of 180 cannabis-dependent adolescent patients, 67% reported experiencing cannabis withdrawal symptoms, and about one-third of those reported using cannabis to relieve or avoid those withdrawal symptoms.[8] A separate sample of adolescent patients studied by the same group[9] included 54 meeting DSM-IV criteria for cannabis dependence; of those, 59% reported cannabis withdrawal.

Winters et al.[5] reported on a clinical group of 659 adolescent cannabis users, of whom 40% had DSM-IV cannabis dependence; among the whole group, 47% reported cannabis withdrawal and/or using cannabis to relieve or avoid that withdrawal. Finally, 7% of a large sample of Australian high school students met DSM-IV criteria for cannabis dependence by the time they had reached age 20; of those with cannabis dependence, three-quarters reported cannabis withdrawal, and 38% of those reporting withdrawal also said that they used cannabis to avoid withdrawal symptoms.[10]

Thus, as found in studies of adults,[7] many cannabis-dependent adolescents report cannabis withdrawal. Many of those also report using cannabis to avoid or relieve withdrawal symptoms, a pattern of use that is "clinically significant."

IDENTIFICATION OF RESEARCH GAPS

The evidence reviewed here suggests that cannabis withdrawal is clinically significant in adolescents. What is missing from the picture now is research supporting DSM-IV's uncertainty about the clinical significance of cannabis withdrawal.

SPECIFIC RESEARCH RECOMMENDATIONS

1. Given the weight of evidence now supporting the clinical significance of a cannabis withdrawal syndrome, the burden of proof must rest with those who would exclude the syndrome from DSM-V. Their argument would be strengthened by studies of cannabis-dependent adolescents showing circumstances in which 1) few report cannabis withdrawal or 2) of those reporting withdrawal, few report using cannabis to avoid or relieve withdrawal. Without such findings, continuing DSM's present exclusion of cannabis withdrawal would be difficult to support.
2. Studies in cannabis-dependent adolescents of the symptoms and time course of cannabis withdrawal, and of withdrawal-precipitated cannabis craving, could be compared with similar studies in adults to determine whether symptoms differ in adolescents and adults.
3. Most of the studies described above examined self-reported symptoms. Directly observed findings could provide stronger conclusions.

Substance Use Disorders and Disruptive Behavior Disorders

STATEMENT OF THE PROBLEM

There is exceptionally strong comorbidity between conduct disorder and substance use disorders among adolescents. Genetic researchers now suggest that conduct–antisocial–substance problems are different behavioral manifestations of the same genetic diathesis. In DSM-V, should a section on substance use disorders be included among, or referenced within, the "Attention Deficit and Disruptive Behavior Disorders" in the section "Disorders Usually First Diagnosed in Infancy, Childhood, or Adolescence"?

REVIEW OF THE LITERATURE

Onset Age

Alcohol dependence often is a disorder of adolescence. Figure 13–1[11] shows that among Americans the incidence of DSM-IV alcohol dependence rises sharply, from age 11 years, peaks at 18, and declines sharply thereafter. Comparable data for other drugs of abuse are not currently available, but clinical experience suggests that they would be similar.

Disorders Comorbid With Adolescent Substance Dependence

Adolescent SD is strongly associated with conduct problems. Conduct disorder (CD) is a disruptive behavior disorder of children and adolescents who have shown in the last year a persistent pattern of behavior in which the basic rights of others, or societal norms or rules, are violated.[12] Some youthful antisocial patients fail to meet the technical criteria for CD because, for example, their behavior was strictly supervised through probation throughout the last year; we refer to such youths as having "serious conduct problems." Earlier CD is a necessary antecedent for a diagnosis of adult antisocial personality disorder (ASPD). Like adult ASPD, adolescent CD is associated strongly with substance problems,[4,13–19] and this is true in both genders[20,21] and in Asian as well as Western countries.[22]

Many youths with CD and SD also meet diagnostic criteria for other disorders. For example, of youths with either CD or attention-deficit/hyperactivity disorder (ADHD), 30%–50% also have the other disorder.[23] The odds of having ADHD rise about 24-fold among youths with CD, compared with those without CD.[24]

The comorbid three-way relationship of CD, SD, and ADHD is complex. Absent CD, ADHD has little or no association with SD. In a large epidemiological sample of adolescent twins, Disney et al.[15] found that "the connection between ADHD and substance use disorders is almost entirely due to a comorbid diagnosis of CD—independent of CD a diagnosis of ADHD has little effect on substance use." Other studies concur.[25–28] Summarizing the data, an NIH Consensus Conference[29] concluded: "Children with ADHD *in combination with conduct disorders* [emphasis added] experience drug abuse, antisocial behavior, and accidents of all sorts." Indeed, ADHD with CD may have different risk factors and a different clinical course than ADHD without CD.[23,30]

Conduct and substance problems run in families and in part have a shared genetic etiology. Our group has shown very significantly more antisocial problems among relatives of our adolescent CD–SUD patients than among relatives of control adolescents.[31] In twin studies estimates of CD's heritability range from about 0.5 to 0.7.[32–36] Analyses of some 1,300 adolescent twin pairs by our group have estimated the heritability of CD at approximately 0.5.[37] The maximum 1-day alcohol consumption by a father significantly predicts the risk for externalizing disorders, substance use, and substance dependence in offspring.[38] Most of the association

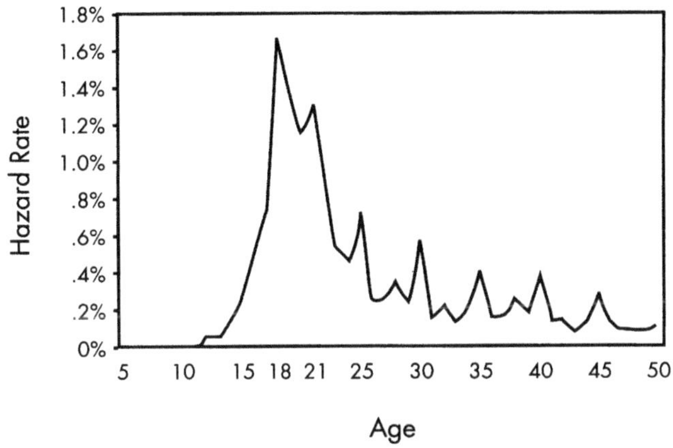

FIGURE 13–1. Age at onset of DSM-IV alcohol dependence, from the National Epidemiologic Survey on Alcohol and Related Conditions, 2003.

Source. Reprinted from Li et al.[11] with permission from the Society of Biological Psychiatry.

of adult alcohol dependence and adolescent conduct problems is of genetic origin,[39] suggesting that a common biology may underlie these tightly linked problems. Non-alcohol drug dependence also shows a genetic association with juvenile conduct problems.[40,41]

Evidence indicates increasingly that among people with CD or ASPD there is a general "vulnerability to the abuse of all categories of drugs,"[42–48] and that the characteristic predisposing to such "general" drug problems may be "disinhibitory psychopathology"—the failure to stop risky behavior—including the failure to refrain from using (and developing dependence on) substances.

That disinhibitory psychopathology is highly heritable, with $h^2 > 0.8$.[49,50] Indeed, a recent twin-family study that considered together CD, alcohol dependence, drug dependence, and ASPD (an extension into adulthood of CD's antisocial behaviors) concluded that "what parents pass on to the next generation is a general vulnerability to [this] spectrum of disorders, with each disorder representing a different expression of this general vulnerability"; that general vulnerability was highly heritable ($h^2 = 0.80$).[51] Our group[52] suggests that a single locus on chromosome 9 may contain one or more genes contributing to both CD and substance dependence.

SUMMARY: RELATIONSHIP TO ADULT SUBSTANCE USE DISORDERS

Since the publication of DSM-IV, new evidence has shown that a) SUDs are often first diagnosed in adolescence, b) those SUDs are often serious enough to bring adolescents into treatment, c) adolescent SUDs are highly associated with conduct disorder (CD, a "disruptive behavior disorder"), and d) a shared genetic etiology contributes to both the SUD and the CD of adolescents.

If the SUDs of adolescents were classified among the disruptive behavior disorders, would that conflict with research evidence from adults? In data from more than 8,000 subjects in the National Comorbidity Survey, Krueger[53] used tetrachoric correlations and confirmatory factor analyses to examine the comorbidity structure of 10 nonpsychotic disorders. He found one major factor of "externalizing disorders," including ASPD and SUDs, and another major factor of "internalizing disorders" with two subfactors. The author noted that the data "organizes common psychopathological variance into internalizing patterns—as well as externalizing patterns involving antisocial behaviors [ASPD] and lifestyles [SUDs]." The research shows that among adults, as in adolescents, antisocial symptoms and symptoms of SUDs are strongly associated.

IDENTIFICATION OF RESEARCH GAPS

a. Except for alcohol dependence, there are currently no good data on age at incidence of substance use disorders.
b. Enlarging the disruptive behavior disorders section of DSM-V to include, or reference, adolescent SUDs could have unforeseen complications .

SPECIFIC RESEARCH RECOMMENDATIONS

1. Find and examine studies of the age at incidence of substance use disorders across adolescence and adulthood. If SUDs usually occur first in adolescence, they should be referenced or listed in the "Disorders Usually First Diagnosed in Infancy, Childhood, or Adolescence" ("Disruptive Behavior Disorders") section.
2. Experts in the nosology of SUDs and disruptive disorders should consider nosological conflicts arising from the possible inclusion of (or reference to) adolescent SUDs in the disruptive behavior disorders.

Reliability of Substance Abuse Diagnoses Among Adolescents

STATEMENT OF THE PROBLEM

Substance abuse may be a diagnosis of special importance among adolescents. Pathological substance use patterns usually begin in adolescence, and so especially among adolescents the less serious substance abuse may be diagnosable before the onset of substance dependence. Unfortunately, reliability of abuse diagnoses may be unacceptably low.

REVIEW OF THE LITERATURE

Structured interviews are intended to produce reliable, valid diagnoses. An important study of adults suggests that we cannot assume reliability for DSM-IV abuse diagnoses. Cottler et al.[54] gave three structured or semistructured diagnostic interviews (Composite International Diagnostic Interview [CIDI], Alcohol Use Disorder and Associated Disabilities Interview Schedule [AUDADIS-ADR], and Schedule for Clinical Assessment in Neuropsychiatry [SCAN]) to each of 420 subjects in Athens, Luxembourg, or St. Louis. Subjects included patients in substance treatment, as well as community volunteers selected in various ways for probable substance use. Regarding dependence, the three diagnostic instruments showed good concordance for alcohol and opioids, fair to good concordance for cocaine and sedatives, and low concordance for amphetamine and cannabis. Agreement on abuse was low for all substances examined. These authors concluded: "The abuse category for all substances warrants further refinement in its conceptualization. If further research continues to find poor reliability or comparability for abuse, its elimination from the nomenclature should be considered."

However, as noted earlier, Martin et al.[6] had two observers watch SCID-guided interviews of adolescent subjects, seeking SUD diagnoses for alcohol, cannabis, sedatives, hallucinogens, and inhalants. Subjects received diagnoses of abuse, dependence, or neither, and three-way kappa statistics for each substance were 0.94. Thus, agreement was excellent.

Moreover, among adolescents substance abuse diagnoses show surprisingly strong discriminative validity. A diagnosis is said to have "discriminative validity" if a group expected to have a high prevalence of the diagnosis actually shows a higher prevalence than some control group; the measured prevalence rates "discriminate" the two groups. For example, using the Composite International Diagnostic Interview—Substance Abuse Module (CIDISAM), Crowley et al.[2] assessed 83 adolescent patients who had serious conduct and substance problems, and 85 control adolescents. The prevalence of DSM-IV substance abuse diagnoses was 30.1% (patients) and 4.7% (controls) for alcohol; 25.3% and 2.4% for cannabis; 14.5% and 0% for hallucinogens; and 9.6% and 0% for cocaine (all values: $P<0.003$). Thus, the diagnoses' discriminative validity was excellent. (There also were, of course, many substance dependence diagnoses, but they are not relevant for this point.)

Cottler et al.[54] studied instrument reliability, comparing results when the same subjects completed three different interview instruments. Martin et al.[6] studied inter-rater reliability from one instrument with both raters seeing the same interview. Crowley et al.[2] studied validity, comparing results obtained when one interview instrument was given to a group of patients and to a separate group of controls. Considered together, their findings suggest that the conceptualization of the abuse diagnosis usefully discriminates adolescents with pathological substance involvement from normal adolescents, but that differences in the instruments' questions or scoring algorithms may contribute to differences in whether a diagnosis is made.

Developers of interview instruments are highly skilled at operationalizing symptom criteria from diagnostic manuals, translating those criteria into a series of diagnostic questions and scoring the responses to generate diagnoses. Apparently, however, the abuse-related questions and algorithms produced by different professional interview-developers produce discrepant results. One must ask whether DSM-IV's symptom criteria for abuse, which do discriminate adolescent patients and controls, are stated with sufficient objectivity to ensure that professional interview-developers will similarly operationalize those criteria. Of course, one must further ask: if the interview products of those highly skilled professionals disagree on abuse diagnoses, how reliable can the diagnoses of busy clinicians be?

A review of DSM-IV's substance abuse criteria reveals areas open to different interpretations, potentially reducing reliability:

a. The terms *recurrent* or *continued* start each criterion. Does *recurrent* mean twice, or three or four times, or more? In the specified 12 months, does *continued* mean twice, or monthly, or daily, or some other frequency?
b. Abuse criterion [1] is "recurrent substance use resulting in a failure to fulfill major role obligations at work, school, or home (e.g., repeated absences or poor work performance related to substance use; substance-related suspensions, or expulsions from school; neglect of children or household)." If one of the listed items, such as "expulsions from school," is "recurrent" (albeit with some uncertain frequency), that would meet the criterion. But what if several of the items had occurred but no single one was recurrent—would the criterion be met? And if so, how many of them must have occurred once to meet the criterion?
c. Abuse criterion [2] is "recurrent substance use in situations in which it is physically hazardous (e.g., driving an automobile or operating a machine when impaired by substance use)." "Operating a machine" is uncommon among substance-involved adolescents, but fighting is common. Would adding an example such as "joining fights when impaired by substance use" increase inter-rater reliability on this criterion with adolescent patients? In another example of uncertainty, the mere use of some substances is immediately dangerous; for example, any occasion of inhalant use may cause a fatal cardiac arrhythmia in susceptible youths. DSM-IV does not make clear whether recurrent inhalant use itself, with no involvement of automobiles or machines, could meet the criterion of "physically hazardous."

IDENTIFICATION OF RESEARCH GAPS

There is good evidence that the criteria for substance abuse do discriminate control youths from those who are pathologically involved with substances, but it appears that the criteria are difficult to reliably operationalize. I am aware of no research in adolescents that has assessed modifications in text phrasing to increase inter-rater reliability of abuse diagnoses.

SPECIFIC RESEARCH RECOMMENDATIONS

1. For the substance abuse criteria, develop altered example situations, altered text descriptions, or altered wording of the current criteria, with the aim of improved inter-rater reliability.
2. Compare inter-rater reliability of the new phrasing against that of the old. Note that this call is not for new abuse criteria, but for improved inter-rater reliability of the current criteria, which have apparent validity.
3. To confirm the validity of the rephrased abuse criteria, perform structured diagnostic interviews of adolescents assessed with a nondiagnostic external validator, such as quantity–frequency (Q-F) of substance use. If the rephrased abuse criteria are valid, adolescents with no diagnoses should have low Q-F values, those with abuse diagnoses should have mid-range Q-F values, and those with dependence diagnoses should have high Q-F values.

Age, Development, and Severity of Dependence

STATEMENT OF THE PROBLEM

A substance use disorder developing in younger adolescents may represent a more severe form of the disorder than one developing in an older adolescent, but DSM-IV provides no procedures by which to consider an adolescent's age in the severity of substance use disorders.

REVIEW OF THE LITERATURE

Miele et al.[55] point out that "inconsistent results in the DSM-IV field trial data led to the elimination of the specific severity guidelines for substance dependence. The dependence diagnosis is now one of the only diagnoses in DSM-IV that does not include a severity specifier. It is difficult to argue that severity is relevant to most other DSM-IV diagnoses but not to alcohol and drug dependence."

The lack of severity specifiers for SUDs raises special developmental issues among adolescents. In a cross-sectional study considering several substances assessed with CIDI-SAM among a community-based sample of more than 3,000 adolescents,[56] there was a dramatic increase in the prevalence of substance dependence (Figure 13–2) and substance abuse as age increased. Similarly, considering only cannabis, von Sydow et al.[57] also showed very sharp increases in prevalence of dependence or abuse during a 42-month follow-up of an epidemiological sample of 14- to 17-year-old youths. The data indicate that a youth with SUD onset at age 12 is much more deviant, at least statistically speaking, than a youth with onset at age 18.

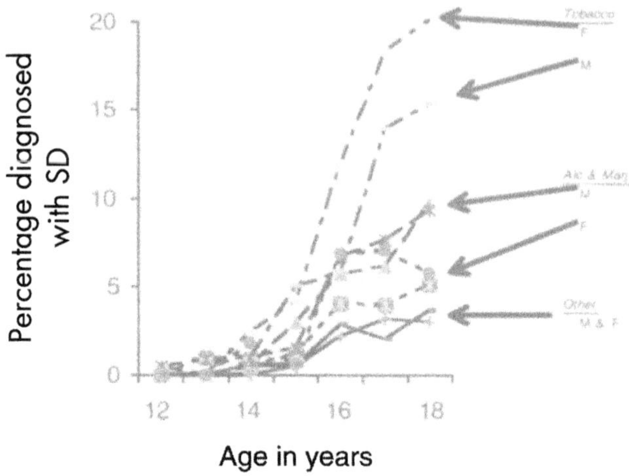

FIGURE 13–2. Percentage of 3,072 community adolescents diagnosed with substance dependence (SD).

F=female (dashed lines); M=male (solid lines); Alc=alcohol; Marj=marijuana; Other=other DSM-IV-defined substance classes.

Source. Redrawn from Young et al.[56]

IDENTIFICATION OF RESEARCH GAPS

Earlier onset of CD symptoms predicts worse posttreatment substance outcomes in adolescents.[58] However, it is not clear at this time whether earlier onset of SUDs also heralds worse substance outcomes, such as earlier relapse after treatment, more substance problems, greater persistence of substance problems, development of abuse or dependence on additional drugs, and so forth.

SPECIFIC RESEARCH RECOMMENDATION

1. Perform secondary analyses of existing prospective or retrospective longitudinal data to determine whether earlier onset of SUDs (between ages 14 and 18) is a severity marker that validly predicts worse course. If adolescent age at onset does predict course, it could be incorporated into DSM-V as a severity marker for adolescents.

Implications of Multi-Substance Dependence for Course and Severity

STATEMENT OF THE PROBLEM

Adolescents often develop substance abuse and/or substance dependence on several different substances, and the number of substances or of diagnostic criteria met reflects overall severity and predicts course. To better reflect severity and predict course, it may be that DSM-V diagnoses should in some way take into account the total number of substances or the total number (across substances) of diagnostic criteria met.

REVIEW OF THE LITERATURE

Our research group has found repeatedly that many adolescent patients qualify for diagnoses of substance abuse or substance dependence on several different substances simultaneously. For example, Young et al.[5] reported that 57 adolescent male patients in residential treatment averaged 1 substance abuse and 3.2 substance dependence diagnoses. Mikulich et al.[9] reported on a sample of 102 adolescent patients that included boys and girls in both residential and outpatient settings; there was an average of 1.9 dependence diagnoses and 1.2 abuse diagnoses. In a study of 847 adolescents admitted for substance treatment, Sakai et al.[59] observed that those with inhalant abuse or dependence had SUD diagnoses on a mean of 4.1 substances; those who had used inhalants without meeting criteria for inhalant abuse or dependence had SUD diagnoses on 3.8 substances, and those without inhalant use had such diagnoses on 2.7 substances.

There is apparently a genetic influence that raises the risk for SUDs, regardless of the drug or drugs to which the individual is exposed. In a report from the Vietnam Era Twin Registry,[60] substance use disorders ran in families, and concordance rates established significant genetic contributions for disorders in most drug categories. One report from that study found that the heritability for different classes of drugs ranged from 0.26 to 0.54. That study further showed that a heritable vulnerability to SUD generally (rather than a vulnerability to SUD on a particular drug) contributed heavily to subjects' drug problems. "There is some characteristic of the individual that imparts vulnerability to the abuse of all drugs."[42] Other authors have commented similarly on common, cross-drug vulnerabilities to substance use disorders.[43–45,47] As noted earlier, Hicks et al.[51] found a common genetic contribution to antisocial, alcohol and other drug problems, and they found 80% heritability for that shared genetic influence. Moreover, Stallings et al.[37] provide suggestive evidence for a genetic locus on chromosome 9 that may contribute to the total number of cross-drug dependence symptoms.

For treatment planning it is essential, of course, to diagnose each substance use disorder independently. Only patients with alcohol use disorders, for example, will be considered for acamprosate treatment, and only those with opioid use disorders may receive methadone maintenance treatment. However, in addition to guiding treatment planning, diagnoses should, when possible, reflect severity and predict course. Regarding severity, Miele et al.[55] noted that "evaluating the severity of [problems from] only one drug may produce a misleading picture of dependence severity in the large proportion of subjects who use multiple substances." Regarding course prediction, we demonstrated that the number of drugs on which an adolescent male patient is dependent at admission significantly predicts (in a 2-year follow-up) both the frequency of substance use and the commission of crimes.[58]

But what phenotype of pathological cross-substance involvement best reflects severity and predicts outcome? Just within our research group we have considered a) the number of substances on which the youth is dependent[4,58,61]; b) the cross-substance number of symptoms of substance dependence[2,61]; c) the number of substances on which the youth has either abuse or dependence diagnoses[59]; d) the cross-substance total number of abuse and dependence symptoms[61]; and e) the cross-substance number of dependence symptoms divided by the number of drugs used more than five times.[59] After an empirical evaluation of 10 competing phenotypes, we also examined f) "dependence vulnerability," defined as the cross-substance dependence symptom count divided by the number of substances used more than five times and expressed in standard deviation units from the means of community adolescents of the same age and gender.[37,62] (We note that regardless of its possible merits for research, [f] appears too complex for clinical application.)

IDENTIFICATION OF RESEARCH GAPS

Research suggests strongly that there are genetic influences contributing to a broad, cross-substance vulnerability to SUDs, and that the extent of patients' pathological cross-substance involvement reflects severity and predicts course. However, there is currently no agreed-upon, clinically practical phenotypic descriptor that could be used in DSM-V to characterize the extent of pathological cross-substance involvement.

SPECIFIC RESEARCH RECOMMENDATIONS

1. Conduct studies to identify and validate a clinically practical phenotypic descriptor that could be used in DSM-V to characterize the extent of pathological cross-substance involvement.
2. Consider using that descriptor in DSM-V to document severity and predict course of substance use disorders. Of course, such a descriptor would supplement, not supplant, current individual-substance diagnoses of abuse or dependence.

Uniform Classifications for Emerging Substances of Abuse

STATEMENT OF THE PROBLEM

Adolescents are often among the first users of new substances appearing on the black market, and clinicians have little guidance on how to classify these new substances.

REVIEW OF THE LITERATURE

I am not aware of a literature addressing this issue. However, I offer two recent examples of the problem.

Since the publication of DSM-IV, "club drugs" have found wide use among adolescents. The substances in this pharmacologically diverse group were categorized together only because of the social circumstances of their introduction to the drug culture—they were used widely in "rave" dance clubs. Responding to growing prevalence in the use of these drugs, at least one structured diagnostic interview was revised to include a new "club drug" category that listed Ecstasy (or 5-methoxy-3,4-methylenedioxyamphetamine; MDMA, a substance with mixed stimulant and hallucinogenic properties[63]), ketamine (an arylcyclohexylamine dissociative anesthetic that is an analogue of phencyclidine[64]), and two illegal sedative-hypnotics,[65] Rohypnol (flunitrazepam) and gamma-hydroxybutyrate (GHB). However, creating this new category in a structured interview meant that information on the diverse club drugs was classed together, rather than with the pharmacologically based categories (hallucinogens, phencyclidine and phencyclidine-like substances, or sedative-hypnotics) used in DSM-IV or in previous editions of that particular interview.

In another example, the cough suppressant Coricidin HBP Cough & Cold tablets, known on the street as "Triple C" and by other names, has found wide favor among adolescents as a substance of abuse.[66] In high doses it frequently produces altered mental states, sometimes including hallucinations. Its main active ingredient, dextromethorphan, is a *d*-isomer opioid, active at the sigma opioid receptor but thought to have little affinity for the mu receptor. An active metabolite blocks *N*-methyl-D-aspartate (NMDA) receptors, as does phencyclidine. Clinicians and researchers have no current guidance on whether to categorize "Triple C" with the opioid drugs or among the "phencyclidine or phencyclidine-like substances."

IDENTIFICATION OF RESEARCH GAPS

Categorization within proper pharmacological groups for emerging substances' syndromes of intoxication, withdrawal, abuse, and dependence may help clinicians to select treatments and predict course, based on knowledge of other members of that drug class. Although DSM-IV provides a substance category of "Other (or Unknown)," its use means that clinicians' selection of treatments or prediction of course may not be illuminated by knowledge of related substances. Unfortunately, once published, diagnostic manuals cannot anticipate drugs that will emerge in the future or guide clinicians and researchers in their categorization.

SPECIFIC RESEARCH RECOMMENDATIONS

1. Regarding substances emerging after the publication of DSM-V, those administering the DSM-V process could begin now to investigate with appropriate agencies (e.g., National Institute on Drug Abuse [NIDA], World Health Organization [WHO]) procedures (e.g., a Web site) to develop and disseminate to clinicians and researchers the "best-fitting" consensus classifications of emerging substances into the appropriate pharmacological categories of DSM-V.
2. Those procedures should then be studied for a) usefulness to clinicians and researchers and b) security from substance users seeking a menu of attractive new substances.

Conclusion

This chapter proposes six areas of adolescent-related research that may help guide the framers of the "Substance-Related Disorders" section of DSM-V. The operational concepts behind DSM-IV's diagnostic criteria for SUD appear to function well among adolescent patients, and this chapter suggests no substantive changes in those criteria. Areas deserving further study include the value of providing criteria for a cannabis withdrawal diagnosis; including or referencing SUD among "Disorders Usually First Diagnosed in Infancy, Childhood, or Adolescence"; altering example situations, text descriptions, or phrasing of the current substance abuse criteria to improve inter-rater reliability; using age at onset (from 14 to 19 years) as a severity marker and predictor of course; using extent of multi-substance involvement as a severity marker and predictor of course; and developing DSM-V-related post-publication procedures for classifying emerging new drugs into DSM-V's categories. Of course, such adolescent research must consider that symptoms may be perceived and reported differently by adolescents and adults, just as they may differ by ethnic or racial groups, or by gender.

References

1. Substance Abuse and Mental Health Services Administration: National Admissions to Substance Abuse Treatment Services: The Treatment Episode Data Set (TEDS) 1992–1996 (Table 3.2). Rockville, MD, Substance Abuse and Mental Health Services Administration, 1998. Available online at http://www.dasis.samhsa.gov/teds96/tbl32. htm.

2. Crowley TJ, Mikulich SK, Ehlers KM, et al: Validity of structured clinical evaluations in adolescents with conduct and substance problems. J Am Acad Child Adolesc Psychiatry 40:265–273, 2001.
3. Mezzich AC, Moss H, Tarter RE, et al: Differences in the pattern and progression of substance use in conduct-disordered adolescents. Am J Addict 3:289–295, 1994.
4. Young SE, Mikulich SK, Goodwin MB, et al: Treated delinquent boys' substance use: onset, pattern, relationship to conduct and mood disorders. Drug Alcohol Depend 37:149–162, 1995.
5. Winters KC, Latimer W, Stinchfield RD: The DSM-IV criteria for adolescent alcohol and cannabis use disorders. J Stud Alcohol 60:337–344, 1999.
6. Martin CS, Pollock NK, Bukstein OG, et al: Interrater reliability of the SCID alcohol and substance use disorders section among adolescents. Drug Alcohol Depend 59:173–176, 2000.
7. Budney AJ, Hughes JR, Moore BA, et al: Review of the validity and significance of cannabis withdrawal syndrome. Am J Psychiatry 161:1967–1977, 2004.
8. Crowley TJ, Macdonald MJ, Whitmore EA, et al: Cannabis dependence, withdrawal, and reinforcing effects among adolescents with conduct symptoms and substance use disorders. Drug Alcohol Depend 50:27–37, 1998.
9. Mikulich SK, Hall SK, Whitmore EA, et al: Concordance between DSM-III-R and DSM-IV diagnoses of substance use disorders in adolescents. Drug Alcohol Depend 61:237–248, 2001.
10. Coffey C, Carlin JB, Degenhardt L, et al: Cannabis dependence in young adults: an Australian population study. Addiction 97:187–194, 2002.
11. Li T-K, Hewitt BG, Grant BF: Alcohol use disorders and mood disorders: a National Institute on Alcohol Abuse and Alcoholism perspective. Biol Psychiatry 56:718–720, 2004.
12. American Psychiatric Association: Diagnostic and Statistical Manual of Mental Disorders, 4th Edition, Text Revision. Washington, DC, American Psychiatric Association, 2000.
13. Clark DB, Kirisci L, Moss HB: Early adolescent gateway drug use in sons of fathers with substance use disorders. Addict Behav 23:561–566, 1998.
14. Costello EJ, Mustillo S, Erkanli A, et al: Prevalence and development of psychiatric disorders in childhood and adolescence. Arch Gen Psychiatry 60:837–844, 2003.
15. Disney ER, Elkins IJ, McGue M, et al: Effects of ADHD, conduct disorder, and gender on substance use and abuse in adolescence. Am J Psychiatry 156:1515–1521, 1999.
16. Grella CE, Hser Y-I, Joshi V, et al: Drug treatment outcomes for adolescents with comorbid mental and substance use disorders. J Nerv Ment Dis 189:384–392, 2001.
17. Kuperman S, Schlosser SS, Kramer JR, et al: Developmental sequence from disruptive behavior diagnosis to adolescent alcohol dependence. Am J Psychiatry 158:2022–2026, 2001.
18. Marmorstein NR, Iacono WG: Major depression and conduct disorder in a twin sample: gender, functioning, and risk for future psychopathology. J Am Acad Child Adolesc Psychiatry 42:225–233, 2003.
19. Taylor J, Malone S, Iacono WG, et al: Development of substance dependence in two delinquency subgroups and nondelinquents from a male twin sample. J Am Acad Child Adolesc Psychiatry 41:386–393, 2002.

20. Heath AC, Bucholz K, Madden PAF, et al: Genetic and environmental contributions to alcohol dependence risk in a national twin sample: consistency of findings in women and men. Psychol Med 27:1381–1396, 1997.
21. Marmorstein NR, Iacono WG: An investigation of female adolescent twins with both major depression and conduct disorder. J Am Acad Child Adolesc Psychiatry 40:299–306, 2001.
22. Chong M-Y, Chan K-W, Cheng ATA: Substance use disorders among adolescents in Taiwan: prevalence, sociodemographic correlates and psychiatric co-morbidity. Psychol Med 29:1387–1396, 1999.
23. Khune M, Schachar R, Tannock R: Impact of comorbid oppositional or conduct problems on attention-deficit hyperactivity disorder. J Am Acad Child Adolesc Psychiatry 36:1715–1725, 1997.
24. Fergusson DM, Horwood LJ, Lynskey MT: Prevalence and comorbidity of DSM-III-R diagnoses in a birth cohort of 15 year olds. J Am Acad Child Adolesc Psychiatry 32: 1127–1134, 1993.
25. Fergusson DM, Lynskey MT, Horwood LJ: Attentional difficulties in middle childhood and psychosocial outcomes in young adulthood. J Child Psychol Psychiatry 38:633–644, 1997.
26. Milberger S, Faraone SV, Biederman J, et al: Familial risk analysis of the association between attention-deficit/hyperactivity disorder and psychoactive substance use disorders. Arch Pediatr Adolesc Med 152:945–951, 1998.
27. Wilens TE, Biederman J, Mick E, et al: Attention deficit hyperactivity disorder (ADHD) is associated with early onset substance use disorders. J Nerv Ment Dis 185:475–482, 1997.
28. Winters KC, August GJ, Realmuto GR: Childhood ADHD, Comorbidity and Risk for Late-Adolescent Drug Abuse. Philadelphia, PA, College on Problems of Drug Dependence, 2004. Available online at http://www.cpdd.vcu.edu. Accessed June 2004.
29. National Institutes of Health Consensus Conference: Diagnosis and Treatment of Attention-Deficit/Hyperactivity Disorder. Bethesda, MD, National Institutes of Health, 1998.
30. Biederman J, Newcorn J, Sprich S: Comorbidity of attention deficit hyperactivity disorder with conduct, depressive, anxiety, and other disorders. Am J Psychiatry 148:564–577, 1991.
31. Miles DR, Stallings MC, Young SE, et al: A family history and direct interview study of the familial aggregation of substance abuse: the adolescent substance abuse study. Drug Alcohol Depend 49:105–114, 1998.
32. Eaves LJ, Silberg JL, Hewitt JK, et al: Analyzing twin resemblance in multisymptom data: genetic applications of a latent class model for symptoms of conduct disorder in juvenile boys. Behav Genet 23:5–19, 1993.
33. Eaves LJ, Silberg JL, Meyer JM, et al: Genetics and developmental psychopathology, 2: the main effects of genes and environment on behavioral problems in the Virginia Twin Study of Adolescent Behavioral Development. J Child Psychol Psychiatry 38:965–980, 1997.
34. Hewitt JK, Silberg JL, Rutter M, et al: Genetics and developmental psychopathology, 1: phenotypic assessment in the Virginia Twin Study of Adolescent Behavioral Development. J Child Psychol Pyschiatry 38:943–963, 1997.

35. Silberg J, Rutter M, Meyer J, et al: Genetic and environmental influences on the co-variation between hyperactivity and conduct disturbance in juvenile twins. J Child Psychol Psychiatry 37:803–816, 1996.
36. Slutske WS, Heath AC, Dinwiddie SH, et al: Modeling genetic and environmental influences in the etiology of conduct disorder: a study of 2682 adult twin pairs. J Abnorm Psychol 106:266–279, 1997.
37. Stallings MC, Corley RP, Hewitt JK, et al: A genome-wide search for quantitative trait loci influencing substance dependence vulnerability in adolescence. Drug Alcohol Depend 70:295–307, 2003.
38. Malone SM, Iacono WG, McGue M: Drinks of the father: father's maximum number of drinks consumed predicts externalizing disorders, substance use, and substance use disorders in preadolescent and adolescent offspring. Alcohol Clin Exp Res 26:1823–1832, 2002.
39. Slutske WS, Heath AC, Dinwiddie SH, et al: Common genetic risk factors for conduct disorder and alcohol dependence. J Abnorm Psychol 107:363–374, 1998.
40. Cadoret RJ, Yates WR, Troughton E, et al: An adoption study of drug abuse/dependency in females. Compr Psychiatry 37:88–92, 1996.
41. Grove WM, Echert ED, Heston L, et al: Heritability of substance abuse and antisocial behavior: a study of monozygotic twins reared apart. Biol Psychiatry 27:1293–1304, 1990.
42. Tsuang MT, Lyons MJ, Meyer JM, et al: Co-occurrence of abuse of different drugs in men: the role of drug-specific and shared vulnerabilities. Arch Gen Psychiatry 55:967–972, 1998.
43. Bierut LJ, Dinwiddie SH, Begleiter H, et al: Familial transmission of substance dependence: alcohol, marijuana, cocaine, and habitual smoking: a report from the Collaborative Study on the Genetics of Alcoholism. Arch Gen Psychiatry 55:982–988, 1998.
44. Goldman D, Bergen A: General and specific inheritance of substance abuse and alcoholism. Arch Gen Psychiatry 55:964–965, 1998.
45. Hettema JM, Corey LA, Kendler KS: A multivariate genetic analysis of the use of tobacco, alcohol, and caffeine in a population based sample of male and female twins. Drug Alcohol Depend 57:69–78, 1999.
46. McGue M, Iacono WG, Legrand LN, et al: Origins and consequences of age at first drink, II: familial risk and heritability. Alcohol Clin Exp Res 25:1166–1173, 2001.
47. Pickens RW, Svikis DS, McGue M, et al: Common genetic mechanisms in alcohol, drug, and mental disorder comorbidity. Drug Alcohol Depend 39:129–138, 1995.
48. Van den Bree MBM, Johnson EO, Neale MC, et al: Genetic and environmental influences on drug use and abuse/dependence in male and female twins. Drug Alcohol Depend 52:231–241, 1998.
49. Krueger RF, Hicks BM, Patrick CJ, et al: Etiologic connections among substance dependence, antisocial behavior, and personality: modeling the externalizing spectrum. J Abnorm Psychol 111:411–424, 2002.
50. Young SE, Stallings MC, Corley RP, et al: Genetic and environmental influences on behavioral disinhibition. Am J Med Genet 96:684–695, 2000.
51. Hicks BM, Krueger RF, Iacono WG, et al: Family transmission and heritability of externalizing disorders. Arch Gen Psychiatry 61:922–928, 2004.

52. Stallings MC, Corley RP, Dennehey B, et al: A genome-wide search for quantitative trait loci influencing antisocial drug dependence in adolescence. Arch Gen Psychiatry 62:1042–1051, 2005.
53. Krueger RF: The structure of common mental disorders. Arch Gen Psychiatry 56:921–926, 1999.
54. Cottler LB, Grant BF, Blaine J, et al: Concordance of DSM-IV alcohol and drug use disorder criteria and diagnoses as measured by AUDADIS-ADR, CIDI and SCAN. Drug Alcohol Depend 47:195–205, 1997.
55. Miele GM, Carpenter KM, Cockerham MS, et al: Substance Dependence Severity Scale (SDSS): reliability and validity of a clinician-administered interview for DSM-IV substance use disorders. Drug Alcohol Depend 59:63–75, 2000.
56. Young SE, Corley RP, Stallings MC, et al: Substance use, abuse and dependence in adolescents: prevalence, symptom profiles and correlates. Drug Alcohol Depend 68: 309–322, 2002.
57. von Sydow K, Lieb R, Hildegard P, et al: The natural course of cannabis use, abuse and dependence over four years: a longitudinal community study of adolescents and young adults. Drug Alcohol Depend 64:347–361, 2001.
58. Crowley TJ, Mikulich SK, Macdonald M, et al: Substance-dependent, conduct disordered adolescent males: severity of diagnosis predicts 2-year outcome. Drug Alcohol Depend 49:225–237, 1998.
59. Sakai JT, Hall SK, Mikulich-Gilbertson SK, et al: Inhalant use, abuse and dependence among adolescent patients: commonly comorbid problems. J Am Acad Child Adolesc Psychiatry 43:1080–1088, 2004.
60. Tsuang MT, Lyons MJ, Eisen SA, et al: Genetic influences on DSM-III-R drug abuse and dependence: a study of 3,372 twin pairs. Am J Med Genet 67:473–477, 1996.
61. Whitmore EA, Mikulich SK, Ehlers KM, et al: One-year outcome of adolescent females referred for conduct disorder and substance abuse/dependence. Drug Alcohol Depend 59:131–141, 2000.
62. Crowley TJ, Mikulich SK, Ehlers K, et al: Discriminative validity and clinical utility of an abuse–neglect interview for adolescents with conduct and substance use problems. Am J Psychiatry 160:1461–1469, 2003.
63. Crowley TJ: Hallucinogen-related disorders, in Comprehensive Textbook of Psychiatry, VI. Edited by Kaplan HI, Sadock BJ. Baltimore, MD, Williams & Wilkins, 1995, pp 831–838.
64. Crowley TJ: Phencyclidine (or phencyclidine-like)-related disorders, in Comprehensive Textbook of Psychiatry, VI. Edited by Kaplan HI, Sadock BJ. Baltimore, MD, Williams & Wilkins, 1995, pp 864–872.
65. O'Brien CP: Drug addiction and drug abuse, in Goodman and Gilman's The Pharmacological Basis of Therapeutics. Edited by Hardman JG, Limbird LE. New York, McGraw-Hill, 2001, pp 621–642.
66. Banerji S, Anderson IB: Abuse of Coricidin HBP Cough & Cold tablets: episodes recorded by a poison center. Am J Health Syst Pharm 58:1811–1814, 2001.

14

ARE SPECIFIC DEPENDENCE CRITERIA NECESSARY FOR DIFFERENT SUBSTANCES?

How Can Research on Cannabis Inform This Issue?

Alan J. Budney, Ph.D.

Cannabis (marijuana) has long been considered a "soft" drug of abuse, as opposed to "hard" drugs such as heroin or cocaine. This distinction raises many questions. Are there other soft drugs (e.g. is nicotine a soft drug? what about alcohol)? What does the distinction of "soft drug" imply? That the substance is not as harmful physically? That it is not addictive (dependence producing) or as addictive as the hard drugs? That it does not have the potential for "physical" dependence? That the general or potential consequences of use or misuse are not as severe?

In this chapter, I use the nonscientific terms "soft" versus "hard drug" intentionally to make the point that the general population and many health care pro-

---

This work was supported in part by National Institute on Drug Abuse grants DA12471, DA12157, DA55186, and T32-DA07242. The author would also like to thank John R. Hughes, Brent A. Moore, and Ryan G. Vandrey for their insights and efforts that contributed to the formulation of the paper reproduced in this chapter.

Reprinted from Budney AJ: "Are Specific Dependence Criteria Necessary for Different Substances? How Can Research on Cannabis Inform This Issue?" *Addiction* 101 (suppl 1): 125–133, 2006. Used with permission of the Society for the Study of Addiction.

fessionals embrace this dichotomy either implicitly or explicitly. The questions raised by this distinction are germane to multiple topics addressed at the *Diagnostic and Statistical Manual of Mental Disorders* (DSM) meeting on the nature of substance use disorders (e.g., dimensional vs. categorical, the role of biological criteria) on which this book is based. Such inquiries also have relevance to the topic I will address; that is, determining whether the construct of substance dependence, as operationalized by the generic dependence criteria of DSM-IV, is adequate or optimal for the diagnosis of the different dependence disorders. To address this question, one needs to determine first the dimensionality of the dependence criteria for each substance. Are the dependence criteria unidimensional—that is, are all items intercorrelated, and does the pattern of correlation yield a single- or multiple-factor solution for each substance? Are the patterns of correlation similar across substances? That is, can the same criteria (phenomenology) be applied reliably to define the various dependence disorders? Finally, do the criteria show differential discriminative function across the different substances?

Because my research and expertise are in the area of cannabis dependence rather than in the more general area of diagnostic validity, stability, or dimensionality, I focus here on cannabis as a means for comment on similarities and differences among the dependence disorders. The rationale for this line of discourse is that if cannabis dependence (a soft drug) can be diagnosed and characterized adequately with the extant generic dependence criteria, then one could argue that the DSM-IV diagnostic guidelines are probably valid and of high utility for other substances with more well-accepted dependence syndromes. I first review and discuss recent studies on cannabis withdrawal. Note that a cannabis withdrawal disorder is not in DSM-IV, and it has been argued recently that it warrants inclusion in future versions of DSM.[1,2] This review will illustrate that cannabis, although considered by many to be different from most other common substances of dependence, is much more similar to than different from the others, even with regard to withdrawal. Second, I review selected studies published since 1994 that examine the validity and internal consistency of cannabis dependence as assessed via DSM criteria. These data will show that the DSM-IV dependence criteria can be applied fairly well to cannabis and yield findings similar to those observed with other substance dependence disorders.

Cannabis Withdrawal and Dependence

Early studies demonstrated that tolerance developed to many of the effects of cannabis.[3] What was unclear, and is of importance to the central question of its dependence potential, was whether withdrawal occurred following cessation of regular cannabis use. Inpatient studies of the 1970s showed that abrupt cessation could produce a wide range of withdrawal effects under certain circumstances.[2,3] However, these effects were characterized as mild, transient, and without serious medical complications and considered "insignificant" when compared to the medical and physiological symptoms associated with severe opiate or alcohol withdrawal.

In contrast, DSM-III-R and the *International Classification of Diseases*, 9th Revision (ICD-9) both included diagnostic categories for cannabis abuse and dependence, recognizing the clinical importance of these disorders. Epidemiological studies showed that approximately 9% of lifetime cannabis users meet the criteria for abuse or dependence and that the rate of significant problems increases with frequency of use.[4–6] What remained in dispute was whether what some might refer to as "physical dependence" (synonymous with "withdrawal") occurred among frequent users of cannabis. This question is highly relevant to determining whether drug-specific dependence criteria are needed to understand, diagnose, and treat substance dependence most effectively. In DSM-IV, only cannabis, hallucinogens, and inhalants do not have associated withdrawal disorders. To some extent, DSM-IV deals with this issue by allowing for dependence diagnoses with or without physiological dependence. Nonetheless, confusion or ambivalence within DSM remains, since the dependence disorders of substances without designated withdrawal syndromes still allow for a diagnosis of "with physiological dependence."

RECENT STUDIES OF CANNABIS WITHDRAWAL

Advances in the understanding of the pharmacology and neurobiology of cannabinoids, and new empirical studies showing that adults sought treatment specifically for problems with cannabis use, rekindled efforts in the 1990s to understand cannabis dependence and withdrawal more clearly. Specific to withdrawal, carefully conducted inpatient laboratory work[7,8] clearly demonstrated abstinence effects when cannabis or oral Δ-9-tetrahydrocannabinol (THC) was discontinued. Outpatient laboratory studies produced concordant findings and demonstrated that the magnitude and time course of cannabis abstinence effects were indicative of a typical substance withdrawal syndrome.[1,9] That is, most effects showed onset within 24–48 hours postcessation, peaked during days 2–4, and returned to baseline within 1–3 weeks. In summary, results across studies were remarkably consistent, particularly given the diverse methodology used across laboratories.

Survey studies from general population and clinical samples have been concordant with the experimental studies, providing convergent validity for the withdrawal syndrome.[2] In the DSM-IV field trials, 25% of individuals who had smoked cannabis at least six times in their lives reported experiencing cannabis withdrawal.[5] Two Australian studies indicated that 20%–32% of long-term cannabis users responded affirmatively to an ICD-10 cannabis withdrawal question.[10,11] Clinical studies of adults seeking treatment for cannabis abuse or dependence showed even higher rates of withdrawal; across studies, 51%–95% of the adults reported cannabis withdrawal during the past year.[12–15] The only clinical study that assessed for specific cannabis withdrawal symptoms reported that 85% of outpatients acknowledged at least four symptoms of at least mild severity,[16] with greater than

70% endorsing the presence of cravings, irritability, nervousness, depressed mood, restlessness, sleep difficulty, and anger.

Cannabis withdrawal among youth that parallels observations from adult studies has also been reported. Withdrawal was endorsed by 15% of adolescents in a community-based sample who met DSM-IV criteria for either cannabis abuse or dependence.[17] In clinical samples of cannabis-abusing youth enrolled in intensive or residential treatment, 40%–67% reported experiencing cannabis withdrawal during prior quit attempts.[18,19] Among adolescents enrolled in outpatient treatment for cannabis, 65% indicated that they had experienced four or more symptoms of withdrawal,[20] and the types of symptoms reported were remarkably similar to those observed with adults.[18,19,21]

As we have argued elsewhere,[2] extant data indicate that cannabis withdrawal warrants designation as a true withdrawal syndrome. That is, abstinence effects a) occur reliably, b) are not exceptionally rare, c) have a specific time course that includes a return to baseline state, d) abate with readministration of the drug, e) are due to deprivation of a specific substance, and f) appear to be clinically significant. Below, I touch only briefly on what remains the most controversial issue regarding cannabis withdrawal, determining whether it is of "clinical significance." The lack of an operational definition of clinical significance, and the absence of studies that directly address this concept, are problematic. Nonetheless, some data suggest that the syndrome has clinical importance. First, DSM-IV requires two to four symptoms for diagnoses of different substance withdrawal syndromes. Extant research indicates that the majority of daily cannabis users report experiencing multiple withdrawal symptoms. Second, quasi-experimental data comparing tobacco withdrawal with cannabis withdrawal suggest that the magnitude and time course of abstinence effects are comparable to those in the well-established tobacco withdrawal syndrome.[21] Third, abstinence symptoms are observable to people living with cannabis users who report withdrawal, and the comments of these observers suggest that symptoms are disruptive to daily living.[1,22] Fourth, some cannabis users report using to "relieve withdrawal symptoms," which suggests that withdrawal contributes to ongoing use of cannabis.[5,23–25] Finally, the majority of individuals enrolled in treatment for cannabis dependence acknowledge withdrawal symptoms, label at least some of them as moderate to severe, and complain that they make cessation more difficult.[12,14,15] In summary, several lines of evidence indicate that cannabis withdrawal can cause significant distress and may undermine successful abstinence; however, an adequate test of whether such distress influences quit attempts or relapse is not yet available.

Table 14–1 lists symptoms that should be considered as a criteria list for a cannabis withdrawal disorder in the next version of DSM. Exactly how many symptoms might need to be endorsed is not clear, but endorsement of at least three and reporting that these cause significant distress could reasonably be considered as sufficient to warrant a diagnosis of cannabis withdrawal.

TABLE 14–1. Proposed withdrawal symptom list for DSM-V

Common symptoms
Anger or aggression
Decreased appetite or weight loss
Irritability
Nervousness/anxiety
Restlessness
Sleep difficulties, including strange dreaming
Less common/equivocal symptoms
Chills
Depressed mood
Stomach pain
Shakiness
Sweating

Before concluding this discussion of cannabis withdrawal, I should note that DSM-IV is not clear about what to do when an individual responds affirmatively to dependence criterion 2a (withdrawal) for a substance that does not have an accepted withdrawal syndrome. That is, should this criterion be assessed and counted in determining dependence diagnoses and severity? The discussion of dependence criterion 2a (p. 194) implies that it can be assessed and counted, yet the listing of dependence criteria (p. 197) indicates that 2a should be assessed using the criteria sets from the drug-specific withdrawal disorder, of which there are none for cannabis.

Finally, and relevant to the issue of whether different diagnostic criteria are needed for different substances, withdrawal symptoms commonly observed in cannabis withdrawal have a great deal of overlap with those of most others. Although each substance withdrawal syndrome has one or two unique symptoms, designation of those specific effects is not necessary for a diagnosis of withdrawal. For example, two of the alcohol withdrawal criteria are grand mal seizures and transient hallucinations, which occur infrequently; however, one can be diagnosed with alcohol withdrawal by manifesting the more commonly observed symptoms of insomnia, anxiety, and nausea, which are shared symptoms of most withdrawal syndromes. Similar scenarios and diagnoses made based solely on withdrawal symptoms shared across substances are highly probable with other substances such as opioids and amphetamines. Hence, the current formulation of withdrawal disorders in DSM lists specific criteria for the different substances, of which a few are unique to that substance; however, withdrawal diagnoses can be made without observation of the unique effects.

A related point to be considered here has been discussed previously by others.[26–28] Historically, withdrawal (and consequently dependence) has been defined by distinct physical or medical conditions observed with severe opioid-dependent individuals, such that establishing alcohol, cocaine, or sedative dependence and withdrawal as true disorders was difficult and took many years.[26] Eventually, it was accepted that such distinct physical symptoms were not necessary to diagnose withdrawal or dependence. Recent studies with animals suggest that the core symptoms of withdrawal may be the emotional and behavioral symptoms associated with abstinence-related neurobiological changes in the limbic system, and these may be more important in precipitating dependence or relapse than what might be thought of as traditional physical symptoms of withdrawal.[28] These emotional and behavioral effects are the withdrawal symptoms that are common across substances, including cannabis. Accordingly, consideration might be given to removing the DSM dependence specifier "with or without physiological dependence," in order to eliminate the implication that physical/medical symptoms of withdrawal are the sole indicators of "physical" dependence. If the reason for the existing specifier is to alert clinicians to potential consequences of withdrawal, then why not change the specifier to indicate this clearly (e.g., designate "with or without significant withdrawal")? This change might have more clinical relevance and would remove the implication that important withdrawal effects are only those that are medical/physical as opposed to emotional/behavioral.

Cannabis Dependence Diagnostic Criteria

Since 1994 a number of investigators have examined the stability and construct validity of the cannabis dependence diagnosis. These studies employ a wide range of sampling strategies and analytical methodologies, each with its own important limitations. Remarkably, with few exceptions, the findings appear to converge and indicate that diagnosis of cannabis dependence using DSM criteria tends to be stable, utilizes the relatively full range of dependence criteria, and appears to be unidimensional, i.e., best defined by a single factor. In summary, the generic DSM dependence criteria seem to perform as well for cannabis as they do for most other substance dependence disorders (see Table 14–2 for DSM-IV-TR criteria). Below I provide a brief review of selected studies on the diagnosis of cannabis and other substance dependence.

EPIDEMIOLOGICAL STUDIES

Morgenstern and colleagues, using the Composite International Diagnostic Interview (CIDI),[29] obtained DSM-IV substance dependence diagnoses in 292 adults enrolled in one of seven inpatient or outpatient substance abuse treatment centers.[30] All participants met criteria for at least one dependence diagnosis; however, substance-specific dependence criteria were assessed for all substances used more than six times. Factor analysis indicated that a one-factor solution provided a good fit for the 202 identified cannabis users, with all seven DSM-IV criteria factor loadings above 0.73 (range: 0.73–091). The other dependence diagnoses (alcohol

TABLE 14–2. DSM-IV-TR substance dependence and abuse criteria

Dependence
Tolerance
Withdrawal
Using for a longer period of time or more than intended
Persistent desire or unsuccessful efforts to quit or cut down
Considerable time spent buying, using, or recovering from the effects
Important activities are given up because of use
Continued use despite persistent or recurrent psychological or physical problems related to use
Abuse
Recurrent use results in failure to fulfill major role obligations
Recurrent use in situations that are physically hazardous
Recurrent legal problems related to use
Continued use despite persistent social or interpersonal problems related to use

cocaine, stimulants, opiates, sedatives, hallucinogens) provided similar factor solutions, with the exception of hallucinogens. The proportion of variance accounted for by the one-factor model was 67.4% for cannabis—the lowest proportion among all the substances other than hallucinogens. However, alcohol (68.1%), sedatives (69.2%), stimulants (71.8%), and cocaine (78.6%) had very comparable proportions. The authors asserted strong support for the DSM-IV approach for diagnosing a unidimensional dependence syndrome across substances, including cannabis.

Feingold and Rounsaville analyzed CIDI data from 394 adults either who met one of the DSM-IV dependence criteria for cannabis or who identified themselves as regular cannabis users during some period of their lifetime.[31] The sample was drawn from multiple sources: inpatient and outpatient drug treatment centers, outpatient psychiatric clinic, and a random sample from the general population. Frequency distribution of the lifetime cannabis dependence criteria spanned the entire range from 0 to 7, but very few individuals (3%) met six or seven criteria. Note that for cannabis, this distribution was skewed to the low end of dependence severity compared with cocaine, alcohol, and opioids, and appeared comparable to that of sedatives and stimulants. A factor analysis constrained to a one-factor solution resulted in factor loadings of 0.55–0.80 for all items, with the exception of withdrawal. This was similar to the factor loadings observed with other substances examined, leading the authors to conclude that the DSM-IV dependence items formed a unidimensional construct within each dependence disorder, including cannabis.

Swift and colleagues assessed 243 long-term cannabis users in Australia, using a "snowball" sampling method to identify networks of cannabis users.[10] Using a semi-structured interview, they found that 57% met DSM-III-R lifetime criteria for dependence. Endorsement of the nine dependence criteria ranged from 5% (withdrawal) to 72% (intoxication during daily activities), indicating that some criteria were much more common than others. Cronbach alpha for the nine dependence items was only 0.59. Principal components factor analysis of the dependence items did not reveal a robust single-factor solution. Rather, a behavioral/compulsive use factor explained 35% of the variance, a tolerance/withdrawal factor explained 16%, and a frequent intoxication factor explained 13%. This study was the only one among the studies reviewed reporting that a one-factor solution did not fit well with the dependence criteria. In a second study, Swift et al. used an abbreviated version of the CIDI to assess DSM-III-R cannabis dependence in a convenience sample of 200 long-term heavy cannabis users at baseline and 1 year later.[11] The great majority (70% and 77%) met criteria for cannabis dependence at times 1 and 2, respectively. The percentage that endorsed each dependence criterion varied from 44% to 60%, suggesting that all symptoms were related to the dependence construct.

Nelson and colleagues used a semistructured interview to assess DSM-IV cannabis dependence in a sample of 519 cannabis users who reported using cannabis at least six times in their lifetime.[32] Participants were drawn from five countries across six sites and included adults from alcohol and drug treatment settings, mental health clinics, general medical clinics, and the general population. Endorsement of the seven dependence items for the past year ranged from 13% to 29%, with the most frequent being "unsuccessful attempts to cut down" and the least frequent being "continued use despite problems." Exploratory principal components factor analyses identified a single-factor solution. Confirmatory factor analyses showed all seven cannabis dependence criteria loading onto the single factor, with factor loadings ranging from 0.82 to 0.93. The authors compared the factor structures across cannabis, opiate, cocaine, and alcohol dependence (each dependence disorder assessed using parallel methods). Although some substances had substantially higher or lower loadings for specific criteria, the authors concluded that the dependence syndromes appeared comparable in structure. Note that the overall number of cannabis dependence items endorsed was skewed toward the lower end of the distribution relative to that for cocaine and opiates and was comparable to that for alcohol.

Swift and colleagues used a large general population sample to identify 722 adults who had used cannabis at least five times during the previous year.[33] Good evidence for the internal consistency of DSM-IV cannabis dependence criteria was obtained using the CIDI to diagnose dependence during the preceding 12 months. Among these cannabis users, an overall Cronbach alpha of 0.75 was observed among the seven dependence items. Among the 150 dependent users i.e., (met at least three criteria), the endorsement rate across criteria was between 10% and 89%, with "withdrawal and persistent desire to control use" being the highest, and "important activities reduced" the lowest. Among the 572 nondependent cannabis users, the range was 0.5%–23%, with "persistent desire to control use" and "withdrawal" being the highest, and "great deal of time spent" being the lowest.

Using the same sample as Swift et al., Teesson and colleagues examined the discriminatory power of the 11 DSM-IV substance abuse and dependence criteria in 722 Australian adults who reported using cannabis more than five times in the past 12 months.[34] One-factor and two-factor models representing alternative hypotheses were tested. The one-factor model assumed that abuse and dependence criteria are reflections of the same underlying factor (i.e., vulnerability to cannabis use disorders), and the two-factor model assumed separate yet correlated factors representing abuse and dependence. Both models fit the data well, and an extremely high correlation was observed between the factors in the two-factor model. Hence, the authors argued for a single underlying dimension. Nine of the 11 criteria had factor loadings of greater than 0.73; only the "legal problems and use in hazardous situations" (both abuse items) showed low reliability/validity. Criterion characteristic curves were then used to determine how well individual items discriminated abuse/dependence. "Withdrawal," "repeated attempts to cut down," "tolerance," and "use larger amounts than intended" were the criteria most likely to determine the presence or absence of a disorder. "Legal problems" and "use in hazardous situations" showed low discriminatory power. Indeed, three of the four abuse criteria were poor discriminators of cannabis use disorder and were associated with more severe, rather than less severe, problems.

Langenbucher and colleagues analyzed CIDI–Substance Abuse Module data on alcohol, cannabis and cocaine abuse and dependence criteria from 372 adults involved in treatment for substance dependence.[35] Factor analysis of the 11 DSM-IV abuse and dependence criterion items yielded similar solutions for the three substances, one main factor and a second weaker factor. The "tolerance" dependence item and "legal problems" abuse item were responsible for the poor fit to a unidimensional solution. Subsequent item response theory analyses showed that diagnostic criteria differed from one another in threshold for discriminating DSM-IV diagnoses, but such between-criteria differences in threshold did not mirror the specifications of DSM-IV. That is, across the three substances, dependence criteria did not reliably discriminate more severe substance problems. A number of the abuse and dependence items provided the same discriminatory information about severity of the problem, and as such the validity of the contention that the dependence criteria reflect a distinct and more severe problem than the abuse criteria was not supported strongly. In summary, the cannabis diagnosis items performed similarly to alcohol and cocaine items in this study; however, for all three substances there appeared to be limitations in the items' discriminatory function, raising questions about the construct validity of the diagnostic criteria.

ADULTS SEEKING TREATMENT FOR CANNABIS DEPENDENCE

Three clinical studies of adults seeking treatment specifically for cannabis dependence provide descriptive information on rates of endorsement of dependence criteria. Unfortunately, no factor-analytical or inter-item correlation analyses of these data have been reported. Budney and colleagues reported on 62 adults seeking outpatient treatment for cannabis dependence.[25] These outpatients endorsed a mean of 6.3 of the 9 DSM-III-R criteria, with the most frequent being "use despite recurrent problems" (97%) and "repeated desire/effort to cut down" (86%) and the least frequent being "reducing/giving up important activities" (41%) and "frequent intoxication or hazardous use" (53%). Rates of endorsement were compared with those from a cocaine treatment sample. The cocaine sample endorsed significantly more criteria on average (7.7 versus 6.3), with significant differences observed for three specific items ("reducing/giving up important activities," "excessive time spent," and "use of larger amounts than intended").

Stephens and colleagues reported similar observations in a much larger sample of adults seeking treatment for cannabis dependence (N=450).[12] These outpatients endorsed a mean of 5.6 of the 7 DSM-IV criteria. Unsuccessful attempts to "quit/cut down" (96%) and "use despite recurrent problems" (95%) were the most frequently endorsed, and "reducing/giving up important activities" (64%) and "tolerance" (68%) were the least frequent. Data from a third sample of 90 adults seeking treatment for cannabis dependence provided further replication of rates of endorsement of cannabis dependence criteria.[36] This sample endorsed a mean of 4.8 of the 7 DSM-IV criteria, with the most frequent being "use despite recurrent problems" (88%) and "repeated desire/effort to cut down" (86%), and the least frequent being "reducing/giving up important activities" (48%) and "withdrawal" (62%). In summary, adults seeking treatment for cannabis endorse the full range of the cannabis dependence criteria, suggesting that the criteria characterize the disorder adequately.

Concluding Comments and Questions for Future Research

This selective review and discussion of the cannabis withdrawal and dependence diagnosis literature provides some insights regarding the validity and utility of using generic versus specific criteria for substance dependence. Here I summarize the primary findings and highlight questions for future research (see Table 14–3).

Adoption of cannabis withdrawal into DSM appears warranted and as such adds to a growing literature indicating that cannabis dependence is most comparable to other substance dependence disorders. Inclusion of cannabis withdrawal would remove the ambiguity in DSM regarding how to utilize withdrawal symptoms reported by cannabis users when formulating a diagnosis. This would also eliminate one of the discrepancies in substance use disorders between the DSM and ICD nosologies. Moreover, recognition of the potential clinical importance of withdrawal syndromes such as cannabis that do not have prominent physical/medical sequelae raises the aforementioned concern about the utility, value, and implication of using the dependence specifier term "with physiological dependence." Would not the use

TABLE 14–3. Summary points

1. Cannabis dependence is more similar to than different from other substance dependence disorders, which lends supports to the use of generic dependence criteria.
2. Adoption of cannabis withdrawal into DSM appears warranted and would remove ambiguity in DSM.
3. Use of a specifier such as "with significant withdrawal" rather than "with physiological dependence" might describe more accurately an important component of the dependence construct and have better clinical utility.
4. Cannabis dependence appears unidimensional (i.e., best defined by one factor) when examined with DSM criteria across multiple studies using diverse methodologies.
5. Cannabis dependence appears to be less "severe" than other major substance dependence disorders such as alcohol, cocaine or opiate dependence.
6. The generic DSM-IV criteria may not discriminate cases in a manner consistent with the underlying constructs of abuse and dependence.
7. Testing whether requiring specific criterion items for particular dependence disorders would enhance sensitivity or specificity of case identification appears warranted.
8. Testing whether the number of criteria required for a dependence diagnosis, and dependence severity indicators, should be substance specific appears warranted.
9. New analytical methods offer exciting opportunities to evaluate and improve our understanding of substance dependence and the criteria we use to define this construct.

of "with significant withdrawal" have more clinical utility, while not contributing inadvertently to the perception that physical/medical symptoms of withdrawal are the sole indicators of "physical dependence"? The differentiation between "physical" and "psychological" dependence is arbitrary and merely contributes to misconceptions about the nature and severity of substance dependence disorders.

If one accepts the assertion that cannabis dependence is more similar to than different from the other major substance dependence disorders, then the research presented here supports the concept of using generic dependence criteria across substances. That said, there appear to be convergent data suggesting that across substances, the generic DSM-IV criteria may not discriminate cases in a way that is consistent with the construct of abuse and dependence as understood implicitly in the context of DSM.[34,35] The factor structure and discriminatory power of the specific criterion items indicate that some items do not perform as would be expected.

Muthén (see Chapter 1, "Should Substance Use Disorders Be Considered Categorical or Dimensional," in this volume) reports similar findings and provides guidance on innovative statistical methods to study further the construct and discriminant validity of the diagnostic criteria. Thus, although the generic dependence criteria perform similarly across substances, it would appear that different generic criteria or use of substance-specific criteria might improve the validity and utility of our dependence diagnostic system. Additional studies are necessary to provide a more well-informed answer to the generic versus specific criteria question.

What is not addressed adequately by existing studies and yet seems critical is whether requiring specific items for a particular dependence diagnosis would improve sensitivity or specificity of case identification, or would enhance clinical practice by focusing attention on important symptoms of a specific dependence disorder. To some extent, this issue is currently addressed by DSM in the features section of the general substance dependence section (pp. 192–193) and in the introductory paragraph for each dependence disorder. Examining how specific dependence criteria algorithms perform compared with the current generic system would provide important empirical data relevant to the question at hand. Related to this issue, if one decided to use specific criteria for each substance or to weight criteria differently for specific substances, what data would be appropriate to guide these decisions: data from samples with a wide range of use and dependence or from clinical samples with a more restricted range? The studies reviewed for the paper on which this chapter is based showed that a specific dependence symptom can load highly in a one-factor solution in one study, whereas the same symptom can have a much lower rank loading in another study. With this in mind, the desired specificity and sensitivity of the diagnostic criteria might differ depending on the purpose of making the diagnosis. Would the same specificity and sensitivity rates be desirable for clinician use in a treatment setting versus use in epidemiological or genetic classification studies?

The cross-substance comparisons reviewed here suggest that cannabis dependence or withdrawal is similar to but typically less "severe" than that associated with major substances such as alcohol, cocaine and opiates. This leads to the question of whether dependence severity should be quantified similarly across substances. That is, would it be valid and useful to designate that severe cannabis dependence might range from four to six symptoms, whereas severe cocaine dependence would require six to seven? Similarly, one must consider whether the dependence cut-off criterion of three or more items is equally valid across all substances. Few data are available that address this issue directly.

Finally, I offer a few reminders of the limitations of the research reviewed herein. Although there appears to be some convergence of findings across the dependence criteria literature, many major methodological differences across studies are apparent. This raises multiple questions. For example, how does the use of samples with varying ranges of cannabis use (e.g., general population with relatively low rates of dependence versus treatment sample with the majority having dependence) differentially affect factor-analytical results? Moreover, none of the large cross-substance comparison studies have examined "pure" samples of participants seeking treatment for a specific substance dependence problem. How do differing methods for assessing symptoms affect outcome? For example, with cannabis, if the wording used to assess withdrawal does not capture the emotional or behavioral aspects of the syndrome (i.e., irritability, sleep difficulties, appetite change), interviewees may provide a negative response either because they have only a traditional understanding of withdrawal as a purely physical phenomenon (shakes, severe nausea or vomiting, etc.) or because they hold the common belief that cannabis cessation does (should) not produce withdrawal. Finally, I remind the reader that one common dependence disorder, nicotine dependence, was not addressed in any of the comparative studies reviewed here. More comment on how the nicotine dependence literature informs the question of using generic versus specific criteria is offered by Hughes in Chapter 15 ("Should Criteria for Drug Dependence Differ Across Drugs?") in this volume.

Conclusion

Cannabis has dependence potential and an associated dependence syndrome that is certainly more similar to than different from the more recognized substance dependence syndromes. The evolution of our knowledge of cannabis, as it has undergone careful study in the human and clinical laboratories, appears to have taken a similar course to most other misused substances. The dependence syndrome of cannabis appears to have the same properties as the other more established dependence syndromes, and DSM-IV captures all aspects of the syndrome. What is not as clear is whether modifying the extant criteria by weighting specific items for specific substances, including or excluding new items, changing the requirements for meeting dependence criteria, or having differing guidelines for characterizing severity across specific dependence syndromes, has validity or utility. That is, the use of generic DSM-IV criteria appears to work as well for cannabis as for other substances, yet the more important question might be: can we do better by developing more sophisticated generic criteria or specific criteria for all substance abuse and dependence disorders? New statistical techniques offer exciting analytical methods to explore and evaluate such questions.

References

1. Budney AJ, Moore BA, Vandrey RG, et al: The time course and significance of cannabis withdrawal. J Abnorm Psychol 112:393–402, 2003.
2. Budney AJ, Hughes JR, Moore BA, et al: A review of the validity and significance of the cannabis withdrawal syndrome. Am J Psychiatry 161:1967–1977, 2004.

3. Compton DR, Dewey WL, Martin BR: Cannabis dependence and tolerance production. Adv Alcohol Subst Abuse 9:129–147, 1990.
4. Hall W, Johnston L, Donnelly N: Epidemiology of cannabis use and its consequences, in The Health Effects of Cannabis. Edited by Kalant H, Corrigall WA, Hall W, et al. Toronto, Ontario, Canada, Centre for Addiction and Mental Health, 1999, pp 69–126.
5. Cottler LB, Schuckit MA, Helzer JE, et al: The DSM-IV field trial for substance use disorders: major results. Drug Alcohol Depend 38:59–69, 1995.
6. Anthony JC, Warner LA, Kessler RC: Comparative epidemiology of dependence on tobacco, alcohol, controlled substances and inhalants: basic findings from the National Comorbidity Survey. Exp Clin Psychopharmacol 2:244–268, 1994.
7. Haney M, Comer SD, Ward AS, et al: Abstinence symptoms following oral THC administration to humans. Psychopharmacology 14:385–394, 1999.
8. Haney M, Ward AS, Comer SD, et al: Abstinence symptoms following smoked marijuana in humans. Psychopharmacology 14:395–404, 1999.
9. Kouri EM, Pope HG: Abstinence symptoms during withdrawal from chronic marijuana use. Exp Clin Psychopharmacol 8:483–492, 2000.
10. Swift W, Hall W, Didcott P, et al: Patterns and correlates of cannabis dependence among long-term users in an Australian rural area. Addiction 93:1149–1160, 1998.
11. Swift W, Hall W, Copeland J: One year follow-up of cannabis dependence among long-term users in Sydney, Australia. Drug Alcohol Depend 59:309–318, 2000.
12. Stephens RS, Babor TF, Kadden R, et al: The Marijuana Treatment Project: rationale, design, and participant characteristics. The Marijuana Treatment Project Research Group. Addiction 97:109–124, 2002.
13. Stephens RS, Roffman RA, Simpson EE: Adult marijuana users seeking treatment. J Consult Clin Psychol 61:1100–1104, 1993.
14. Copeland J, Swift W, Rees V: Clinical profile of participants in a brief intervention program for cannabis use disorder. J Subst Abuse Treat 20:45–52, 2001.
15. Budney AJ, Higgins ST, Radonovich KJ, et al: Adding voucher-based incentives to coping skills and motivational enhancement improves outcomes during treatment for marijuana dependence. J Consult Clin Psychol 68:1051–1061, 2000.
16. Budney AJ, Novy P, Hughes JR: Marijuana withdrawal among adults seeking treatment for marijuana dependence. Addiction 94:1311–1322, 1999.
17. Young SE, Corley RP, Stallings MC, et al: Substance use, abuse and dependence in adolescence: prevalence, symptom profiles and correlates. Drug Alcohol Depend 68:309–322, 2002.
18. Crowley TJ, Macdonald MJ, Whitmore EA, et al: Cannabis dependence, withdrawal, and reinforcing effects among adolescents with conduct disorder symptoms and substance use disorders. Drug Alcohol Depend 50:27–37, 1998.
19. Mikulich SK, Hall SK, Whitmore EA, et al: Concordance between DSM-III-R and DSM-IV diagnoses of substance use disorders in adolescents. Drug Alcohol Depend 61:237–248, 2001.
20. Vandrey R, Budney AJ, Kamon JL, et al: Cannabis withdrawal in adolescent treatment seekers. Drug Alcohol Depend 78:205–210, 2005.
21. Vandrey RG, Budney AJ, Moore BA, et al: A cross-study comparison of cannabis and tobacco withdrawal. Am J Addict 14:54–63, 2005.

22. Budney AJ, Hughes JR, Moore BA, et al: Marijuana abstinence effects in marijuana smokers maintained in their usual living environment. Arch Gen Psychiatry 58:917–924, 2001.
23. Coffey C, Carlin JB, Degenhardt L, et al: Cannabis dependence in young adults: an Australian population study. Addiction 97:187–194, 2002.
24. Winters KC, Latimer W, Stinchfield RD: The DSM-IV criteria for adolescent alcohol and cannabis use disorders. J Stud Alcohol 60:337–344, 1999.
25. Budney AJ, Radonovich KJ, Higgins ST, et al: Adults seeking treatment for marijuana dependence: a comparison to cocaine-dependent treatment seekers. Exp Clin Psychopharmacol 6:419–426, 1998.
26. Edwards G: Withdrawal symptoms and alcohol dependence: fruitful mysteries. Br J Addict 85:447–461, 1990.
27. Hughes JR, Higgins ST, Bickel WK: Nicotine withdrawal versus other drug withdrawal syndromes: similarities and dissimilarities. Addiction 89:1461–1470, 1994.
28. Koob GF, LeMoal M: Drug addiction, dysregulation of reward, and allostasis. Neuropsychopharmacology 24:97–129, 2001.
29. Cottler LB, Robins LN, Helzer JE: The reliability of the CIDI-SAM: a comprehensive substance abuse interview. Br J Addict 84:801–814, 1989.
30. Morgenstern J, Langenbucher J, Labouvie EW: The generalizability of the dependence syndrome across substances: an examination of some properties of the proposed DSM-IV dependence criteria. Addiction 89:1105–1113, 1994.
31. Feingold A, Rounsaville B: Construct validity of the dependence syndrome as measured by DSM-IV for different psychoactive substances. Addiction 90:1661– 1669, 1995.
32. Nelson CB, Rehm J, Üstün TB, et al: Factor structures for DSM-IV substance disorder criteria endorsed by alcohol, cannabis, cocaine and opiate users: results from the WHO reliability and validity study. Addiction 94:843–855, 1999.
33. Swift W, Hall W, Teesson M: Characteristics of DSM-IV and ICD-10 cannabis dependence among Australian adults: results from the National Survey of Mental Health and Wellbeing. Drug Alcohol Depend 63:147–153, 2001.
34. Teesson M, Lynskey M, Manor B, et al: The structure of cannabis dependence in the community. Drug Alcohol Depend 68:255–262, 2002.
35. Langenbucher JW, Labouvie E, Martin CS, et al: An application of item response theory analysis to alcohol, cannabis, and cocaine criteria in DSM-IV. J Abnorm Psychol 113:72–80, 2004.
36. Budney AJ, Moore BA, Higgins ST, et al: Clinical trial of abstinence-based vouchers and cognitive-behavior therapy for marijuana dependence. J Consult Clin Psychol 74: 307–316, 2006.

15

SHOULD CRITERIA FOR DRUG DEPENDENCE DIFFER ACROSS DRUGS?

John R. Hughes, M.D.

Syndromal criteria for drug dependence in the 1980 *Diagnostic and Statistical Manual of Mental Disorders,* 3rd Edition (DSM-III), differed across drugs.[1] The conceptualization that all drugs had several common features[2,3] led to the use of the same criteria for dependence for all drugs and was adopted in DSM-III-R[4] in 1987, in the *International Classification of Diseases,* 10th Revision (ICD-10),[5] in 1992 and continued in DSM-IV[6] in 1994. These "generic" criteria were based mainly on observations of those dependent on alcohol and opiates.[7] Although several studies and reviews have examined whether these criteria are applicable to other drugs of dependence,[8–17] none have directly addressed the question of whether generic or drug-specific criteria have more utility.

In this chapter, I review existing data that bear on this question by examining the specific example of nicotine versus alcohol and opiate use/dependence (specif-

---

Writing of this article was supported by Senior Scientist Award DA-00490 from the National Institute on Drug Abuse. I thank Jack Henningfield for helpful comments.

Reprinted from Hughes JR: "Should Criteria for Drug Dependence Differ Across Drugs?" *Addiction* 101 (suppl 1):134–141, 2006. Used with permission of the Society for the Study of Addiction.

ically, the review focuses on nicotine dependence via cigarettes, as this is the most common form[18]). However, a similar exercise could occur comparing marijuana versus sedative dependence or hallucinogen versus amphetamine dependence, and so forth.

Do Experts Act as If All Drug Use/Dependence Is the Same?

There are many examples of scientists treating different drug use/dependencies as if they were similar.[19] For example, the U.S. National Institute on Drug Abuse (NIDA) has for many years included nicotine within its mandate to treat "drug abuse" (http://www.nida.nih.gov). The U.S. Surgeon General collated several lines of evidence that nicotine dependence was similar to other drug dependencies.[16] The U.S. Food and Drug Administration (FDA) sought to regulate nicotine as a drug dependency.[20]

On the other hand, many experts appear to recognize differences in drug use/dependence. For example, the terms *drug abuse* and *drug dependence* usually exclude nicotine. Among articles with the term *drug abuse* or *drug dependence* in their titles in the journal *Addiction* in 1994, 73% discussed illicit drugs, 60% discussed alcohol, but only 20% discussed nicotine.[21] Also, several of the most widely used interviews for psychiatric diagnosis—for example, the Structured Clinical Interview for DSM-IV Axis I Disorders (SCID)—include alcohol and illicit drugs but not nicotine.[22] As another example, the World Health Organization's Mental Health Survey reported worldwide rates of "drug dependence" yet failed to even mention that these did not include nicotine, evidently assuming that readers would know that the term did not refer to nicotine dependence.[23]

Similarities Between Nicotine and Alcohol/Opiate Use and Dependence

This common exclusion of nicotine dependence from consideration when discussing drug dependence is probably due to several differences between nicotine and non-nicotine drug dependencies (Table 15–1). To help put these differences into context, I begin this chapter with a discussion of similarities between nicotine and alcohol/opiate dependence. The more commonly listed similarities are that both nicotine and non-nicotine drugs induce a) self-administration in nonhumans, b) subjective effects, c) compulsive use, d) impaired control, e) continued use despite harmful effects, f) high and rapid rates of relapse after an attempt to stop, g) tolerance, h) withdrawal, and i) rapid reinstatement upon lapsing.[16] In addition, both nicotine and non-nicotine drugs of dependence j) cause dependence via effects on

TABLE 15–1. Similarities and differences between nicotine and alcohol/opiate dependence

Similarities	Differences	Unclear if similar or different
Compulsive use*	Dependence rare in adult non-daily users	Frequency and rapidity of release
Continued use despite harm*	Does not cause other mental disorders	Incidence of spontaneous remission
Highly conditionable Impaired control over drug use	Forgo activities to use rare* High intensity of use	Nondopaminergic neurotransmitter systems involved
Influenced by genotype	Little euphoria Lots of time with drug rare*	Rate of postdependence controlled use
Mediated via dopamine release	No behavioral intoxication	
Rapid relapse	Prosocial beneficial effects	
Rapid reinstatement		
Serves as reinforcer in nonhumans		
Subjective effects		
Tolerance*		
Withdrawal*		

*DSM/ICD criteria.

dopaminergic systems, k) are highly conditionable, and l) are influenced by genotype.[16] Finally, the strong association of nicotine dependence with non-nicotine drug dependence[24–26] and the fact that much of the heritability of non-nicotine drug use is shared with that for nicotine use[27] support a commonality notion. These similarities are not trivial and have been described in more detail elsewhere.[16,28–31]

Differences Between Nicotine Versus Alcohol and Opiate Dependence

Comparing drug dependencies is common (Table 15–2), but can be misleading because the tendency is to attribute differences in dependencies to differences in the pharmacology of the drugs. In reality, the differences may be more due to the preexisting characteristics of people who chose to become dependent on one drug versus another. For example, those who become dependent on illicit drugs differ from those who become dependent on nicotine in sex ratio, age, employment, and so forth.[12] Unfortunately, most studies comparing drugs confuse between- and within-person variability. One method to minimize this confusion is to compare various dependencies within the same person—for example, among those who simultaneously have both alcohol and nicotine dependence, do self-rated compulsion to use and inability to quit alcohol and nicotine appear to be similar?[32]

The major difference between nicotine and alcohol/ opiate dependencies is that nicotine dependence almost never causes adverse behavioral outcomes.[33] Although it is possible that a smoker would lose a job or become divorced over his or her smoking, this appears to be rare. In addition, unlike alcohol and opiate dependence, nicotine dependence does not appear to be a proximal cause of violence, child neglect, and so forth. This difference was recognized by ICD-9, when it included tobacco dependence under "non-dependent abuse of drugs" because "tobacco differs from other drugs of dependence in its psychotoxic effects.[34,p.199] Also consistent with this notion, nicotine is the only drug of dependence in DSM that does not have a) a diagnosis of intoxication, b) any drug-induced mental disorders and c) an abuse diagnosis.[35] In fact, this lack of behavioral harm has been thought to contribute to the development of nicotine dependence because it allow users to imbibe large amounts of nicotine for long periods of time without interference in life tasks.[36] This lack of behavioral harm also is probably a major reason that nicotine dependence was for so long not recognized as a dependence.[36] This is because the recognition of drug disorders is mainly via psychiatrists and other behavioral clinicians whose responsibility is for behavioral, not physical, abnormalities. Also, one can argue that much of society's response to drug problems is a reaction to behavioral, not physical, harm from drug use.[37] This relative lack of adverse behavioral outcomes does not mean that nicotine dependence is not clinically significant. Clinical significance is defined in DSM-IV-TR[35] as "present distress…or disability…or…significantly increased risk of suffering death…or an important loss of freedom" (p. xxxi). Clearly, nicotine dependence applies to the latter two.

A second, related difference is that although some nicotine users describe nicotine as producing euphoria,[38] most smokers describe the subjective effects of nicotine in terms of improving their functioning (i.e., improved concentration; decreased stress, anxiety, or depression; decreased anger or hunger).[39] It is controversial whether these effects represent the reversal of withdrawal effects[40–42] or true enhancement effects.[16,39,40,43] Either way, most smokers describe their reason for using nicotine much more as drug use to improve function than as drug use to produce a pleasant state.[44]

A third difference is the intensity of use. Few adult cigarette users are nondaily smokers.[18] In daily smokers, nicotine is self-administered over 200 times/day (20 cigarettes/day times 10 puffs/cigarette), 365 days/year. Smoking may be one of the most frequent and enduring behaviors in humans.[36] Thus, the chance for automa-

TABLE 15–2. Rankings of dependence criteria

Criterion	Basis	Nicotine	Alcohol	Opiate	Cocaine
Dependence among users (Anthony et al. 1999)	Data	4	3	1	2
Difficulty abstaining (Hunt et al. 1971[54])	Data	4	4	4	4
Liking by non-abusers (U.S. Surgeon General 1988)	Data	2	3	2	4
Prevalence of dependence (Anthony et al. 1994[12])	Data	4	3	1	2
Self-reported addictiveness (Kozlowski et al. 1989[32])	Data	4	1	3	2
Animal self-administration (U.S. Surgeon General 1988)	Subjective	2	2	3	4
Behavioral disruption (Hughes 2001[36])	Subjective	1	4	3	2
Tolerance (Kalant et al. 1971[78])	Subjective	3	4	4	3
Withdrawal (Hughes and Howard 94[21])	Subjective	2	4	3	1

ticity factors[45] to become prominent in nicotine dependence may be much greater than for other drugs of dependence.

A fourth difference is that it appears that dependence is rare among adult nondaily users of nicotine,[46] whereas it is common among nondaily users of alcohol and opiates.[35] This could be because nicotine dependence may be more related to physical dependence (i.e., withdrawal) and physical dependence may require daily dosing; however, whether or not this is true is unclear.[47]

A fifth difference is that the neurobiological effects of nicotine and non-nicotine drugs differ. For example, opiates produce an overflow of dopamine outside the nucleus accumbens that is associated with euphoria and potentiates drug reinforcement, whereas this effect is very small with nicotine.[48] Also, nicotine has the ability to potentiate the reinforcing effects of non-drug reinforcers; this has not been demonstrated for opiates.[48] Also, unlike opiates, nicotine desensitizes receptors, increases receptor number, and has biphasic effects on receptors.[22]

Some comparisons of nicotine versus alcohol/opiate dependencies have been used to argue that nicotine dependence appears to be so dissimilar to other drug dependencies that it is not really a drug dependence.[49,50] This logic is false, because as long as a drug dependence conforms to the central feature of drug dependence (i.e., in DSM-IV-TR: continued "the use of substance despite significant substance-related problems"[35,p.192]), exactly how that is manifested does not challenge the validity of its standing as a drug dependence per se. Many plants and animals in the same phylum on the surface appear very different but are grouped together due to sharing a central feature.

Similarities or Differences?

There are several areas in which it is unclear whether nicotine dependence does or does not differ from alcohol/opiate dependencies. Although the most popular theories of nicotine, alcohol, and opiate dependence posit dopamine release as a common pathway,[51] recent work has suggested that nicotine's effects on nondopaminergic systems, such as noradrenergic and glutaminergic systems may be as important in nicotine dependence[52]; however, nondopaminergic systems also appear important in alcohol and opiate dependence.[53] An early study suggested the relapse curves from attempts to stop nicotine, alcohol, and opiates are similar[54]; however, this study was of a small selected group of subjects, and a replication has not been published. Although cross-study comparisons suggest that the rates of spontaneous remissions for nicotine versus alcohol and opiate dependencies appear roughly similar,[55] studies have not examined the rates of remission between nicotine and alcohol/opiate dependencies within the same population using similar definitions of remission. Whether the rate of conversion from dependence to controlled drug use is similar between nicotine and alcohol/opiate dependence also has not been examined.[55] Although high rates of reinstatement after a lapse were first described for alcohol and opiates,[2] the rapidity and inevitability of nicotine reinstatement are as great as, and may actually be greater than, those for alcohol and opiates.[56]

Are Some Generic Dependence Criteria Not Applicable to Nicotine?

Four of the DSM/ICD generic criteria appear to be readily applicable to nicotine: withdrawal, compulsive use, difficulty controlling use, and use despite harm.[29] On the other hand, because the DSM/ICD criteria were developed based mainly on observations of alcohol and opiate users, four criteria do not appear to apply.[29] First, although *tolerance* can refer to tolerance to the aversive effects of the drug, in discussions of drug dependence it refers more often to a diminution in reinforcing or subjective effects over time and a resultant escalation of use over time. Adult nicotine users do not readily endorse the concept that they have to use more nicotine than they did a few years ago to obtain the same positive subjective effects,[57,58] and most do not report increasing use of tobacco after the initial period of use.[16] Second, the generic dependence criterion "using more than intended" typically refers not to using for longer periods of time but to using more than intended on a given occasion.[16] Again, few nicotine users endorse this criterion.[57,58] Third and fourth, the criteria "spending a great deal of time obtaining, using, or recovering from the drug" and "giving up activities to use the drug" are also rarely endorsed.[57,58] This is in part because nicotine is legal and widely available and because it rarely has intoxication effects. The inapplicability of these four criteria is evidenced by the fact that most structured interviews for nicotine dependence have had to use idiosyncratic proxies for these criteria[59,60] (e.g., smoking daily has been used as a proxy for tolerance). Although one could state that the above are not problems with criteria but rather problems with operationalization of criteria, another view is that if one cannot adequately operationalize a criterion, then the criterion is problematic.

If certain generic criteria are not really applicable to nicotine dependence, what would be the major harms in including these criteria in the diagnosis of nicotine dependence? One harm would be that including such items introduces "noise" to the diagnosis decreasing its specificity and sensitivity. Another harm is that if one is using a threshold of number of criteria to make a diagnosis, then having these less relevant criteria effectively changes the threshold across drugs. If one assumes, as argued above, that among the seven DSM criteria, only withdrawal, difficulty controlling use, and use despite harm apply to nicotine dependence, and if one assumes all seven criteria apply to alcohol and opiate dependence, then to fulfill criteria for nicotine dependence, a patient must meet three of three relevant criteria, whereas to fulfill criteria for alcohol/opiate dependence a patient must meet three of seven relevant criteria.

Another potential harm is that maintaining generic criteria may give a false sense of commonality across drugs of dependence. This can lead to invalid statements that impede understanding, policy formation, and treatment. For example, because most non-nicotine drug dependencies cause behavioral harm that results in social problems, accepted treatment for these dependencies includes a significant psychosocial therapy.[61] Many health organizations have reasoned that since smoking is a form of drug dependence, then, as with other drug dependencies, all smokers must have psychosocial therapy and thus require such therapy to obtain medications, treatment reimbursement, and so forth. In fact, most smokers have no social harm from smoking, do not believe they need psychosocial therapy, and will not attend such therapy.[62] More importantly, several meta-analyses have shown that although psychosocial therapy increases quit rates, it is not essential for smokers to quit, and that medications double quit rates independently of whether psychosocial therapy occurs.[63] Thus, generalizing from the treatment of alcohol/ opiate dependence to that for nicotine dependence produced a policy that inhibits smokers from being able to obtain treatment.

Are There Dependence Criteria That Apply Only to Nicotine?

So far in this chapter I have focused on whether the existing DSM/ICD criteria developed for alcohol/opiate dependence apply to nicotine. The converse question is whether there are non-DSM/ICD criteria that would be applicable to nicotine but would not be applicable to alcohol/opiate dependence.

Most of the scales to measure nicotine dependence do not include DSM/ICD criteria.[13,16,64–66] In many public health publications, simple consumption—cigarettes/day—is used as a measure of dependence. In fact, consumption measures are fairly good predictors of ability to abstain, comorbidity, and other outcomes and have outperformed the DSM criteria.[67] In contrast, simple consumption is a poor measure of alcohol and opiate dependence.[68] The most widely used measure of nicotine dependence is the Fagerstrom Test for Nicotine Dependence (FTND).[69] Among its items, the time to the first cigarette is the most robust predictor of ability to abstain and response to treatment.[66]

Interestingly, most clinical studies of nicotine dependence use not DSM or ICD criteria but non-DSM measures. For example, among the 23 clinical trials on nicotine dependence identified by *Index Medicus* in 2004, 18 used a measure of dependence. Of these 18, none used a DSM or ICD measure and 16 used either a consumption or a Fagerstrom measure. Clearly, nicotine researchers are not seeing value in the DSM/ICD system as it is currently proposed. This is probably because the above non-DSM/ICD measures have been validated in several prospective predictive validity tests whereas, strikingly, DSM nicotine dependence performed poorly in validity tests.[64–66] In fact, one study found that both simple cigarettes/day and FTND outperformed DSM in predicting inability to stop smoking.[67]

Conclusion

The use of generic criteria in DSM/ICD was based on an observation of the commonality in the expression of drug dependence across drugs of dependence.[70] Importantly, this commonality is consistent with several other lines of evidence: the association of dependence on one drug with dependence on other drugs,[11] the fact that a shared genotype predicts use of several drugs,[27] and common neurobiological[51] and behavioral[71] causes of drug dependencies.

On the other hand, as documented in this chapter, experts do treat drug dependencies as different and the manifestation of dependence does differ across drugs. In addition, it is implausible that each and every drug of dependence should produce the exact same clinical dependence profile. For this to be true, one would have to assume each drug has the same pharmacological effect or that expression of drug dependence, whatever the inciting drug, occurs via a common final pathway.

The purpose of this review was to discuss the pros and cons of using generic versus drug-specific criteria for dependence. Because drug dependencies have both commonalities and differences, the real question is whether there are sufficient differences to warrant abandoning the generic criteria. In the next subsection, I discuss empirical studies that could be done to determine whether sufficient diversity exists.

SUGGESTIONS FOR FUTURE STUDIES

First, existing and future data sets could be analyzed to further test whether the profile of the rates of endorsement of existing DSM/ICD dependence criteria differs across drugs. For example, is withdrawal very common with nicotine dependence but very rare with cocaine dependence? Although such studies have been conducted,[9–15,17,72] these typically examine across-person rather than within-person dependencies (and are subject to the confounds described earlier) and have used proxies rather than actual DSM/ICD criteria. A finding that the incidences of criteria differ substantially across drugs would suggest that the expression of dependence is not common but rather drug specific.

Second, these same data sets could be used to test whether nicotine dependence has a similar factor structure to non-nicotine dependencies. This review could locate only one comparison of the factor structure of multiple drug dependencies.[9] A finding that drug dependencies have different factor structures would argue for drug-specific criteria.

However, as stated earlier, the important question is not whether there are differences among drugs of dependence but whether these differences are large enough to warrant abandoning the generic criteria now being used. Even if large differences in the above two analyses were found, this would probably not be sufficient. The crucial test would be to show that using drug-specific criteria improves the validity and utility of drug dependence diagnoses to a clinically significant degree.

The major issue in this crucial analysis will be determining the validity and utility criteria. Validation tests proposed for diagnoses have included natural history (e.g., rates of spontaneous remission), familial aggregation, and laboratory tests.[73] Given the rapid progress in genetics in recent years, another important validation tests would be whether the dependence criteria show strong heritabilities.[74] For clinicians, however, one of the most important validation tests is the ability to predict abstinence. Another very important validation test is differential response to treatment (i.e., the extent to which making a diagnosis of dependence allows one to select the best treatment). For example, the drug-specific criteria of time-to-first-cigarette predicts need for treatment and need for higher doses of nicotine medications.[75] Given the small overlap between time-to-first-cigarette and the generic DSM/ICD criteria,[76] it is unclear if generic criteria would do similarly. In summary, the accumulation of evidence that non-generic criteria outperform generic criteria in predicting abstinence or response to treatment would be the most compelling evidence for abandoning generic criteria for nicotine dependence.

CONCLUDING REMARKS

In this chapter, I have focused on the case of nicotine versus non-nicotine drug dependencies and used alcohol and opiate dependence as examples of the latter. Clearly, one could undertake a similar comparison of generic versus drug-specific criteria for cannabis versus other drug dependencies, for cocaine versus alcohol dependence, and so forth, and several authors have already done so.[9,10,12–15,72]

Although abandoning the generic criteria could mean developing specific criteria for each of the 11 drugs of dependence in the existing DSM, the generic system could be changed piecemeal. For example, nicotine could be the only drug to have specific criteria. The major liability with this solution would be that it would suggest nicotine dependence is not a "classical" or "typical" dependence, and some might interpret this to mean it is not a "true" dependence.[49,50] Another possibility is to divide drugs into classes (e.g., stimulants, sedatives and hallucinogens) and have different criteria for different classes.

Finally, a decision on generic versus drug-specific criteria is similar to a decision on whether to keep one disorder or split it into two disorders.[77] Thus, perhaps a first task is to suggest what evidence would be needed to warrant a switch to drug-specific criteria.

The question of generic versus drug-specific criteria in DSM/ICD inevitably raises the question of the utility of the notion of commonalities across drugs.[3,13,37] Currently, many researchers and clinicians believe there is substantial common etiology and expression of dependence across drugs. On the other hand, most social systems believe drug dependencies differ in their manifestations; for example, note the large differences in how governments respond to nicotine versus opioid dependence. However, if a diagnostic system is meant to be "atheoretical" (and one can debate if this is desirable), then it should use the best diagnostic indicators, independent of their implications for theoretical systems.

References

1. American Psychiatric Association: Diagnostic and Statistical Manual of Mental Disorders, 3rd Edition. Washington, DC, American Psychiatric Association, 1980.
2. Edwards G: The alcohol dependence syndrome: a concept as stimulus to inquiry. Br J Addict 81:171–183, 1986.
3. Levinson PR, Gernstein DR, Maloff DRE: Commonalities in Substance Abuse and Habitual Behavior. Lexington, MA, Lexington Books, 1983.
4. American Psychiatric Association: Diagnostic and Statistical Manual of Mental Disorders, 3rd Edition, Revised. Washington, DC, American Psychiatric Association, 1987.

5. World Health Organization: International Statistical Classification of Diseases and Related Health Problems, 10th Revision. Geneva, Switzerland, World Health Organization, 1992.
6. American Psychiatric Association: Diagnostic and Statistical Manual of Mental Disorders, 4th Edition. Washington, DC, American Psychiatric Association, 1994.
7. Rounsaville BJ, Alarcon RD, Andrews G, et al: Basic nomenclature issues for DSM-V, in A Research Agenda for DSM-V. Edited by Kupfer DJ, First MB, Regier DA. Washington, DC, American Psychiatric Association, 2002, pp 1–29.
8. Cottler LB: Comparing DSM-III-R and ICD-10 substance use disorders. Addiction 88:689–696, 1993.
9. Kosten TR, Rounsaville BJ, Babor TF, et al: Substance-use disorders in DSM-III-R: evidence for the dependence syndrome across different psychoactive substances. Br J Psychiatry 151:834–843, 1987.
10. Kandel D, Chen K, Warner LA, et al: Prevalence and demographic correlates of symptoms of last year dependence on alcohol, nicotine, marijuana and cocaine in the U.S. population. Drug Alcohol Depend 44:11–29, 1997.
11. Anthony JC, Chen C-N, Storr CL: Drug dependence epidemiology. Clin Neurosci 5:55–68, 2005.
12. Anthony JC, Warner LA, Kessler RC: Comparative epidemiology of dependence on tobacco, alcohol, controlled substances, and inhalants: basic findings from the National Cormorbidity Survey. Exp Clin Psychopharmacol 2:244–268, 1994.
13. West R: Theory of Addiction. Oxford, England, Blackwell, 2006.
14. Langenbucher JW, Labouvie E, Martin CS, et al: An application of item response theory analysis to alcohol, cannabis, and cocaine criteria in DSM-IV. J Abnorm Psychol 113:72–80, 2004.
15. Henningfield JE: Symptoms of substance dependence associated with use of cigarettes, alcohol, and illicit drugs—United States, 1991–92. MMWR Morb Mortal Wkly Rep 44:830–839, 1995.
16. U.S. Department of Health and Human Services: The Health Consequences of Smoking: Nicotine Addiction: A Report of the U.S. Surgeon General. Washington, DC, US Government Printing Office, 1988.
17. Langenbucher JW, Morgenstern J, Miller KJ: DSM-III, DSM-IV and ICD-10 as severity scales for drug dependence. Drug Alcohol Depend 39:139–150, 1995.
18. Giovino GA: Epidemiology of tobacco use in the United States. Oncogene 21:7326–7340, 2002.
19. Jaffe JH: Tobacco use as a mental disorder: the rediscovery of a medical problem. NIDA Res Monogr 17:202–219, 1977.
20. Kessler DA, Barnett PS, Witt A, et al: The legal and scientific basis for FDA's assertion of jurisdiction over cigarettes and smokeless tobacco. JAMA 277:405–409, 1997.
21. Hughes JR, Howard TS: Nicotine don't get no respect (letter). JAMA 271:585, 1994.
22. Skodol AE, Bender DS: Diagnostic interviews for adults, in Handbook of Psychiatric Measures. Edited by Rush AJ, Pincus HA, First MB, et al. Washington, DC, American Psychiatric Association, 2000, pp 45–71.
23. Hughes JR: Nicotine dependence and WHO mental health surveys. JAMA 292:1021–1022, 2004.

24. Hughes JR: Clinical implications of the association between smoking and alcoholism, in Alcohol and Tobacco: From Basic Science to Policy (NIAAA Research Monograph No 30). Edited by Fertig J, Fuller R. Rockville, MD, National Institute on Alcoholism and Alcohol Abuse, 1996, pp 171–185.
25. Kandel DB, Huang F-Y, Davies M: Comorbidity between patterns of substance use dependence and psychiatric syndromes. Drug Alcohol Depend 64:233–241, 2001.
26. Grant BF, Hasin DS, Chou SP, et al: Nicotine dependence and psychiatric disorders in the United States: results from the National Epidemiologic Survey on Alcohol and Related Conditions. Arch Gen Psychiatry 61:1107–1115, 2004.
27. Madden PAF, Heath AC: Shared genetic vulnerability in alcohol and cigarette use and dependence. Alcohol Clin Exp Res 26:1919–1921, 2002.
28. Royal College of Physicians of London: Nicotine Addiction in Britain. London, The Lavenham Press, 2000.
29. Hughes JR: Smoking as a drug dependence: a reply to Robinson and Pritchard. Psychopharmacology (Berl) 113:282–283, 1993.
30. Stolerman IP, Jarvis MJ: The scientific case that nicotine is addictive. Psychopharmacology (Berl) 117:2–10, 1995.
31. West RJ: Nicotine addiction: a re-analysis of the arguments. Psychopharmacology (Berl) 108:408–410, 1992.
32. Kozlowski LT, Wilkinson DA, Skinner W, et al: Comparing tobacco cigarette dependence with other drug dependencies. JAMA 261:898–901, 1989.
33. Benowitz NL: Nicotine Safety and Toxicity. New York, Oxford University Press, 1998.
34. World Health Organization: Manual of the International Statistical Classification of Diseases, Injuries and Causes of Death, 9th Revised Edition. Geneva, Switzerland, World Health Organization, 1977.
35. American Psychiatric Association: Diagnostic and Statistical Manual of Mental Disorders, 4th Edition, Text Revision. Washington, DC, American Psychiatric Association, 2000.
36. Hughes JR: Why does smoking so often produce dependence? A somewhat different view. Tob Control 10:62–64, 2001.
37. Peele S: Diseasing of America: Addiction Treatment Out of Control . Lexington, MA, Lexington Books, 1989.
38. Pomerleau CS, Pomerleau OF: Euphoriant effects of nicotine in smokers. Psychopharmacology (Berl) 108:460–465, 1992.
39. Warburton DM, Revell A, Walters AC: Nicotine as a resource, in Pharmacology of Nicotine. Edited by Rand MJ, Thurau K. London, England, ICSU Press, 1988, pp 359–373.
40. Hughes JR: Distinguishing withdrawal relief and direct effects of smoking. Psychopharmacology (Berl) 104:409–410, 1991.
41. Parrott AC: Cigarette-derived nicotine is not a medicine. World J Biol Psychiatry 4:49–55, 2003.
42. Heishman SJ: What aspects of human performance are truly enhanced by nicotine? Addiction 93:317–320, 1998.
43. Glautier S: Measures and models of nicotine dependence: positive reinforcement. Addiction 99:30–50, 2004.

44. Piper ME, Piasecki TM, Federman EB, et al: A multiple motives approach to tobacco dependence: the Wisconsin Inventory of Smoking Dependence Motives (WISDM-68). J Consult Clin Psychol 72:139–154, 2004.
45. Tiffany ST: A cognitive model of drug urges and drug-use behavior: role of automatic and nonautomatic processes. Psychol Rev 97:147–168, 1990.
46. Shiffman S, Paty JA, Gnys M, et al: Nicotine withdrawal in chippers and regular smokers: subjective and cognitive effects. Health Psychol 14:301–309, 1995.
47. DiFranza JR, Savageau JA, Fletcher K, et al: Measuring the loss of autonomy over nicotine use in adolescents. Arch Pediatr Adolesc Med 156:397–403, 2002.
48. Balfour DJK: The neurobiology of tobacco dependence: a preclinical perspective on the role of the dopamine projections to the nucleus. Nicotine Tob Res 6:899–912, 2004.
49. Frenk H, Dar R: A Critique of Nicotine Addiction. Norwell, MA, Kluwer Academic Publishers, 2000.
50. Atrens DM: Nicotine as an addictive substance: a critical examination of the basic concepts and empirical evidence. J Drug Issues 31:325–394, 2001.
51. Koob GF, LeMoal M: Drug addiction, dysregulation of reward, and allostasis. Neuropsychopharmacology 24:97–129, 2001.
52. Laviolette SR, van der Kooy D: The neurobiology of nicotine addiction: bridging the gap from molecules to behaviour. Neurosci Nat Rev 5:55–65, 2004.
53. Littleton J: Conceptualizing addiction. Receptor regulation as a unitary mechanism for drug tolerance and physical dependence—not quite as simple as it seemed! Addiction 96:87–101, 2001.
54. Hunt WA, Barnett LW, Branch LG: Relapse rates in addiction programs. J Clin Psychol 27:455–456, 1971.
55. Klingemann H, Sobell L, Barker J, et al: Promoting Self-Change From Problem Substance Use: Practical Implications for Policy, Prevention and Treatment. Dordrecht, The Netherlands, Kluwer Academic Publishers, 2001.
56. Kenford SL, Fiore MC, Jorenby DE, et al: Predicting smoking cessation: who will quit with and without the nicotine patch. JAMA 271:589–594, 1994.
57. Breslau N, Kilbey MM, Andreski P: DSM-III-R nicotine dependence in young adults: prevalence, correlates and associated psychiatric disorders. Addiction 89:743–754, 1994.
58. John U, Meyer C, Hapke U, et al: Nicotine dependence and lifetime amount of smoking in a population sample. Eur J Public Health 14:182–185, 2004.
59. Breslau N: The idiosyncratic definition of nicotine dependence. Arch Gen Psychiatry 54:973–974, 1997.
60. Kandel DB, Chen K: Extent of smoking and nicotine dependence in the United States: 1991–93. Nicotine Tob Res 2:263–274, 2000.
61. American Psychiatric Association: Practice Guideline for the Treatment of Patients With Substance Use Disorders: Alcohol, Cocaine, Opioids. Washington, DC, American Psychiatric Press, 1995.
62. Hughes JR: Pharmacotherapy for smoking cessation: unvalidated assumptions, anomalies and suggestions for further research. J Consult Clin Psychol 61:751–760, 1993.
63. Hughes JR, Shiffman S, Callas P, et al: A meta-analysis of the efficacy of over-the-counter nicotine replacement. Tob Control 12:21–27, 2002.
64. Piper ME, McCarthy DE, Baker TB: Assessing tobacco dependence: a guide to measure evaluation and selection. Nicotine Tob Res 8:339–351, 2006.

65. West R: Defining and assessing nicotine dependence in humans, in Understanding Smoking and Nicotine Addiction. Edited by Goode J. London, England, Wiley (in press).
66. Colby SM, Tiffany ST, Shiffman S, et al: Measuring nicotine dependence. Drug Alcohol Depend 59:523–539, 2000.
67. Breslau N, Johnson EO: Predicting smoking cessation and major depression in nicotine-dependent smokers. Am J Public Health 90:1122–1127, 2000.
68. Mirin SM, Batki SLBO, Isabell PG, et al: Practice guideline for the treatment of patients with substance use disorders; alcohol, cocaine, opioids. Am J Psychiatry 152:1–59, 1995.
69. Fagerstrom K-O, Schneider NG: Measuring nicotine dependence: a review of the Fagerstrom Tolerance Questionnaire. J Behav Med 12:159–182, 1989.
70. Edwards G, Gross MM: Alcohol dependence: provisional description of a clinical syndrome. Br Med J 1:1058–1061, 1976.
71. Robinson TE, Berridge KC: Mechanisms of action of addictive stimuli: incentive-sensitization and addiction. Addiction 96:103–114, 2001.
72. Cottler LB, Schuckit MA, Helzer JE, et al: The DSM-IV field trial for substance use disorders: major results. Drug Alcohol Depend 38:59–69, 1995.
73. Robins E, Guze SB: Establishment of diagnostic validity in psychiatric illness: its application to schizophrenia. Am J Psychiatry 126:983–987, 1970.
74. Lessov CN, Martin NG, Statham DJ, et al: Defining nicotine dependence for genetic research: evidence from Australian twins. Psychol Med 34:865–879, 2004.
75. Fagerstrom K-O: Time to first cigarette; the best single indicator of tobacco dependence? Monaldi Arch Chest Dis 59:91–94, 2003.
76. Hughes JR, Oliveto AH, Riggs R, et al: Concordance of different measures of nicotine dependence: two pilot studies. Addict Behav 29:1527–1539, 2004.
77. Zimmerman M, Spitzer RL: Classification in psychiatry, in Kaplan and Sadock's Comprehensive Textbook of Psychiatry, Vol II, 8th Edition. Edited by Sadock BJ, Sadock VA. Philadelphia, PA, Lippincott Williams & Wilkins, 2004, pp 1003–1034.
78. Kalant H, LeBlanc AE, Gibbins RJ: Tolerance to, and dependence on, some non-opiate psychotropic drugs. Pharmacol Rev 23(3):135–191, 1971.

16

SHOULD ADDICTIVE DISORDERS INCLUDE NON-SUBSTANCE-RELATED CONDITIONS?

Marc N. Potenza, M.D.

Statement of the Problem

In this chapter, I examine the data supporting whether or not the scope of addictions should extend beyond substance use disorders (SUDs). Specifically, within *Diagnostic and Statistical Manual of Mental Disorders* (DSM), should specific mental health disorders be grouped together with SUDs within the category of addictions? If so, which mental health disorders? What additional information is needed to move forward in the appropriate categorization of disorders meeting a definition of addiction?

Reprinted from Potenza MN: "Should Addictive Disorders Include Non-Substance-Related Conditions?" *Addiction* 101 (suppl 1):142–151, 2006. Used with permission of the Society for the Study of Addiction.

Review of the Literature

ADDICTION AND DSM

The nomenclature system within the text revision of the fourth edition of DSM (DSM-IV-TR; American Psychiatric Association[1]) currently lacks the term *addiction.* Substance use disorders (SUDs) are categorized according to the specific problematic substance within separate groupings: abuse, dependence, withdrawal and intoxication. Of these categories, dependence might be most likened to addiction, and one could consider changing the nomenclature to replace "dependence" with "addiction." As described in greater detail below, there exist both pros (e.g., limiting confusion regarding the use of the term *dependence*—physical dependence versus DSM-defined, diagnostic dependence) and cons (e.g., the stigma generally associated with the term *addiction*) of making such a change.

DEFINING ADDICTION

In order to determine whether addictions should extend beyond SUDs, it is important to have a definition for the term *addiction.* Derived from the Latin *addicere,* meaning "bound to" or "enslaved by," the term was used initially without a specific reference to substance use. Over the past several centuries, it has become identified increasingly with impaired control over substance use behaviors.[2] Nonetheless, there has been a recent shift returning toward consideration of non-substance-related disorders as addictive in nature.[3,4] A central element cited typically in defining addiction is "loss of control" over a behavior, with associated adverse consequences,[2,3,5] although "impaired control" has been cited as a more appropriate description.[2] Arguments have been forwarded to move toward the use of *addiction* rather than the current term *dependence,* given confusion over different definitions of dependence. For example, physical dependence can be achieved upon chronic administration of a drug (e.g., a beta-blocker for hypertension) and can include aspects of tolerance and withdrawal but is generally not associated with the harmful effects of an addiction (e.g., drug-seeking and drug-using that interfere with major areas of life functioning—see definition of core elements of addiction in the next paragraph). In other words, a change in terminology might shift the focus of the disorder from chronic use of a substance and the associated physical dependence to the harmful effects of the addictive process on the individuals, their friends, families, society, and so forth. Thus, more precise terminology might help to reduce controversy over such interventions as methadone maintenance that are associated with physical dependence but reduce the impact of addiction, and would be consistent with the shift, following DSM-III, away from aspects of physical dependence as the core features of substance dependence.

One description of the core elements of addiction includes (modified from reference 3): 1) craving state prior to behavioral engagement, or a compulsive engagement; 2) impaired control over behavioral engagement; and 3) continued behavioral engagement despite adverse consequences. If one adopts these components as core elements of addiction, other behavioral disorders, particularly those currently classified as impulse-control disorders (ICDs), warrant consideration as addictions. Consistently, the National Institute on Drug Abuse (NIDA), a research funding agency in the United States, has recently cited as important the study of nondrug behaviors/disorders (pathological gambling, obesity) in understanding substance dependence.[6]

IMPULSIVITY AND IMPULSE-CONTROL DISORDERS

The core elements proposed above for addiction share features with a definition proposed for impulsivity[7]: "a predisposition toward rapid, unplanned reactions to internal or external stimuli without regard to the negative consequences of these reactions to the impulsive individual or others." When this definition is applied, impulsivity has relevance to a broad array of psychiatric disorders, including substance use, antisocial and borderline personality disorders, bipolar disorder, attention-deficit/hyperactivity disorder, and ICDs.[7] ICDs are currently grouped together in DSM-IV-TR in the category of "Impulse-Control Disorders Not Elsewhere Classified," and include pathological gambling (PG), kleptomania, pyromania, intermittent explosive disorder, trichotillomania, and ICD not otherwise specified. Similarly, the ICDs are not grouped with SUDs in the *International Classification of Diseases and Related Health Problems,* 10th Revision (ICD-10),[8] in which PG and other ICDs are grouped in the section of "Disorders of Adult Personality and Behavior" under the heading of "Habit and Impulse Disorders." Additional ICDs have been proposed, including compulsive shopping, compulsive computer use, and compulsive sexual behaviors.[9,10] ICDs are particularly relevant to the discussion in this chapter, as ICDs such as PG have been described as "behavioral addictions" or "addictions without the drug" because they share similar features with substance dependence.[11,12] The ICDs do not include obsessive-compulsive disorder (OCD), another disorder characterized by repetitive interfering behaviors. As discussed later, the relationship between OCD and ICDs is currently incompletely understood.

ICDs are poorly understood in comparison to other psychiatric disorders. Assessments of ICDs have largely been excluded from major psychiatric epidemiological surveys: no ICDs were assessed in the National Comorbidity Survey,[13] and only the St. Louis site of the Epidemiologic Catchment Area (ECA) study included measures of PG.[14] As such, our understanding of how ICDs fit into the structure of common psychiatry disorders is limited,[15,16] and such information would be helpful in determining the most appropriate categorization of PG and other ICDs. One reason for exclusion of ICDs from these studies is that psychometrically validated instruments for assessing these disorders are largely lacking; for example, the Structured Clinical Interview for DSM-IV Axis I Disorders (SCID) does not contain modules for any ICD.[17] However, a SCID-compatible module for PG has been described recently,[18] and further psychometric testing of this instrument and development of others will be important. The availability of such instruments could facilitate the inclusion of PG and other ICD measures into routinely conducted national surveys such as the National Household Survey on Drug Abuse, as was recommended congressionally.[19]

The importance of assessing and treating ICDs is highlighted by recent studies suggesting high rates of ICDs in co-occurrence with other psychiatric disorders. For example, a recent study of 204 consecutive psychiatric inpatient admissions observed that following screening, over 30% of patients were identified as having a current ICD, in contrast to the less than 2% of patients who were diagnosed with an ICD on admission.[20] Given that symptoms of ICDs such as PG have been associated with worse treatment outcome in substance use and other psychiatric domains,[21] the findings suggest the need for improved identification and treatment of ICDs. Brief screening instruments would be particularly helpful for this purpose.[10]

Arguably, PG represents the ICD that has been most studied to date. As such, the remainder of the chapter will focus on PG and provide data relevant to its potential inclusion with substance dependence within a category of addictions.

DIAGNOSTIC CRITERIA

The current diagnostic criteria for PG share many features with those for substance dependence.[1] Similar inclusionary criteria exist for interference in major areas of life functioning, tolerance, withdrawal, and repeated unsuccessful attempts to cut back or quit. Some differences between the structuring/defining of gambling and SUDs currently exist and warrant consideration in DSM-V—for example, a category for gambling less severe than PG yet still problematic (problem gambling), similar to the DSM structuring of substance abuse versus substance dependence.[22]

CLINICAL CHARACTERISTICS AND SOCIAL FACTORS

Multiple similarities in clinical characteristics have been cited. High rates of PG have been observed in adolescents and young adults and low rates in older adults,[23,24] mirroring the patterns seen in SUDs.[25] The natural histories of PG and SUDs suggest that many people recover on their own following peaks of problem behaviors in adolescence and early adulthood.[26] Like those with SUDs, individuals with PG generally score high on measures of impulsiveness.[27,28] Data suggest that other features of SUDs (e.g., Cloninger's and Babor's typologies of alcoholic individuals, severity of PG associated with early age at onset) might be similarly applicable to PG.[29,30] As these typologies have clinically relevant implications,[31] these and other possible subtypes of PG (e.g., those based on specific types or patterns of gambling) warrant further examination.[32] Gender differences also appear similar between PG and SUDs. As with most SUDs, women are less likely than men to experience PG.[33] The gender-related phenomenon of "telescoping" (in which women have a later initial engagement in the addictive behavior but a foreshortened time period from first engagement to addiction) appears applicable to both PG and SUDs.[33–36] Both SUDs and PG are thought to impact a large social network; for example, it has been suggested that each person with PG influences 8–10 other people.[37] Data suggest that specific racial/ethnic groups, including African Americans and Native Americans, might have higher rates of PG, similar to the findings of higher rates of some SUDs within these groups.[38] Cultural attitudes may influence gambling behaviors. Certain forms of gambling have relatively greater popularity in specific cultures (e.g., the mahjong and pachinko forms of gambling in Asian groups). Differences in cultural attitudes may also influence treatment approaches and treatment-seeking for PG.[39] Social acceptedness of behaviors can influence behavioral engagement; for example, recent changes in attitudes toward tobacco smoking have been associated with a decline in consumption.[40] Changes in the use of heroin by military personnel during and following the Vietnam War suggest the importance of multiple factors (social acceptedness, drug availability, stress) in influencing substance use behaviors. Substantial changes in the social acceptedness and availability of legalized gambling have occurred recently.[41] Although it is not possible to derive a causal relationship, concurrent with the increased availability and social acceptance of gambling there has been an apparent increase in rates of PG.[23] Given the probable strong influence of multiple environmental factors (e.g., socioeconomic status, cultural expectations) on gambling and substance use behaviors in general, and specifically on differences observed between racial and ethnic groups, the extent to which these findings suggest similar diagnostic groupings for PG and SUDs should be considered cautiously.[38]

CO-OCCURRING DISORDERS

Studies of multiple clinical samples suggest high rates of co-occurrence between SUDs and PG in both directions.[10,42] Limited data exist from nationally representative samples to investigate the co-occurrence of PG with other psychiatric disorders, as studies investigating gambling behaviors have generally had limited psychiatric assessments,[24] and those investigating psychiatric disorders had limited or no gambling assessments.[12] Data from the St. Louis ECA study indicate that problem gamblers (those with one or more symptoms of PG) were more likely than nongamblers to use tobacco and alcohol, meet criteria for abuse or dependence for these substances, and meet criteria for multiple other psychiatric disorders, including antisocial personality, mood, anxiety, and psychotic disorders.[13] Among the strongest associations were those for antisocial personality disorder and alcohol use, suggesting that problem gambling is linked closely to externalizing behaviors.[13,14] A recently conducted survey of more than 43,000 individuals found that a broad range of Axis I and Axis II disorders co-occurred frequently with PG.[43] Direct investigation of how PG and other ICDs fit into the structure of mental health disorders is needed.[14]

The ECA study found no association (odds ratio of 0.6) between problem gambling and OCD.[13] This finding seems particularly relevant given a proposed categorization of PG as an obsessive-compulsive spectrum disorder.[44] The lack of a significant association between PG and OCD has also been observed in large samples of individuals with OCD.[10] As such, these data do not support a strong link between OCD and PG and do not support their c.ategorization together. As specific ICDs (such as trichotillomania) appear to co-occur frequently with OCD, more study is needed to determine the extent to which ICDs are related to one another and SUDs.

PERSONALITY FEATURES AND BEHAVIORAL MEASURES

Individuals with PG and SUDs have been shown to perform similarly on personality and neurocognitive assessments of impulsivity. Both groups have been shown to score highly on self-reported measures of impulsiveness and sensation-seeking.[27,28,45] In contrast, individuals with OCD tend to score high on measures of harm avoidance. Although both PG and OCD subjects score highly on measures of compulsivity, high scores in PG subjects appear limited to impaired control over mental activities and urges/worries about losing control over motor behaviors.[46] In contrast, in OCD subjects the high scores tend to generalize across more domains, including those on which SUD groups score lower (e.g., washing).[47]

PG and SUD groups have demonstrated rapid temporal discounting of rewards, and those with both PG and SUDs tend to show the steepest discounting rates.[45,48–50] Similar to individuals with OCD[51] and SUDs,[45,52] individuals with PG have shown disadvantageous performance on the Iowa Gambling Task (IGT),[53] a paradigm that, by strict definition, does not involve gambling but rather assesses risk–reward decision-making. In people with SUDs, poor performance on the IGT correlates with real-life measures of adverse functioning.[52]

BIOCHEMISTRY

Multiple transmitter systems have been similarly implicated in ICDs and SUDs.[8,54] Many biochemical similarities involving serotonergic systems have been observed across disorders linked by impaired impulse control. Low levels of the serotonin metabolite 5-hydroxyindoleacetic acid have been found in the cerebrospinal fluids of individuals with PG and alcoholism.[54] Levels of platelet monoamine oxidase, considered a peripheral marker of serotonin function, are decreased in subjects with PG, and similar findings have been observed in individuals with SUDs and behaviors characterized by impaired impulse control.[54] Behavioral responses to the partial serotonin 5-HT_1/5-HT_2 agonist *m*-chlorophenylpiperazine (m-CPP) have been found to distinguish individuals with impaired impulse control, including those with PG and alcohol abuse/dependence, from those without.[54] Specifically, affected individuals report a euphoric response following m-CPP administration, whereas unaffected subjects do not. Individuals with impulsive aggression have shown blunted activation of the ventromedial prefrontal cortex (vmPFC) in response to m-CPP and another serotonergic drug (fenfluramine).[55,56] These findings are similar to those observed in alcoholic individuals following challenge with m-CPP.[57] Further research is needed to examine the extent to which these findings are applicable to PG, other ICDs, and other SUDs. Additional biological information, such as that gleaned from biochemical, neuroimaging, and genetic studies, is anticipated to have a crucial and expanding role over time in understanding and categorizing disorders appropriately.

NEUROCIRCUITRY

Few neuroimaging studies have been performed involving subjects with PG or formal ICDs. Evidence to date suggests similarities between PG, SUDs, and other disorders characterized by impaired impulse control. Decreased activation of vmPFC has been observed in PG subjects during the presentation of gambling cues[28] or performance of the Stroop Color–Word Interference Task.[58] Diminished activation of left vmPFC similarly distinguished PG and bipolar subjects from control subjects during Stroop performance,[58,59] and diminished activation of this region has been associated with impulsive aggression in depressed subjects.[60] These findings suggest that vmPFC is involved in impulse regulation across a spectrum of diagnostic disorders. vmPFC has been implicated as a critical component of decision-making circuitry in risk–reward assessment, with abnormal function demonstrated in association with SUDs.[52,61]

A brain circuit central to addiction involves the dopaminergic mesolimbic pathway linking the ventral tegmental area to the nucleus accumbens (NAc) or ventral striatum.[62] Developmental models of motivational neurocircuitry underlying PG and SUDs have included dopaminergic activity within the NAc as a focal point.[63,64] Emerging brain imaging data suggest that similar components of the mesolimbic pathway are involved in PG and SUDs. During a guessing task that simulated gambling, subjects with PG showed less ventral striatal activation than did control subjects, and gambling severity correlated inversely with ventral striatal activation.[65] Similarly, adults with alcohol dependence versus those without have been found to activate ventral striatum less robustly in anticipation of working for monetary reward,[66] and similar findings have been observed in subjects with a family history of alcoholism versus subjects without a family history of alcoholism.[67] In that healthy adolescents versus young adults also showed diminished ventral striatal activation during task performance, the findings might help to explain the high rates of addiction observed during adolescence.[68] Diminished ventral striatal activation in addiction also appears relevant to craving states. In a study of gambling urges in PG and cocaine cravings in cocaine dependence (CD), diminished activation of ventral striatum similarly distinguished addicted (PG, CD) from control subjects during viewing of the respective gambling or drug videotapes.[69]

A "reward deficiency" model of addiction was proposed that is consistent with the recently obtained imaging data.[70] This model could account for the pattern of rapid discounting of rewards that is observed in PG and SUDs. That is, small, immediate rewards have been found to activate preferentially brain regions implicated in PG and SUDs, including the ventral striatum and vmPFC.[65,71]

Whereas neuroimaging data suggest similarities between PG and SUDs, they suggest differences between PG and OCD. Multiple cue provocation studies have found increased activity of cortico-striatal-thalamo-cortical circuitry in OCD.[72] In contrast, relatively decreased activation of these brain regions was observed during gambling urges in PG.[28]

GENETICS

The best support for genetic contributions to PG and SUDs comes from studies of the Vietnam Era Twin Registry.[73] These studies indicate heritable contributions to PG[74] and shared environmental and genetic contributions to PG and alcohol dependence[75] and PG and antisocial behaviors.[76] These findings are similar to those suggesting common genetic contributions to a range of drug use disorders.[77]

Molecular genetic studies have suggested similarities between PG and SUDs. For example, the D2A1 allele of the D_2 dopamine receptor gene *(DRD2)* has been reported to increase in frequency from nonaddicted to PG and co-occurring PG and SUD groups.[78] Similarly, the gene has been implicated in PG with and without SUDs.[79] More conclusive data from genomewide studies are emerging and similarly implicate genetic factors in PG and SUDs.[80] As genetic factors have been associated with positive outcome for treatment of SUDs,[81] genetic sampling should be considered in treatment trials in PG and other ICDs.

TREATMENT

Pharmacological treatments for PG and other ICDs are at an early stage of testing.[9] No drugs are currently approved by the U.S. Food and Drug Administration (FDA) for the treatment of PG or other ICDs, and of the small number of placebo-controlled trials performed to date, they have generally been short-term, involved small samples, and excluded individuals with co-occurring disorders.[82] As with SUDs, serotonin reuptake inhibitors have shown mixed results in the treatment of PG.[9] The mu opioid receptor antagonist naltrexone has FDA approval for the treatment of opioid and alcohol dependence. Naltrexone is thought to mediate its therapeutic effects in treating addictive disorders through opioid receptor–mediated, indirect modulation of activity within the mesolimbic dopaminergic system.[82] Naltrexone has been found to be superior to placebo in the treatment of PG.[82] As in SUDs, naltrexone appears to target addictive urges in PG, as the drug was most efficacious in individuals with strong gambling urges at treatment onset.[83] Data with nalmefene provide further support for a role of opioid receptor antagonism in the treatment of PG[84] and additional evidence for a link between PG and SUDs.[85]

Behavioral treatments are at an early stage of testing for PG and other ICDs.[86] As in SUDs, 12-step self-help groups have long been a mainstay of gambling treatment, with data suggesting high initial dropout rates but improvement related to continued attendance.[87] Existing data support roles for several therapist-driven techniques (motivational interviewing, motivational enhancement, cognitive-behavioral therapy) in the treatment of PG.[88,89] These interventions have largely been modeled after those that have been shown to be effective in the treatment of SUDs.[90,91] As data suggest that in the treatment of SUDs combined behavioral and pharmacological intervention is generally more effective than either alone,[92] the investigation of such approaches is needed in PG and other ICDs.

ALTERNATIVE MODELS

An alternative hypothesis has posited that PG represents a mood spectrum disorder.[93] Consistent with this model, high rates of depressive disorders have been observed in conjunction with PG,[13,42] shared genetic contributions to PG and major depression have been found,[94] similar brain activation patterns have been observed between PG and bipolar subjects during Stroop performance,[58,59] and similar pharmacotherapies have been emerging as effective treatments for PG and bipolar disorder.[82,95] However, many of the clinical features central to PG (e.g., the diagnostic criteria) are more similar to SUDs than to depression, with the exception of gambling to relieve a dysphoric mood.[1] Several of the links between PG and mood disorders also apply to SUDs,[96] suggesting the need for further research in the area of co-occurring disorders to identify common contributions to ICDs, SUDs, and mood disorders. Other models (e.g., conceptualization of PG along antisocial/conduct or attention-deficit spectra) could also be considered, and additional studies into the underlying biologies of these psychiatric disorders and their overlap with PG, other ICDs, and SUDs should help generate more precise diagnostic categorization.

CONCLUSIONS

Existing data suggest that 1) PG shares many features with SUDs (supporting their grouping together as addictions); 2) PG does not share as many features with OCD (not supporting the grouping of PG with OCD as an obsessive-compulsive spectrum disorder); and 3) PG and mood disorders share features (suggesting the need for more investigation into the underlying mechanisms). The current categorization of PG as an ICD is not inconsistent with these other categorizations, and increased impulsivity or disadvantageous risk–reward decision-making appears to be a common link across PG, other ICDs, and SUDs.

Identification of Research Gaps and Specific Recommendations

RESEARCH GAP 1: ASSESSING AND CATEGORIZING ICDS

Although substantial data exist for the inclusion of PG within the framework of addictions, less data are available for other ICDs. More work is needed to characterize the formal ICDs currently grouped together in DSM, as well as those currently under various stages of consideration (compulsive shopping, compulsive computer use, compulsive sexual behaviors). Other disorders characterized by impaired impulse control (e.g., attention-deficit/hyperactivity disorder and binge-eating disorder) should be examined further with respect to their relationship with formal ICDs and SUDs. Empirically validated instruments for assessment of ICDs are needed, such that these disorders can be routinely assessed in large epidemiological studies and ongoing surveys of risk behaviors (e.g., National Household Survey on Drug Abuse, Monitoring the Future, and Centers for Disease Control and Prevention Youth Risk Behavior Survey). Information from such studies would be helpful in monitoring the relationship over time between ICDs and other psychiatric disorders, including SUDs. Formal analysis of where PG and other ICDs fit within the structure of common psychiatric disorders is needed. Such studies should help to clarify the extent to which disorders such as PG, other ICDs, major depression, SUDs, and other psychiatric disorders should be grouped together or separately. Longitudinal assessments would be important in gathering more information on the natural histories of PG and other ICDs with respect to SUDs and other psychiatric disorders. Specific questions investigating the relationship between risk behaviors (e.g., does one usually gamble when drinking or smoking and vice versa) would help to define aspects that have until now been largely only associated. Inclusion of subsyndromal measures is important given concerns regarding the most appropriate threshold for diagnosing PG and the observation of increased psychopathology in groups engaging in subsyndromal levels of gambling. Such information would be helpful in determining the extent to which additional diagnostic categories (e.g., problem gambling) should be considered in DSM-V, as well as the extent to which public health guidelines that currently exist for alcohol consumption should be considered for gambling. The readiness of psychiatrists, other health care providers and patients to define PG and other ICDs as addictions warrants consideration. For example, the term *addiction* has historically carried negative connotations, and resistance might be encountered regarding incorporation of the term into DSM. Additionally, given the small amount of data on ICDs other than PG, should PG be removed from its current categorization as an ICD or would the entire category be moved with less data to justify a shift?

RESEARCH GAP 2: SPECIAL POPULATIONS

Most research performed to date in PG has involved predominantly or exclusively Caucasian men, generating a deficiency in our understanding of other groups. As with SUDs, in studies in which subgroups have been identified, differences have often been observed. As with SUDs, certain groups (adolescents and young adults, males) appear to have higher rates of PG. Other groups also warrant specific consideration: women may be considered in some ways more susceptible than men to PG and SUDs given the telescoping phenomenon, and older adults, despite lower rates of PG and SUDs, may be particularly vulnerable, given the limited abilities to regain lost money. More research is needed to substantiate links among PG, other ICDs, and SUDs across specific populations, and to investigate the specific factors that influence addictive behaviors within these groups (environmental, biochemical, neural, genetic). Both risk (e.g., experiencing of stressful life events) and protective factors (e.g., school attendance or community involvement) should be better characterized for specific populations to assess the extent to which similar processes contribute to PG, other ICDs and SUDs. Research into the applicability of current diagnostic criteria across specific groups (e.g., age and gender) should be performed similarly or concordantly in order to investigate the importance of differences (e.g., in inclusionary criteria or thresholding thereof) across ICDs and SUDs for specific populations.

RESEARCH GAP 3: NEUROCOGNITION/NEUROIMAGING

Recent advances in neuroscience have resulted in the rapid acquisition of large amounts of data. However, few ICDs have been studied using these techniques. Specific investigations using brain imaging (magnetic resonance imaging [MRI], functional MRI [fMRI], positron emission tomography [PET], single photon emission computed tomography [SPECT]) are needed involving subjects with PG and other ICDs. Structural MRI studies are needed to examine PG and ICD subjects and the relationship between brain structure and symptom severity and other clinical characteristics. Functional imaging studies, particularly those using paradigms targeting impulsivity and risk–reward decision-making, seem particularly salient to PG, other ICDs, and SUDs. Studies investigating patterns of brain connectivity (e.g., using diffusion tensor imaging or independent component analysis techniques) would be helpful in identifying whether similar neural circuits are disrupted in ICDs and SUDs. Ligand-based studies of neurotransmitter systems implicated in PG and other ICDs are needed to evaluate the extent to which specific neurotransmitter systems are similarly dysregulated in ICDs and SUDs. These studies would be of particular relevance to providing an empirical basis for the testing of specific pharmacological treatments across ICDs and SUDs. Using similar assessments and paradigms across multiple, theoretically linked diagnostic groups would facilitate the identification of common elements across diagnostic groups.

Genetic factors, particularly commonly occurring, functional allelic variants known to influence brain activity, should be examined in conjunction with neuroimaging in PG, other ICDs, and SUDs.

The inclusion of personality or neurocognitive measures (e.g., those targeting aspects of impulsivity and compulsivity) would allow for further assessment that could be used in conjunction with imaging methods and treatment trials to better explore PG and other ICDs and their relationships to SUDs and other psychiatric disorders. Incorporation of such measures into treatment studies of ICDs and SUDs could help to determine the extent to which similar pathological processes should be targeted across SUDs and ICDs.

Given the high rates of co-occurrence between PG and other psychiatric disorders, including SUDs, future imaging studies of individuals with these co-occurring disorders are important. Incorporation of imaging modalities into behavioral and pharmacological treatment studies of ICDs and SUDs could help to identify the extent to which similar brain activation changes are associated with effective outcome across disorders.

RESEARCH GAP 4: GENETICS

Few large-scale genetic studies have included measures of PG and other ICDs. A more thorough investigation of existing data from the Vietnam Era Twin Registry could characterize further the relationship between PG, SUDs, and other psychiatric disorders. Additional twin studies beyond the exclusively older male Vietnam Era Twin Registry group are needed to examine women and sociocultural influences on expression of PG, other ICDs, SUDs, and other psychiatric disorders, as well as to estimate genetic and environmental contributions to the disorders within a current environmental context. Genomewide, molecular genetic studies using current strategies (e.g., affected sibling-pair designs) are needed for probands with PG and other ICDs to identify specific genetic contributions to the disorders and determine the extent to which they are similar to or distinct from SUDs.

Genetic factors contributing to specific stages of progression of PG and other ICDs should be identified and compared with those identified in similar studies of SUDs. Genetic studies should employ measures of environmental influences given data supporting gene × environment interactions in the development of psychiatric disorders. Identification of specific genes similarly contributing to PG, other ICDs, and SUDs could facilitate targeting of specific therapies across disorders. Identification of specific genetic factors relating similarly to treatment outcome with similar behavioral or pharmacological therapies across disorders would suggest the correction of similar pathological processes across ICDs and SUDs.

Conclusion

Pathological gambling and other impulse-control disorders have historically received relatively little attention from the mental health research and treatment communities. As such, substantial gaps of knowledge exist in the biological, phenomenological, and clinical characteristics of ICDs and in the relationship between specific ICDs and other disorders. As recent studies have suggested that ICDs are relatively common,[19] it is important not only to understand better the basic mechanisms underlying the disorders, but also to advance prevention and treatment strategies.[9] Examinations should carefully investigate the relationship between ICDs and other psychiatric disorders, given the high rates of co-occurrence observed between ICDs and other disorders in population-based and clinical samples.[19,43] The improved understanding of the relationship between ICDs and other psychiatric disorders, particularly SUDs, has important implications not only for the categorization of ICDs but also for improving prevention and treatment strategies.[85]

References

1. American Psychiatric Association: Diagnostic and Statistical Manual of Mental Disorders, 4th Edition, Text Revision. Washington, DC, American Psychiatric Association, 2000.
2. Maddux JF, Desmond DP: Addiction or dependence? Addiction 95:661–665, 2000.
3. Shaffer HJ: Strange bedfellows: a critical view of pathological gambling and addiction. Addiction 94:1445–1448, 1999.
4. Holden C: "Behavioral" addictions: do they exist? Science 294:980–982, 2001.
5. West R: Theories of addiction. Addiction 96:3–13, 2001.
6. National Institute on Drug Abuse, National Institute of Mental Health, National Institute of Diabetes and Digestive and Kidney Diseases: Reward and decision-making: opportunities and future directions. Neuron 36:189–192, 2002.
7. Moeller FG, Barratt ES, Dougherty DM, et al: Psychiatric aspects of impulsivity. Am J Psychiatry 158:1783–1793, 2001.
8. World Health Organization: International Statistical Classification of Diseases and Related Health Problems, 10th Revision. Geneva, Switzerland, World Health Organization, 1992.
9. Potenza MN, Hollander E: Pathological gambling and impulse control disorders, in Neuropsychopharmacology: Fifth Generation of Progress. Edited by Nemeroff JC, Charney D, Davis K, et al. Baltimore, MD, Lippincott Williams & Wilkins, 2002, pp 1725–1742.
10. Grant JE, Potenza MN: Impulse control disorders: clinical characteristics and pharmacological management. Ann Clin Psychiatry 16:27–34, 2004.
11. Potenza MN, Fiellin DA, Heninger GR, et al: Gambling: an addictive behavior with health and primary care implications. J Gen Intern Med 17:721–732, 2002.
12. Blanco C, Moreyra P, Nunes EV, et al: Pathological gambling: addiction or obsession? Semin Clin Neuropsychiatry 6:167–176, 2001.

13. Kessler RC, McGonagle KA, Zhao S, et al: Lifetime and 12-month prevalence of DSM-III-R psychiatric disorders in the United States: results from the National Comorbidity Survey. Arch Gen Psychiatry 51:8–19, 1994.
14. Cunningham-Williams RM, Cottler LB, Compton WM III, et al: Taking chances: problem gamblers and mental health disorders: results from the St. Louis Epidemiologic Catchment Area Study. Am J Public Health 88:1093–1096, 1998.
15. Krueger RF: The structure of common mental disorders. Arch Gen Psychiatry 56:921–926, 1999.
16. Kendler KS, Prescott CA, Neale MC: The structure of genetic and environmental risk factors for common psychiatric and substance use disorders in women and men. Arch Gen Psychiatry 60:929–937, 2003.
17. First MB, Spitzer RL, Gibbon M, et al: Structured Clinical Interview for DSM-IV, Patient Edition. Washington, DC, American Psychiatric Press, 1995.
18. Grant JE, Steinberg MA, Kim SW, et al: Preliminary validity and reliability testing of a structured clinical interview for pathological gambling. Psychiatry Res 128:79–88, 2004.
19. James KC: National Gambling Impact Study Commission: Final Report to Congress, 1999. Available online at http://govinfo.library.unt.edu/ngisc/reports/fullrpt.html. Accessed January 26, 2007.
20. Grant JE, Levine L, Kim D, et al: Prevalence of impulse control disorders in adult psychiatric inpatients. Am J Psychiatry 162:2184–2188, 2005.
21. Potenza MN, Levinson-Miller C, Poling J, et al: Gambling risk behaviors in alcohol dependent individuals with co-occurring disorders. Alcohol Clin Exp Res 28:1154, 2004.
22. Toce-Gerstein M, Gerstein DR, Volberg RA: A hierarchy of gambling disorders in the community. Addiction 98:1661–1672, 2003.
23. Shaffer HJ, Hall MN, Vander Bilt J: Estimating the prevalence of disordered gambling behavior in the United States and Canada: a research synthesis. Am J Public Health 89:1369–1376, 1999.
24. Gerstein D, Hoffmann J, Larison C, et al: Gambling Impact and Behavior Study. 1999. Available online at http://www.norc.org/online/gamb-fin.htm. Accessed March 27, 1999.
25. Wagner FA, Anthony JC: From first drug use to drug dependence: developmental periods of risk for dependence upon marijuana, cocaine, and alcohol. Neuropsychopharmacology 26:479–488, 2002.
26. Slutske WS, Jackson KM, Sher KJ: The natural history of problem gambling from age 18 to 29. J Abnorm Psychol 112:263–274, 2003.
27. Blaszczynski A, Steel Z, McConaghy N: Impulsivity in pathological gambling: the antisocial impulsivist. Addiction 92:75–87, 1997.
28. Potenza MN, Steinberg MA, Skudlarski P, et al: Gambling urges in pathological gamblers: an fMRI study. Arch Gen Psychiatry 60:828–836, 2003.
29. Potenza MN, Steinberg MA, McLaughlin SD, et al: Illegal behaviors in problem gambling: analysis of data from a gambling helpline. J Am Acad Psychiatry Law 28:389–403, 2000.
30. Lynch WJ, Maciejewski PK, Potenza MN: Psychiatric correlates of gambling in adolescents and young adults grouped by age of gambling onset. Arch Gen Psychiatry 61: 1116–1122, 2004.

31. Johnson BA, Roache JD, Javors MA, et al: Ondansetron for reduction of drinking among biologically predisposed alcoholic patients. JAMA 284:963–971, 2000.
32. Dowling N, Smith D, Thomas T: Electronic gaming machines: are they the "crack cocaine" of gambling? Addiction 100:33–45, 2005.
33. Potenza MN, Steinberg MA, McLaughlin SD, et al: Gender-related differences in the characteristics of problem gamblers using a gambling helpline. Am J Psychiatry 158:1500–1505, 2001.
34. Randall CL, Robert JS, Del Boca FK, et al: Telescoping of landmark events associated with drinking: a gender comparison. J Stud Alcohol 60:252–260, 1999.
35. Lynch WJ, Roth ME, Carroll ME: Biological basis of sex differences in drug abuse: preclinical and clinical studies. Psychopharmacology (Berl) 164:121–137, 2002.
36. Tavares H, Zilberman ML, Beites FJ, et al: Gender differences in gambling progression. J Gambl Stud 17:151–160, 2001.
37. Lobsinger C, Beckett L: Odds on the Break Even: A Practical Approach to Gambling Awareness. Canberra, Australia, Relationships Australia, 1996.
38. Cunningham-Williams RM, Cottler LB: The epidemiology of pathological gambling. Semin Clin Neuropsychiatry 6:155–166, 2001.
39. Petry NM: Gambling participation and problems among Southeast Asian refugees. Psychiatr Serv 54:1142–1148, 2003.
40. Slovic P: Smoking: Risk, Perception and Policy. Thousand Oaks, CA, Sage Publications, 2001.
41. Potenza MN, Kosten TR, Rounsaville BJ: Pathological gambling. JAMA 286:141–144, 2001.
42. Crockford DN, el-Guebaly N: Psychiatric comorbidity in pathological gambling: a critical review. Can J Psychiatry 43:43–50, 1998.
43. Petry NM, Stinson FS, Grant BF: Co-morbidity of DSM-IV pathological gambling and other psychiatric disorders: results from the National Epidemiologic Survey on Alcohol and Related Conditions. J Clin Psychiatry 66:564–574, 2005.
44. Hollander E, Wong CM: Obsessive-compulsive spectrum disorders. J Clin Psychiatry 56(suppl):3–6, 1995.
45. Petry NM: Substance abuse, pathological gambling, and impulsiveness. Drug Alcohol Depend 63:29–38, 2001.
46. Blanco C, Grant J, Potenza MN, et al: Impulsivity and compulsivity in pathological gambling. Poster presentation at College on Problems of Drug Dependence, San Juan, PR, June 15, 2004. Available online at http://biopsych.com:81/cpdd04_web/FMPro. Accessed October 25, 2004.
47. Sumnall HR, Wagstaff GF, Cole JC: Self-reported psychopathology in polydrug users. Psychopharmacology (Berl) 18:75–82, 2004.
48. Petry NM, Casarella T: Excessive discounting of delayed rewards in substance abusers with gambling problems. Drug Alcohol Depend 56:25–32, 1999.
49. Petry NM: Delay discounting of money and alcohol in actively using alcoholics, currently abstinent alcoholics, and controls. Psychopharmacology (Berl) 154:243–250, 2001.
50. Petry NM: Pathological gamblers, with and without substance use disorders, discount delayed rewards at high rates. J Abnorm Psychol 110:482–487, 2001.

51. Cavedini P, Riboldi G, D'Annucci A, et al: Decision-making heterogeneity in obsessive-compulsive disorder: ventromedial prefrontal cortex function predicts different treatment outcomes. Neuropsychologia 40:205–211, 2002.
52. Bechara A: Risky business: emotion, decision-making, and addiction. J Gambl Stud 19:23–51, 2003.
53. Cavedini P, Riboldi G, Keller R, et al: Frontal lobe dysfunction in pathological gambling. Biol Psychiatry 51:334–341, 2002.
54. Potenza MN: The neurobiology of pathological gambling. Semin Clin Neuropsychiatry 6:217–226, 2001.
55. Siever LJ, Buchsbaum MS, New AS, et al: d,1-Fenfluramine response in impulsive personality disorder assessed with [18F]fluorodeoxyglucose positron emission tomography. Neuropsychopharmacology 20:413–423, 1999.
56. New AS, Hazlett EA, Buchsbaum MS, et al: Blunted prefrontal cortical 18-fluorodeoxyglucose positron emission tomography response to meta-chlorophenylpiperazine in impulsive aggression. Arch Gen Psychiatry 59:621–629, 2002.
57. Hommer D, Andreasen P, Rio D, et al: Effects of m-chlorophenylpiperazine on regional brain glucose utilization: a positron emission tomographic comparison of alcoholic and control subjects. J Neurosci 17:2796–2806, 1997.
58. Potenza MN, Leung H-C, Blumberg HP, et al: An fMRI Stroop study of pathological gamblers. Am J Psychiatry 160:1990–1994, 2003.
59. Blumberg HP, Leung HC, Skudlarski P, et al: A functional magnetic resonance imaging study of bipolar disorder: state- and trait-related dysfunction in ventral prefrontal cortices. Arch Gen Psychiatry 60:601–609, 2003.
60. Dougherty RS, Deckersbach T, Marci C, et al: Ventromedial prefrontal cortex and amygdala dysfunction during an anger induction positron emission tomography study in patients with major depressive disorder with anger attacks. Arch Gen Psychiatry 61:795–804, 2004.
61. London ED, Ernst M, Grant S, et al: Orbitofrontal cortex and human drug abuse: functional imaging. Cereb Cortex 10:334–342, 2000.
62. Nestler EJ, Aghajanian G: Molecular and cellular basis of addiction. Science 278:58–63, 1997.
63. Chambers RA, Potenza MN: Neurodevelopment, impulsivity and adolescent gambling. J Gambl Stud 19:53–84, 2003.
64. Chambers RA, Taylor JR, Potenza MN: Developmental neurocircuitry of motivation in adolescence: a critical period of addiction vulnerability. Am J Psychiatry 160:1041–1052, 2003.
65. Reuter J, Raedler T, Rose M, et al: Pathological gambling is linked to reduced activation of the mesolimbic reward system. Nat Neurosci 8:147–148, 2005.
66. Hommer D: Motivation in alcoholism (slides). Presented at the International Conference on Applications of Neuroimaging to Alcoholism, New Haven, CT, January 2004. Available online at http://info.med.yale.edu/ctna/ICANA_files/ICANA_PDF-slides/Hommerfmri.pdf. Accessed January 12, 2005.
67. Hommer D, Bjork JM, Knutson B, et al: Motivation in children of alcoholics. Alcohol Clin Exp Res 28:22A, 2004.

68. Bjork JM, Knutson B, Fong GW, et al: Incentive-elicited brain activation in adolescents: similarities and differences from young adults. J Neurosci 24:1793–1802, 2004.
69. Potenza MN, Gottschalk C, Skudlarski P, et al: Neuroimaging studies of behavioral and drug addictions: gambling urges in pathological gambling and cocaine cravings in cocaine dependence. Presentation at the 157th annual meeting of the American Psychiatric Association, New York City, May 1–6, 2004.
70. Blum K, Cull JG, Braverman ER, et al: Reward deficiency syndrome. Am Sci 84:132–145, 1996.
71. McClure SM, Laibson DI, Loewenstein G, et al: Separate neural systems value immediate and delayed monetary rewards. Science 306:503–507, 2004.
72. Saxena S, Rauch SL: Functional neuroimaging and the neuroanatomy of obsessive-compulsive disorder. Psychiatr Clin North Am 23:1–19, 2000.
73. Shah KR, Eisen SA, Xian H, et al: Genetic studies of pathological gambling: a review of methodology and analyses of data from the Vietnam Era Twin (VET) Registry. J Gambl Stud 21:177–201, 2005.
74. Eisen SA, Lin N, Lyons MJ, et al: Familial influences on gambling behavior: an analysis of 3359 twin pairs. Addiction 93:1375–1384, 1998.
75. Slutske WS, Eisen S, True WR, et al: Common genetic vulnerability for pathological gambling and alcohol dependence in men. Arch Gen Psychiatry 57:666–674, 2000.
76. Slutske WS, Eisen S, Xian H, et al: A twin study of the association between pathological gambling and antisocial personality disorder. J Abnorm Psychol 110:297–308, 2001.
77. Tsuang MT, Lyons MJ, Meyer JM, et al: Co-occurrence of abuse of different drugs in men. Arch Gen Psychiatry 55:967–972, 1998.
78. Comings DE: The molecular genetics of pathological gambling. CNS Spectr 3:20–37, 1998.
79. Comings DE, Gade-Andavolu R, Gonzalez N, et al: The additive effect of neurotransmitter genes in pathological gambling. Clin Genet 60:107–116, 2001.
80. Gelernter J: Recent findings from a genome-wide linkage scan for cocaine dependence. Neuropsychopharmacology 29:s26, 2004.
81. Oslin DW, Berrettini W, Kranzler HR, et al: A functional polymorphism of the mu-opioid receptor gene is associated with naltrexone response in alcohol-dependent patients. Neuropsychopharmacology 28:1546–1552, 2003.
82. Grant JE, Kim SW, Potenza MN: Advances in the pharmacological treatment of pathological gambling disorder. J Gambl Stud 19:85–109, 2003.
83. Kim SW, Grant JE, Adson DE, et al: Double-blind naltrexone and placebo comparison study in the treatment of pathological gambling. Biol Psychiatry 49:914–921, 2001.
84. Grant JE, Potenza M, Hollander E, et al: A multicenter investigation of fixed-dose nalmefene in the treatment of pathological gambling. Neuropsychopharmacology 29: s122, 2004.
85. Tamminga CA, Nestler EJ: Pathological gambling: focusing on the addiction, not the activity. Am J Psychiatry 163:180–181, 2006.
86. Petry NM, Roll JM: A behavioral approach to understanding and treating pathological gambling. Semin Clin Neuropsychiatry 6:177–183, 2001.
87. Petry NM: Patterns and correlates of Gamblers Anonymous attendance in pathological gamblers seeking professional treatment. Addict Behav 28:1049–1062, 2003.

88. Petry NM, Ledgerwood D, Molina C: Behavioral Treatments for Problem and Pathological Gambling. Washington, DC, American Public Health Association, 2004.
89. Hodgins DC, Currie SR, el-Guebaly N: Motivational enhancement and self-help treatments for problem gambling. J Consult Clin Psychol 69:50–57, 2001.
90. Carroll KM, Connors GJ, Cooney NL, et al: A Cognitive Behavioral Approach: Treating Cocaine Addiction. Rockville, MD, National Institute on Drug Abuse, 1998.
91. Miller WR: Motivational Enhancement Therapy With Drug Abusers. Manual available online at http://motivationalinterview.org/clinical/METDrugAbuse.PDF. Accessed January 15, 2005.
92. Rounsaville BJ: Can psychotherapy rescue naltrexone treatment of opioid addiction? in Integrating Behavioral Therapies With Medications in the Treatment of Drug Dependence. Edited by Onken LS, Blaine JD, Boren JJ. Rockville, MD, National Institute on Drug Abuse, 1995, pp 37–52.
93. Moreyra P, Ibanez A, Saiz-Ruiz J, et al: Categorization, in Pathological Gambling: A Clinical Guide to Treatment. Edited by Grant JE, Potenza MN. Washington, DC, American Psychiatric Publishing, 2004, pp 55–68.
94. Potenza MN, Xian H, Shah K, et al: Shared genetic contributions to pathological gambling and major depression in men. Arch Gen Psychiatry 62:1015–1021, 2005.
95. Hollander E, Pallanti S, Allen A, et al: Does sustained-release lithium reduce impulsive gambling and affective instability versus placebo in pathological gamblers with bipolar spectrum disorders? Am J Psychiatry 162:137–145, 2005.
96. Charney DS (ed): Impact of substance abuse on the diagnosis, course and treatment of mood disorders. Biol Psychiatry 56:703–818, 2004.

17

SHOULD THE SCOPE OF ADDICTIVE BEHAVIORS BE BROADENED TO INCLUDE PATHOLOGICAL GAMBLING?

Nancy M. Petry, Ph.D.

Core features define conditions listed as substance use disorders. They include ingestion of a substance to the extent that its use is harmful and continued consumption of the substance despite knowledge of its harm. Substance use along with other behaviors that occur in excess despite their deleterious impacts are referred to colloquially as "addictions." These include, but are not limited to, excessive gambling, Internet use, eating, sex, and shopping. Only one of these excessive behaviors—pathological gambling—currently carries a diagnosis in the *Diagnostic and Statistical Manual of Mental Disorders* (DSM).[1] Discussions are under way regarding the classification of such conditions in general, and pathological gambling in particular, within a common framework of addictive disorders. In this chapter,

---

Preparation of the report reproduced in this chapter was supported by National Institutes of Health grants R01-MH60417, R01-MH60417-suppl, R01-DA13444, R01-DA018883, RO1-DA016855, RO1-DA14618, P50-AA03510, P50-DA09241, and M01-RR06192, and the Patrick and Catherine Weldon Donaghue Medical Research Foundation.

Reprinted from Petry NM: "Should the Scope of Addictive Behaviors Be Broadened to Include Pathological Gambling?" *Addiction* 101 (suppl 1):152–160, 2006. Used with permission of the Society for the Study of Addiction.

I examine issues that need to be explored in order to determine whether nonpharmacological conditions should be considered within the same classification system as substance use disorders. Pathological gambling is used as the exemplar because it is the disorder with the most scientific research.

Pathological Gambling

HISTORY AND CLASSIFICATION

Pathological gambling was introduced into DSM in the third edition (DSM-III).[2] Over the past 25 years, the criteria for this disorder have changed, and knowledge has expanded about its etiology, comorbidity and treatment. Despite advances in understanding the disorder, important issues remain to be addressed, including its diagnosis and classification, the focus of this chapter. Essential features and diagnostic criteria of pathological gambling are described first across the versions of DSM in which the disorder was included. Data related to the criteria are then detailed, with an emphasis on features and phenomenology that are shared with, as well as distinct from, those of substance use disorders.

DSM-III

When pathological gambling was first introduced into DSM, it was listed as a "Disorder of Impulse Control, Not Elsewhere Classified." Essential features of this class of conditions were 1) not resisting impulses or temptations to engage in an act that is harmful to oneself or others, 2) rising tension before the act, and 3) pleasure or liberation during the behavior, with guilt or regret later.

Pathological gamblers continue to wager even when they know that it is not in their best interests to keep betting. They describe rising anxiety or excitement prior to gambling.[3] Wagering may engender excitement, pleasure, or relief from tension, but it can be followed by guilt or remorse. Individuals who do not fit into this classification but who bet from time to time do not seem to experience these same emotions with gambling. For example, social gamblers appear able to not gamble or to quit betting once losses begin to mount, and any regret or guilt they experience is mild and transitory.

As shown in Table 17–1, one would need to experience a chronic and progressive inability to resist impulses to gamble and at least three of seven other symptoms to receive a diagnosis. Most criteria addressed financial issues related to obtaining gambling money from legal sources (criteria 2 and 7) and illegal venues (criteria 1, 4), and poor accounting of money (criterion 5). Only two criteria (3 and 6) did not focus on finances; they assessed negative impacts of gambling on family and work. An exclusionary criterion was that pathological gambling could not be related to antisocial personality disorder.

TABLE 17–1. Criteria for pathological gambling across versions of the *Diagnostic and Statistical Manual of Mental Disorders* (DSM)

Criterion	Item number in versions		
	DSM-III	DSM-III-R	DSM-IV
Chronically unable to resist gambling impulses	Mandatory		
Arrests for (admits to*) illegal acts (forgery, fraud, embezzlement, etc.) to obtain gambling money	1	8*	
Fails to honor debts or other financial responsibilities	2		
Family or spouse relationship difficulties related to gambling	3		
Borrows money from illegal sources (e.g., loan sharks) to gamble	4		
Not able to account for money (extensive monetary losses or gains, if claimed)	5		
Absences from work because of gambling	6		
Relies on others to provide money for desperate financial situations		7	10
Preoccupied with gambling or with ways to obtain money to gamble		1	1
Gambles more money, or wagers over a longer period of time, than intended		2	
Needs to increase the amounts or frequency of gambling to obtain desired excitement		3	2
Feels restless or irritable if not able to gamble		4	4
Consistently losing money and going back again to try to win back losses ("chasing")		5	6
Tries repeatedly to reduce or stop gambling		6	3
Often gambles when expected to meet social or occupational obligations		7	
Sacrifices or jeopardizes important social, occupational or recreational activities to gamble		8	9
Continues gambling even though unable to pay debts, or regardless of social, occupational or legal problems that the person knows to be exacerbated by gambling		9	
Gambles to escape from problems or to relieve negative moods			5
Lies to family members, therapist, or others to conceal the extent of involvement with gambling			7

No known studies evaluated these criteria as they apply to pathological gamblers, and the items as well as the diagnostic threshold seemed to be based on clinical impressions. The population evaluated at that time consisted almost exclusively of men who wagered on illegal forms of gambling.[4] The associated features described in DSM-III seemed to depict this picture: "These individuals are most often overconfident, somewhat abrasive, very energetic, and 'big spenders.'"

DSM-III-R

Modifications to the criteria for DSM-III-R[5] included removal of chronic and progressive inability to resist gambling impulses, and a requirement of endorsing at least four of nine criteria (Table 17–1, middle column) for a diagnosis. The criteria were changed substantially in this version relative to DSM-III. In particular, emphasis on money was reduced and replaced with assessment of the impact of gambling on psychosocial functioning. Many of these criteria were similar to those for psychoactive substance dependence.[1,p.181] In fact, the only unique criterion for pathological gambling was related to "chasing" lost money (criterion 5). In DSM-III-R, the restriction upon concurrent diagnoses with antisocial personality disorder was removed. Mood disorders were considered in the differential diagnosis, with the relationship between manic or hypomanic episodes mentioned.

DSM-IV

DSM-IV[1] included 10 criteria for pathological gambling (Table 17–1, right column), with a threshold of five or more items needed for a diagnosis. Criteria 1–4, 6 and 9 are similar to those in DSM-III-R. The fifth and seventh criteria have no parallel in earlier versions. Criteria 8 and 10 are similar to ones in DSM-III, which were subsequently removed in DSM-III-R. The exclusion of "manic episodes" as accounting more effectively for gambling behavior is made explicit in DSM-IV.

Some parallels between substance dependence disorders and pathological gambling remained in DSM-IV. Five of the seven dependence criteria have almost identical criteria in pathological gambling, but the others no longer have a parallel item. These include items related to escaping negative moods, chasing losses, lying to others, committing illegal acts, and relying on others for bailouts.

The number of criteria necessary for a diagnosis of pathological gambling has risen from three to four to five across the three DSM versions. More criteria have been added in each revision, but the proportion needed for a diagnosis has increased, with the result that obtaining a diagnosis may have become more stringent across the revisions, and possibly more difficult than substance use disorders.

INSTRUMENTS FOR ASSESSING PATHOLOGICAL GAMBLING AND PREVALENCE RATES

Prevalence rates of pathological gambling vary with the definitions and instruments used to define the disorder. Early studies, and a recent nationally representative study in the United States, relied on the South Oaks Gambling Screen (SOGS)[6] to assess prevalence rates. This instrument was developed during the era of DSM-III, and of the 20 items, 9 relate to sources of borrowing money. When the SOGS is used, rates of pathological gambling are estimated to be 1.6%–4.0% in the United States[7,8] and 0.8%–6.0% in other countries.[9,10] Although widely utilized, the SOGS may overdiagnose relative to instruments that are tied more closely to DSM-IV criteria. Three recent national surveys in the United States used DSM-IV-based instruments, alone or in combination with the SOGS. In a survey by Welte et al.,[8] rates of pathological gambling were 4.0% with the SOGS and 2.0% with a DSM-IV-based instrument. Two other national surveys, using DSM-IV-based instruments, found rates of 0.4%[11] and 0.8%.[12]

Limited data exist regarding psychometric properties of these instruments. The 17-item National Opinion Research Center DSM Screen for Gambling Problems (NODS) is based directly on DSM-IV criteria and covers some criteria in two forms.[12] Internal consistency is 0.79 when affirmative responses to the 10 DSM-IV criteria are examined, and 0.84 for the full scale.[13] Principal component analysis identified three factors. Four items reflecting negative behavioral consequences loaded on factor 1, and the second factor consisted of items related to preoccupation and impaired control. Items associated with family, social, and employment problems loaded on both factors 1 and 2. Tolerance, withdrawal, and relief gambling loaded on factor 3. Toce-Gerstein et al.[14] inspected responses to NODS items among 399 people who responded affirmatively to at least one DSM pathological gambling criterion in the Gerstein et al.[12] survey. Most people who met only one or two criteria reported chasing losses. Those who endorsed three to four items affirmed most often items related to lying, escape, and preoccupation. Individuals who met diagnostic criteria also reported loss of control, withdrawal, risking social relationships, and financial bailouts. Only the most severely disturbed gamblers committed illegal acts to support gambling.

The survey of more than 43,000 respondents[11,15] used a 15-item DSM-based instrument. Internal consistency of symptom items ($\alpha = 0.92$) and criteria for pathological gambling ($\alpha = 0.80$) was adequate.

Although these two national surveys[11,12] utilized different instruments, they found somewhat similar prevalence rates. The proportion of pathological gamblers identified in the surveys[12,15] who endorsed the various criteria are shown in Table 17–2. Of the five most commonly endorsed criteria, two have parallel items in substance use diagnoses: preoccupation and tolerance. Chasing, lying, and escape questions were also reported by relatively high proportions of gamblers in both surveys.

TABLE 17–2. Proportions of pathological gamblers endorsing DSM-IV criteria

	Gerstein et al.[12] $n=63$	Blanco et al.[15] $n=187$
Preoccupation	87.3%	97.8%
Chasing	84.1%	89.8%
Lying	77.8%	80.8%
Tolerance	57.2%	78.5%
Escape	84.1%	66.5%
Loss of control	65.1%	67.3%
Bailout	53.9%	50.1%
Withdrawal	71.4%	48.4%
Risked relationships	61.9%	37.0%
Illegal acts	19.0%	18.0%

These criteria have no direct parallel criteria in drug dependence diagnoses, although aspects of the behavioral patterns may be considered somewhat analogous.

While proportions of pathological gamblers who endorsed the DSM criteria were in some ways similar between the samples, some variations were also noted. These differences may relate to the manner in which the criteria were worded, the samples to whom surveys were administered, or the use of in-person versus telephone interviews. To the extent that some diagnostic criteria for substance use and pathological gambling disorders are related, the phenomenology, clinical features, and comorbidity may be strengthened artificially. That is, if a criterion is engagement in a behavior to such an extent that it adversely impacts one's family relationships, then individuals who have poor family relationships may be likely to endorse the negative impact of alcohol and gambling, and possibly other behaviors, on family relations.

In sum, defining features of pathological gambling are not yet well established and have varied across versions of DSM. Some criteria associated with substance use disorders are common in pathological gamblers, but others have no direct parallels in the dependence criteria.

COMORBIDITIES AND DEMOGRAPHIC FEATURES

Pathological gambling is highly comorbid with substance use disorders. For example, over 70% of individuals identified with pathological gambling had an alcohol use disorder, and over 30% had a drug use disorder.[11] High comorbidity may suggest that the disorders are part of the same spectrum and should be classified accordingly. However, substance use disorders are not the only psychiatric conditions that occur with pathological gambling. Significant odds ratios of pathological gambling are also noted with mood, anxiety, and personality disorders.[11] Thus, comorbidities do not lend support for or refute the notion that these disorders should be classified together as addictive disorders. Many psychiatric conditions co-occur,[16] and parallels in diagnostic criteria may explain comorbidities, at least in part.

In terms of demographics, younger age, male gender, minority ethnicity, and low socioeconomic status increase risk for drug use disorders and pathological gambling.[10,17,18] However, these characteristics are related to many psychiatric conditions and thus may not be useful for determining classifications.

PHYSIOLOGY AND BIOLOGY

Some physiological substrates may be similar with respect to gambling and substance use disorders. Rugle and Melamed[19] reported frontal lobe dysfunction in pathological gamblers relative to control subjects. Regard et al.[20] also found impaired concentration, memory, and executive functioning in gamblers. Similar deficits have been reported in substance abusers.[21] Some studies of neural processing are finding that gains and losses may be processed differentially in certain brain regions, primarily the frontal lobe.[22,23] In a functional magnetic resonance imaging study of controls, Gehring and Willoughby[24] found that choices made subsequent to losses may be riskier and associated with greater brain activity than choices made after gains. Petry[25] showed that substance abusers who also have a gambling problem performed more poorly on this gain–loss task than substance abusers without gambling problems, and both groups performed more poorly than controls. Cavedini et al.[26] replicated these results, noting that even "pure" pathological gamblers performed more poorly on this task than controls. On another decision-making task assessing preferences for sooner, smaller (vs. later), larger monetary rewards, both substance abusers and gamblers had similar deficits, with an additive effect noted in individuals with both disorders.[27,28] Performance on this task is linked to impulsivity.[29] However, no known studies have conducted brain imaging of gamblers participating in this task, so effects on particular brain regions and their association with substance use disorders are speculative.

Studies investigating neurotransmitters are also limited. Perhaps of greatest interest to the putative link with substance use disorders is dopamine, which is associated with reward and reinforcement and implicated in drug use disorders.[30] Two studies evaluated cerebrospinal fluid (CSF) levels of dopamine in gamblers, but they produced different results. Roy et al.[31] found no differences between gamblers and controls in plasma, urinary, or CSF dopamine levels, but Bergh et al.[32] found a decrease in dopamine and an increase in its metabolites in the CSF of gamblers.

Opioids are another class of abused drugs, and the relationship between endogenous opioids and gambling has been investigated. Shinohara et al.[33] found elevated levels of beta-endorphin in gamblers in Japan, which peaked during winning periods. Blaszczysnski et al.[34] found low plasma levels of beta-endorphin in horse race pathological gamblers but no differences relative to controls among poker machine players. In their study, betting did not alter beta-endorphin levels.

Other neurotransmitter systems have also been studied. Serotonin is of interest because low levels of this neurotransmitter are linked to impulsive behaviors.[35] Moreno et al.[36] found some evidence of a hypoactive serotonergic system in gamblers. Two other studies[37,38] reported decreased platelet monoamine oxidase activity, and another[39] found low CSF levels of a serotonin metabolite. While these data suggest the possibility of a serotonin deficiency, and possibly postsynaptic hypersensitivity of serotonin receptors, other studies found no serotonin abnormalities in gamblers.[31,32,40]

In terms of norepinephrine (NE), Roy et al.[31] found lower plasma levels of an NE metabolite, 3-methoxy-4-hydroxyphenylglycol (MHPG), and greater urinary outputs of NE in gamblers relative to controls, but no changes in CSF NE levels. Roy et al.[41] found correlations between personality measures of extroversion and CSF levels of MHPG, plasma levels of MHPG, and urinary NE output.

While studies show abnormalities in neurotransmitter levels in pathological gamblers compared with controls, most reports were conducted in very small samples. Some allowed for inclusion of individuals with comorbid conditions, thereby reducing the ability to isolate specific effects of pathological gambling. Discrepant results across studies may also be related to different techniques used to obtain CSF and measure metabolites. Thus, neurotransmitter abnormalities that may share features between substance use and pathological gambling disorders should be considered speculative relationships. In other research, genes are being evaluated, as they may influence expression of neurochemicals.

GENETICS

Pathological gambling clearly has a genetic component, and it may share some genetic links with substance use disorders. Adults identified as pathological gamblers are more likely than nonpathological gamblers to report having a parent with a gambling problem.[42] Winters and Rich[43] noted greater similarity of gambling behaviors in 42 monozygotic twin pairs compared with 50 dizygotic twin pairs, but this effect was noted only in men and for specific types of wagering.

Only one other twin study of pathological gambling exists. Eisen et al.[44] reported that familial factors (inheritance or shared childhood experiences) explained 62% of the variance in developing pathological gambling in a sample of 6,718 male members of the Vietnam Era Twin Registry. Further, a linear relationship was observed between alcohol abuse or dependence and severity of disordered gambling in this sample. Slutske et al.,[45] using biometric modeling, found that 12%–20% of the genetic variation in the risk for disordered gambling was accounted for by genetic variation in common with the risk for alcohol dependence. Although these data suggest a role of familial factors in pathological gambling, it clearly is a multifaceted disorder, with environmental factors also important.

A molecular genetics study[46] found an association between the Taq-A1 allele of the D_2 dopamine receptor gene and gambling. This allele is also associated with impulsive, compulsive and addictive behaviors.[47] Other studies suggest a role for the D_1 and D_4 receptor genes[48,49] in pathological gambling. The *DRD4* sequence is related to attention-deficit disorder, Tourette's disorder, and substance abuse.[49] Pérez de Castro et al.[50] found that the less efficient variant of this polymorphism in *DRD4* was common among female, but not male, gamblers. A polymorphism in the MAO-A gene was found among men with severe gambling problems.[51] These results suggest that genetic contributions may differ between genders, with serotonergic dysfunction more common in men and dopaminergic dysregulation in women. However, more research with larger samples is needed to confirm these findings.

Another study of 139 gamblers and 139 controls[52] found that *DRD2, DRD4,* and the dopamine transporter gene *DAT1* were associated with pathological gambling, accounting for about 8% of the variance. The 16 genes tested, including those for dopamine, serotonin, and NE, together accounted for 15%–21% of the variance. The authors concluded that dopamine, serotonin, and NE all play a role in the disorder, but none are unique to it. Rather, they all are associated with a range of psychiatric conditions. Individuals who inherit a threshold number of these genes may be at increased risk of developing impulsive, compulsive and substance use problems.

TREATMENTS AND OUTCOMES

Pathological gambling and substance abuse share some commonalities in course and outcomes. Both usually begin in adolescence or early adulthood, although excessive wagering may emerge in a subset of individuals during middle age.[53] They both have waxing and waning courses.[54,55] About 60% of individuals identified as lifetime pathological gamblers do not meet current criteria.[7] Similarly, a proportion of substance abusers overcome drug and alcohol problems.[56] Natural recovery may be common in both disorders.[57,58] Motivation to change is an important construct associated with cessation of gambling[59] and substance abuse.[60] Skills deficits in managing situations that are high risk for use of substances or wagering are also noted in both disorders.[61,62]

Given these similarities, many psychosocial treatments applied to pathological gamblers were adapted from substance use disorder treatments, including 12-step, motivational, and cognitive-behavioral therapies and even pharmacotherapies.[10] However, similar therapies do not necessarily lend support for similar etiologies, as many of these therapies are used in other psychiatric conditions as well. One type of psychotherapy appears unique for pathological gambling. A cognitive therapy focusing on altering irrational gambling cognitions shows potential efficacy,[63,64] and it has no direct parallel in treatment of substance use or other psychiatric disorders.

Advantages of Expansion to Addictive Disorders

The studies reviewed in this chapter provide some support for reclassifying substance use and pathological gambling under the umbrella of addictive disorders. Comorbidity is high, presenting features have parallels, demographic features share commonalities, and physiology and genetics have some overlap. Some advantages might stem from an addictive disorders classification.

Although awareness of pathological gambling is low in most mental health fields, substance abuse treatment programs seem more likely than general mental health treatment programs to inquire about gambling histories in their patients. Classification of pathological gambling and substance use disorders within the same framework might further increase awareness of the disorder. It might also extend treatments to pathological gamblers within the context of drug abuse treatment clinics.

If pathological gambling were classified along with substance use disorders, the number of criteria needed for a diagnosis might be reduced, and this may lead to a more accurate classification of individuals. Another potential advantage is that a subdiagnostic condition (e.g., gambling abuse) may be considered. Epidemiological studies indicate that a larger proportion of the population has a subthreshold condition than those who meet full diagnostic criteria,[7,12] and the disorder appears to exist along a continuum.[15] Inclusion of less severe forms of disorders in DSM may be appropriate clinically[65]; it may also encourage more research and treatment efforts. Reclassification of the disorders may reduce balkanization of these disorders, which appear, at least on some levels, to share similar features.

Funding and research efforts may also increase by combining these disorders within the same classification system. Currently in the United States, the National Institute on Drug Abuse (NIDA) and National Institute on Alcohol Abuse and Alcoholism (NIAAA) fund drug and alcohol research, respectively, but not gambling research, unless the gambling co-occurs with substance use. Thus, there remains a somewhat artificial distinction between research that focuses exclusively on pathological gambling substance abusers and that which includes all pathological gamblers, with or without substance use problems. It is unclear, however, which institute, NIDA or NIAAA, would consider the disorder under its jurisdiction.

Disadvantages of Expansion to Addictive Disorders

Despite potential advantages of reclassification, disadvantages can also be highlighted. An obvious, albeit possibly artificial, rationale for keeping the disorders distinct relates to the lack of ingestion of a substance with pathological gambling.

Substance abusers often experience significant relief once the acute effects of withdrawal subside, but adverse effects of pathological gambling persist long-term, especially related to financial matters.

Although few data yet support the criteria that define presenting features of pathological gambling, it appears that criteria may not be as similar between pathological gambling and substance use disorders as they are across drug use disorders. The phenomenon of chasing, the most common in pathological gamblers, has no direct parallel in substance use disorders. The impact of pathological gambling on finances does not have such a strong component in drug use disorders. Conversely, direct negative impacts of some forms of drug use on health are not as relevant in gambling, although global health is poor in gamblers.[66]

Including pathological gambling as an addictive disorder along with substance use disorders might increase stigmatization. Pathological gamblers might feel uncomfortable in group sessions with substance abusers. They might withdraw from treatment prematurely if they do not feel the therapy is addressing their unique needs. Clinics that treat primarily substance abusers might not be as experienced with, or receive a sufficient number of, treatment-seeking gamblers to have groups dedicated to them.

Finally, expansion to a category of addictive disorders ultimately might lead to a catch-all of "disorders," some of which might be inappropriate for diagnosis. For example, television, work, exercise, and chocolate addictions have been described.[67–70] One must be cautious of where to draw the line between simply an excessive behavior pattern and a bona fide psychiatric disorder.

Reclassification of all excessive behaviors might also inadvertently impede understanding of some of these conditions. For example, over two-thirds of Americans are overweight, but does this statistic suggest that most Americans are addicted to food? Conversely, a subset of the population might be considered addicted to purging, and another subset to not eating (anorexia). These actual eating disorders, and others that might eventually be considered legitimate psychiatric disorders, might be better understood within the context of eating disorders than within the context of addictive disorders. Similarly, excessive Internet use is often related to pornography viewing[71] and as such might (or might not) be better understood within the context of a sexual disorder than as a behavioral addiction.

Summary

Although only limited data exist about some of these conditions, the pros and cons of altering classification systems should be considered prior to deciding whether pathological gambling is better categorized as an impulse control or addictive disorder. Societal interest with excessive behavior patterns cannot be separated entirely from science or medicine, but weighing the evidence along with the costs and benefits of changing is necessary for advancing the field as a whole. Society and individuals may benefit from expanding scientific classification systems to include other excessive behavior patterns.[72] Diagnosis of nicotine dependence may be a case in point; it allowed for and encouraged medical and psychological treatment for one of the most cost-effective and life-saving interventions in health care. Further consideration of other nonpharmacological addictions as diagnoses, whether they are included alongside or separate from pharmacological addictions, may similarly stimulate assessment and treatment, and ultimately even prevention efforts.

References

1. American Psychiatric Association: Diagnostic and Statistical Manual of Mental Disorders, 4th Edition. Washington, DC, American Psychiatric Association, 1994.
2. American Psychiatric Association: Diagnostic and Statistical Manual of Mental Disorders, 3rd Edition. Washington, DC, American Psychiatric Association, 1980.
3. Lesieur H: The Chase: Career of the Compulsive Gambler. Oxford, England, Anchor, 1977.
4. Mark ME, Lesieur HR: A feminist critique of problem gambling research. Br J Addict 87:549–565, 1992.
5. American Psychiatric Association: Diagnostic and Statistical Manual of Mental Disorders, 3rd Edition, Revised. Washington, DC, American Psychiatric Association, 1987.
6. Lesieur HR, Blume SB: The South Oaks Gambling Screen (the SOGS): a new instrument for the identification of pathological gamblers. Am J Psychiatry 144:1184–1188, 1987.
7. Shaffer HJ, Hall MN, Vander Bilt J: Estimating the prevalence of disordered gambling behavior in the United States and Canada: a research synthesis. Am J Public Health 89:1369–1376, 1999.
8. Welte J, Barnes G, Wieczorek W, et al: Alcohol and gambling pathology among U.S. adults: prevalence, demographic patterns and comorbidity. J Stud Alcohol 62:706–712, 2001.
9. Orford J, Sproston K, Erens B: SOGS and DSM-IV in the British Gambling Prevalence Survey: reliability and factor structure. International Gambling Studies 3:53–65, 2003.
10. Petry NM: Pathological Gambling: Etiology, Comorbidity, and Treatment. Washington, DC, American Psychological Association, 2005.
11. Petry NM, Stinson FS, Grant BF: Comorbidity of DSM-IV pathological gambling and psychiatric disorders: results from the National Epidemiologic Survey on Alcohol and Related Conditions. J Clin Psychiatry 66:564–574, 2005.
12. Gerstein DR, Volberg RA, Toce MT, et al: Gambling Impact and Behavior Study: Report to the National Gambling Impact Study Commission. Chicago, IL, National Opinion Research Center, 1999.
13. Hodgins DC: Using the NORC DSM Screen for Gambling Problems (NODS) as an outcome measure for pathological gambling: psychometric evaluation. Addict Behav 29:1685–1690, 2004.
14. Toce-Gerstein M, Gerstein DR, Volberg RA: A hierarchy of gambling disorders in the community. Addiction 98:1661–1672, 2003.

15. Blanco C, Hasin DS, Petry NM, et al: Sex differences in subclinical and DSM-IV pathological gambling: results from the National Epidemiologic Survey on Alcohol and Related Conditions. Psychol Med 36:943–953, 2006.
16. Kessler RC, McGonagle KA, Zhao S, et al: Lifetime and 12-month prevalence of DSM-III-R psychiatric disorders in the United States: results from the National Comorbidity Study. Arch Gen Psychiatry 51:8–19, 1994.
17. Furr-Holden CDM, Anthony JC: Epidemiologic differences in drug dependence: a US–UK cross-national comparison. Soc Psychiatry Psychiatr Epidemiol 38:165–172, 2003.
18. National Research Council: Pathological Gambling: A Critical Review. Washington, DC, National Academy Press, 1999.
19. Rugle L, Melamed L: Neuropsychological assessment of attention problems in pathological gamblers. J Nerv Ment Dis 181:107–112, 1993.
20. Regard M, Knoch D, Gütling E, et al: Brain damage and addictive behavior: a neuropsychological and electroencephalogram investigation with pathologic gamblers. Cog Behav Neurol 16:47–53, 2003.
21. Goldstein RZ, Leskovjan AC, Hoff AL, et al: Severity of neuropsychological impairment in cocaine and alcohol addiction: association with metabolism in the prefrontal cortex. Neuropsychologia 42:1447–1458, 2004.
22. Bechara A, Damasio H, Tranel D, et al: Deciding advantageously before knowing the advantageous strategy. Science 275:1293–1295, 1997.
23. Breiter HC, Aharon I, Kahneman D, et al: Functional imaging of neural responses to expectancy and experience of monetary gains and losses. Neuron 30:619–639, 2001.
24. Gehring WJ, Willoughby AR: The medial frontal cortex and the rapid processing of monetary gains and losses. Science 295:2279–2282, 2002.
25. Petry NM: Substance abuse, pathological gambling, and impulsivity. Drug Alcohol Depend 63:29–38, 2001.
26. Cavedini P, Riboldi G, Keller R, et al: Frontal lobe dysfunction in pathological gambling patients. Biol Psychiatry 51:334–341, 2002.
27. Petry NM: Pathological gamblers, with and without substance use disorders, discount delayed rewards at high rates. J Abnorm Psychol 110:482–487, 2001.
28. Petry NM, Casarella T: Excessive discounting of delayed reinforcers in substance abusers with gambling problems. Drug Alcohol Depend 56:25–32, 1999.
29. Alessi SM, Petry NM: Pathological gambling severity is associated with impulsivity in a delay discounting procedure. Behav Processes 64:345–354, 2003.
30. Koob GF: Drug of abuse: anatomy, pharmacology and function of reward pathways. Trends Pharmacol Sci 13:177–184, 1992.
31. Roy A, Adinoff B, Roehrich L, et al: Pathological gambling: a psychobiological study. Arch Gen Psychiatry 45:369–373, 1988.
32. Bergh C, Eklund T, Sodersten P, et al: Altered dopamine function in pathological gambling. Psychol Med 27:473–475, 1997.
33. Shinohara K, Yanagisawa A, Kagota Y, et al: Physiological changes in Pachinko players: beta-endorphin, catecholamines, immune system substances and heart rate. Appl Human Sci 18:37–42, 1999.
34. Blaszczynski AP, Wintor SW, McConaghy N: Plasma endorphin levels in pathological gambling. Journal of Gambling Behavior 2:3–14, 1986.

35. Oreland L, Ekblom J, Garpenstrand H, et al: Biological markers, with special regard to platelet monoamine oxidase (trbc-MAO), for personality and personality disorders. Adv Pharmacol 42:301–304, 1998.
36. Moreno I, Sáiz-Ruiz J, López-Ibor JJ: Serotonin and gambling dependence. Hum Psychopharmacol 6:S9–S12, 1991.
37. Blanco C, Orensanz-Muñoz L, Blanco-Jerez C, et al: Pathological gambling and platelet MAO activity: a psychobiological study. Am J Psychiatry 153:119–121, 1996.
38. Carrasco JL, Sáiz-Ruiz J, Hollander E, et al: Low platelet monoamine oxidase activity in pathological gambling. Acta Psychiatr Scand 90:427–431, 1994.
39. Nordin C, Eklundh T: Altered CSF 5-HIAA disposition in pathological male gamblers. CNS Spectr 4:25–33, 1999.
40. Roy A, Linnoila M: CSF studies on alcoholism and related behaviours. Prog Neuropsychopharmacol Biol Psychiatry 13:505–511, 1989.
41. Roy A, DeJong J, Linnoila M: Extraversion in pathological gamblers: correlates with indexes of noradrenergic function. Arch Gen Psychiatry 46:679–681, 1989.
42. Volberg RA, Steadman HJ: Prevalence estimates of pathological gambling in New Jersey and Maryland. Am J Psychiatry 166:1618–1619, 1989.
43. Winters KC, Rich T: A twin study of adult gambling behavior. J Gambl Stud 14:213–225, 1998.
44. Eisen SA, Lin N, Lyons MJ, et al: Familial influences on gambling behavior: an analysis of 3359 twin pairs. Addiction 93:1375–1384, 1998.
45. Slutske WS, Eisen S, True WR, et al: Common genetic vulnerability for pathological gambling and alcohol dependence in men. Arch Gen Psychiatry 57:666–673, 2000.
46. Comings DE, Rosenthal RJ, Lesieur HR, et al: A study of the dopamine D2 receptor gene in pathological gambling. Pharmacogenetics 6:223–234, 1996.
47. Blum K, Sheridan PJ, Wood RC, et al: Dopamine D2 receptor gene variants: association and linkage studies in impulsive-addictive compulsive behavior. Pharmacogenetics 5:121–141, 1995.
48. Comings DE, Gade R, Wu S, et al: Studies of the potential role of the dopamine D1 receptor gene in addictive behaviors. Mol Psychiatry 2:44–56, 1997.
49. Comings DE, Gonzalez N, Wu S, et al: Studies of the 48 bp repeat polymorphism of the DRD4 gene in impulsive, compulsive, addictive behaviors: Tourette syndrome, ADHD, pathological gambling, and substance abuse. Am J Med Genet 88:358–368, 1999.
50. Pérez de Castro I, Ibáñez A, Torres P, et al: Genetic association study between pathological gambling and a functional DNA polymorphism at the D4 receptor. Pharmacogenetics 7:345–348, 1997.
51. Ibáñez A, Pérez de Castro I, Fernández-Piqueras J, et al: Genetic association study between pathological gambling and DNA polymorphic markers at MAO-A and MAO-B genes. Mol Psychiatry 5:105–109, 2000.
52. Comings DE, Gade-Andavolu R, Gonzalez N, et al: The additive effect of neurotransmitter genes in pathological gambling. Clin Genet 60:107–116, 2001.
53. Petry NM: A comparison of young, middle age, and older adult treatment-seeking pathological gamblers. Gerontologist 42:92–99, 2002.

54. Slutske WS, Jackson KM, Sher KJ: The natural history of problem gambling from age 18 to 29. J Abnorm Psychol 112:263–274, 2003.
55. Muthén BO, Muthén LK: The development of heavy drinking and alcohol-related problems from ages 18–37 in a U.S. national sample. J Stud Alcohol 61:290–300, 2000.
56. Institute of Medicine: Broadening the Base of Treatment for Alcohol Problems. Washington, DC, National Academy of Sciences, 1990.
57. Hodgins DC, el-Guebaly N: Natural and treatment-assisted recovery from gambling problems: a comparison of resolved and active gamblers. Addiction 95:777–789, 2000.
58. Sobell LC, Cunningham JA, Sobell MB: Recovery from alcohol problems with and without treatment: prevalence in two population surveys. Am J Public Health 86:966–972, 1996.
59. Petry NM: Stages of change in treatment-seeking pathological gamblers. J Consult Clin Psychol 73:312–322, 2005.
60. Prochaska JO, Velicer WF, Rossi JS, et al: Stages of change and decisional balance for 12 problem behaviors. Health Psychol 13:39–46, 1994.
61. Chaney EF, O'Leary MR, Marlatt GA: Skill training with alcoholics. J Consult Clin Psychol 46:1092–1104, 1978.
62. McCormick RA: The importance of coping skill enhancement in the treatment of the pathological gambler. J Gambl Stud 10:77–86, 1994.
63. Ladouceur R, Sylvain S, Boutin C, et al: Cognitive treatment of pathological gambling. J Nerv Ment Dis 189:774–780, 2001.
64. Sylvain C, Ladouceur R, Boisvert JM: Cognitive and behavioral treatment of pathological gambling: a controlled study. J Consult Clin Psychol 65:727–732, 1997.
65. Kessler RC, Merikangas KR, Berglund P, et al: Mild disorders should not be eliminated from the DSM-V. Arch Gen Psychiatry 60:1117–1122, 2003.
66. Pietrzak R, Molina C, Ladd GT, et al: Health and psychosocial correlates of problem gambling in the elderly. Am J Geriatr Psychiatry 13:510–519, 2005.
67. Flowers CP, Robinson B: A structural and discriminant analysis of the Work Addiction Risk Test. Educ Psychol Meas 62:517–526, 2002.
68. McIlwraith R, Jacobvitz RS, Kubey R, et al: Television addiction: theories and data behind the ubiquitous metaphor. Am Behav Sci 35:104–121, 1991.
69. Terry A, Szabo A, Griffiths M: The exercise addiction inventory: a new brief screening tool. Addiction Research and Theory 12:489–499, 2004.
70. Tuomisto T, Hetherington MM, Morris MF, et al: Psychological and physiological characteristics of sweet food "addiction." Int J Eat Disord 25:169–175, 1999.
71. Griffiths M: Excessive Internet use: implications for sexual behavior. Cyberpsychol Behav 3:537–552, 2000.
72. West R: Theory of Addiction. London, England, Blackwell, 2006.

18

CHARACTERISTICS OF NOSOLOGICALLY INFORMATIVE DATA SETS THAT ADDRESS KEY DIAGNOSTIC ISSUES FACING THE DSM-V AND ICD-11 SUBSTANCE USE DISORDERS WORKGROUPS

Linda B. Cottler, Ph.D.
Bridget F. Grant, Ph.D.

Over the past two decades, many nosological issues have been addressed by the *Diagnostic and Statistical Manual of Mental Disorders* (DSM) and *International*

L.B.C. acknowledges the support of the National Institute on Drug Abuse of the National Institutes of Health (grants DA005585, DA005688, DA014854, DA015984, DA07313, and GB67741).

Reprinted from Cottler LB, Grant BF: "Characteristics of Nosologically Informative Data Sets That Address Key Diagnostic Issues Facing the DSM-V and ICD-11 Substance Use Disorders Workgroups." *Addiction* 101 (suppl 1):161–169, 2006. Used with permission of the Society for the Study of Addiction.

Classification of Diseases (ICD) substance use disorders workgroups. Numerous sources of material were utilized to make final decisions for DSM-IV, such as ongoing consultation with more than 50 expert advisors, a literature review of published articles on specific topics, and secondary data analyses with funding from the MacArthur Foundation. Even with those efforts, a number of key questions remained requiring focused field trials, which were funded by the American Psychiatric Association.[1] However, there are lingering issues that have not been resolved by consultation, literature review, and statistical analyses. These will be revisited, or addressed de novo, by the DSM workgroup. The spectrum of these lingering points is broad owing to the number of substances classified under the diagnostic umbrella of substance use disorders.

Salient issues for DSM-V have been addressed in the chapters by Saunders and Schuckit (see introduction to this volume) and Schuckit and Saunders (see Chapter 19, "Empirical Basis of Substance Use Disorders," in this volume). Among them are the following: is the cookie-cutter approach still valid? In other words, can the same set of criteria apply for all substances, for all age groups, and for users from all cultures? Is there coherence in the abuse and dependence syndrome? Are dependence and abuse two distinct concepts, or do abuse and dependence represent one spectrum, with abuse being the milder form of dependence? Should DSM develop separate research and clinical diagnostic criteria, as did the tenth revision of the ICD? A related topic concerns dimensional and categorical approaches to diagnoses and whether there should be a dichotomous approach, or if there could be a mild, moderate, or severe subtype, with use of a number of criteria as a diagnostic approach. Related to this, as Helzer et al. discuss in this volume (see Chapter 2, "Should There Be Both Categorical and Dimensional Criteria for the Substance Use Disorders in DSM-V?"), certain risk factors, such as family history or a biomarker, might be utilized to determine the certainty of a diagnosis. The revision process may also evaluate the pros and cons of including quantity/frequency in the criteria. Further, revisions should inspect the redundancy in the criteria; if two or more items seem to co-occur to such an extent that they are actually measuring the same construct, they should be candidates for merging or paring. Similarly, if the data show that one or more criteria are too common to discriminate nonproblem from problem users, such criteria should be reconsidered. The literature has evolved since the last revision on the issue of diagnostic orphans, and the data published should be put to good use to decide on the cut points for diagnoses. An issue that signals a return to the DSM-III alcohol dependence concept is whether there should be a requirement for either tolerance or withdrawal, including how restrictive or inclusive the withdrawal syndromes should be. The workgroup may determine whether assessments should separately assess impairment criteria for each substance use disorder, or whether the criteria themselves contain enough adjectives to describe the clinical severity of each behavior. The workgroup will most probably discuss the mélange of adjectives to describe addictive behaviors, such as "persistent," "recurrent," and "maladaptive." Finally, data will also be presented on the necessity of adding new drug categories and criteria. Candidates will most probably be 3,4-methylenedioxymethamphetamine (MDMA) abuse/dependence, caffeine abuse/dependence, cannabis withdrawal, and steroid abuse.

Characteristics of Optimally Informative Data Sets

The aforementioned persistent issues will be tackled by the DSM-V and ICD-11 committees. Fortunately, relevant empirical data are available to be used as the foundation for resolving these key nosological issues, especially data from a handful of studies specifically funded for such tasks through the National Institute on Drug Abuse (NIDA) and the National Institute on Alcohol Abuse and Alcoholism (NIAAA) (Table 18–1). Studies such as these exist solely for the purpose of nosological inquiry. Moreover, the assessments used in these studies were developed for interdiagnostic system comparisons for several or all substance categories; diagnostic comparisons between clinicians and nonclinicians; test–retest reliability of symptoms and diagnoses, with protocols for understanding reasons for unreliability; cross-cultural comparisons of disorders; evaluation of the relevance of adopted criteria for "new" drugs; and other nosological uses. Although small in number, these studies are rich in content, and some are international in scope. Data for reanalyses will also include projects that the institutes have funded, with these issues secondary to other goals of the research. These studies, funded by NIDA and NIAAA, will be able to generate useful information because they were designed with methods and assessment instruments identical to those of the primarily nosological studies (Table 18–2). The data sets will be able to assist the workgroups as the points mentioned above are analyzed individually.

One general population study is of particular relevance for assisting in decisions underlying DSM-V and ICD-11 revisions. The NIAAA National Epidemiologic Survey on Alcohol and Related Conditions (NESARC), recently released to the scientific community, is the largest (n=43,093) survey of DSM-IV alcohol, drug and mental disorders conducted in the United States.[2] Briefly, NESARC is a nationally representative sample of the adult population of the United States, targeting adults not institutionalized, 18 years and older, who reside in the 50 states and the District of Columbia. NESARC was a face-to-face survey with an overall response rate of 81%. Because of its sample and detailed coverage of substance use disorders, and because of the quantity and frequency of alcohol and risk factors, it is ideally suited for many of the topics of interest to the workgroup.

Workgroups have learned that the decisions underlying the revision process for the *Diagnostic and Statistical Manual* must be evidence-based. The characteristics of databases used for such nosological decisions are listed in Table 18–3, and de-

TABLE 18–1. Data sets specifically funded for nosological work on substance use disorders

Name	Diagnostic systems/substance	Assessment	Study characteristics	Sample
Clinical implications of drug abuse diagnoses Rounsaville, PI DA 005592	DSM-IV and -III-R All substances and personality disorders	SCID	Test–retest design Clinical validity	*N*=400 Users in and out of treatment (18–60 years old)
Reliability and validity of DSM and ICD substance use disorders Cottler, PI DA 005585	DSM-III, -III-R, -IV ICD-10 All substances	SAM SCAN ASI Urine Collaterals	Test, 1-week retest SCAN validity Discrepancy protocol interview	*N*=1,000 Users in treatment Users from ECA Pain patients, adolescents (18–44 years old)
DSM-IV field trials Schuckit, PI, and Cottler, Coord, Center MacArthur and APA funding	DSM-III, -III-R, -IV ICD-10 All substances	SAM	San Diego, Denver, Vermont, Philadelphia, St. Louis	*N*=600 Users in treatment and from general population (18–54 years old)
Validating epidemiological measures of alcohol and drug dependence Langenbucher, PI DA 005688	DSM-III, -IV ICD-10 Alcohol, opiates, cannabis, and cocaine	SAM CIDI	Treatment sample from drug abuse treatment units in NY, NY, CT, PA, and MA Validity of DSM-IV and ICD-10 with secondary data analysis of community subjects	*N*=370 National Comorbidity Survey Secondary data analysis

TABLE 18–1. Data sets specifically funded for nosological work on substance use disorders *(continued)*

Name	Diagnostic systems/substance	Assessment	Study characteristics	Sample
Validating epidemiological measures of alcohol dependence Hasin, PI AA 008910	DSM-IV All substances	AUDADIS PRISM	Test–retest design	*N*=296 Clinic sample
St. Louis WHO Reliability and Validity Study Cottler, PI WHO funded	DSM-III, -III-R, -IV ICD-10 All substances	CIDI AUDADIS SCAN	Three-instrument design Discrepancy interview protocol	*N*=150 In and out of treatment (18–40 years old)
Tri-City Study of MDMA Use, Abuse and Dependence Cottler, PI DA 014854	DSM-IV All substances (and steroids) MDMA, GHB, Rohypnol, and ketamine separated	SAM for club drugs RBA SCAN Hair samples STD testing	Test, 1-week retest SCAN validity Discrepancy interview protocol Debriefing interview Ethnographic substudy of withdrawal symptoms	*N*=650 St. Louis, Miami, and Sydney Community sample (15–35 years old)

TABLE 18–1. Data sets specifically funded for nosological work on substance use disorders *(continued)*

Name	Diagnostic systems/substance	Assessment	Study characteristics	Sample
MDMA use, abuse and dependence in Taiwan Cottler, PI NIDA contract	DSM-IV All substances (and steroids) MDMA, GHB, Rohypnol, and ketamine separated, urine	SAM for club drugs RBA SARS Hair	Test and validity SAM clinician interview Discrepancy interview protocol Debriefing interview fMRI study	*N*=150 Community sample from Taipei (18–30 years old)
Reliability and validity of inhalants Ridenour, PI DA 015984	DSM-IV and marijuana, cocaine, hallucinogens, and separate criteria for four categories of inhalants	SAM for inhalants RBA SCAN Urine	Test, 1-week retest SCAN validity Discrepancy interview protocol Debriefing interview	*N*=150 Community sample (12–25 years old)
PRISM comorbidity diagnosis for drug abuse treatment Hasin, PI DA 010919	DSM-IV All substances	PRISM	Test–retest	*N*=285 Clinic samples

Note. APA=American Psychiatric Association; ASI=Alcohol Severity Index; AUDADIS=Alcohol Use Disorder and Associated Disabilities Interview Schedule; CIDI=Composite International Diagnostic Interview; DSM=*Diagnostic and Statistical Manual of Mental Disorders*; ECA=Epidemiologic Catchment Area; fMRI=functional magnetic resonance imaging; GHB=gamma-hydroxybutyrate; ICD=*International Classification of Diseases*; MDMA = methylenedioxymethamphetamine; NIDA = National Institute on Drug Abuse; PI=primary investigator; PRISM=Psychiatric Research Interview for Substance and Mental Disorders; RBA=relative binding affinity; SAM=Substance Abuse Module; SCAN=Structured Clinical Assessment in Neuropsychiatry; SCID=Structured Clinical Interview for DSM; STD=sexually transmitted disease; WHO=World Health Organization.

TABLE 18–2. Data sets informative to DSM-V and ICD-11 workgroups, but not exclusively funded for such

Name	Diagnostic systems/substance	Assessment	Study characteristics	Sample
Alcohol in Israel: G×E effects Hasin, PI AA013654 + NIDA supplement	DSM-IV All substances and primary and secondary substance–induced MDD, PTSD, panic, GAD, ASP	AUDADIS PRISM Family history	Random household survey in Israel G×E interactions	N=2,500 General household sample (20–65 years old)
Australian Twin Study Heath, PI AA 007728	DSM-IV (PCP, hallucinogens, inhalants excluded)	SSAGA Genotyping, QTL mapping	Adult twins in Australia	N=13,000 Twins and spouses and relatives
Alcohol dependence: general population validity Hasin, PI AA 008159	DSM-IV All substances and major depression, ASP	AUDADIS	Baseline, 1- and 10-year follow-up of pre-screened heavy drinkers + supplementary evaluation of 9/11/01 exposure and response	N=962 Household sample (18–65 years old)
Missouri Adolescent Female Twins Study (MOAFTS) Heath, PI AA 00922	DSM-IV (PCP, hallucinogens, inhalants excluded) and psychiatric disorders	SSAGA	Female twins, parents Telephone and in person Cohort sequential design, birth records	N=3,000 female twins, 2,000 male twins (13–25 years old)

TABLE 18–2. Data sets informative to DSM-V and ICD-11 workgroups, but not exclusively funded for such *(continued)*

Name	Diagnostic systems/substance	Assessment	Study characteristics	Sample
COGA Begleiter, PI AA 008401	DSM-IV ICD-10	SSAGA Segregation and linkage analysis	Family study of high-risk drinkers Six sites: St. Louis, San Diego, Brooklyn, Iowa City, Farmington, Indianapolis	*N*=10,000 2,000 children and adolescents
Course of drug use disorders: effects of comorbidity Hasin, PI DA 008409	DSM-IV All substances and psychiatric disorders, and ASP and borderline	PRISM	Baseline and 6-, 12-, and 18-month follow-up	*N*=960 Methadone maintenance patients and dual-diagnosis inpatients (18+ years)

Note. ASP=antisocial personality disorder; AUDADIS=Alcohol Use Disorder and Associated Disabilities Interview Schedule; COGA=Collaborative Studies on the Genetics of Alcoholism; DSM=*Diagnostic and Statistical Manual of Mental Disorders*; E=environmental; G=genetic; GAD=generalized anxiety disorder; ICD=*International Classification of Diseases*; MDD=major depressive disorder; NIDA = National Institute on Drug Abuse; PCP=phencyclidine; PI=primary investigator; PRISM=Psychiatric Research Interview for Substance and Mental Disorders; PTSD=posttraumatic stress disorder; SSAG=Semistructured Assessment for the Genetics of Alcoholism.

TABLE 18–3. Characteristics of optimally informative data sets for DSM-V and ICD-11 workgroups on substance use disorders

1. The assessment should be true to the current nomenclature and nosology being studied.
2. The assessment should be flexible regarding potentially new rearrangements of scoring algorithms.
3. All substances and their consequences should be assessed individually.
4. Older versions of criteria should be collected in tandem with newer versions to evaluate the net cast by each system and version.
5. The "full version" rather than a "shortened screener version" should be used (i.e., no skip-outs).
6. The sample should be one that is generalizable in the broadest sense (i.e., diverse age, gender, ethnicity).
7. Diagnostic algorithms for scoring the disorders should be accessible for review.
8. Data sets with mixed methods for collection of data (survey and ethnography), as well as data sources (key informants, medical records, family history, hair or urine tests, or imaging), should be utilized as they offer dimensional diagnostic approaches.
9. Assessments should be reliable and valid concerning diagnoses and criteria.
10. Data sets must stretch the limits of the criteria to allow for the potential discovery of new drug classifications, new criteria, or new diagnoses.

scribed in detail below. Although all databases have some flaws, those in Table 18–3 come closest to achieving all of the ideal characteristics.

THE ASSESSMENT USED SHOULD BE TRUE TO THE NOMENCLATURE AND NOSOLOGY BEING STUDIED

To be useful, data must first and foremost be true to the nosology (classification) and nomenclature (terminology) being considered for revisions. Many studies of substance use disorders in the field, or already completed, were conducted with assessments that did not accurately elicit the diagnostic criteria because of inaccurate terminology or frequency thresholds. In others, diagnostic criteria were lumped together for all substances and not assessed independently. The World Mental Health–Composite International Diagnostic Interview (WMH-CIDI), administered to more people around the world than any other psychiatric interview as part of the World Health Organization World Mental Health Survey Initiative,[3] has significant limitations. Because of time constraints in the survey, the questions on DSM-IV substance dependence were skipped altogether if abuse was negative.

Thus, in the National Comorbidity Survey–Replication (NCS-R) study,[4] alcohol and "drug" dependence are only considered among the select group of people who have already met criteria for abuse. This same procedure has been used in the recent National Institute of Mental Health–sponsored NCS-A adolescent study, the NCS-2, a 10-year follow-up of the original NCS conducted in 1990–1992,[5] and the National Study of African American Life and the National Study of Latino and Asian Americans.[6] People who are negative for dependence represent those correctly classified as negative, and those misclassified who a) have not yet used drugs or alcohol or b) have used drugs or alcohol but do not meet criteria for abuse or dependence, in addition to those who c) have used drugs or alcohol and do not meet the criteria for abuse but who do meet the criteria for dependence. A sizeable proportion of users (34%), primarily women and minorities, have met criteria for current alcohol dependence without abuse and are missed with this skip pattern.[7] Similar underestimation has been found for drug dependence.[8] Whether dependence and abuse are distinct, or whether abuse and dependence represent one spectrum, with abuse being the milder form of substance use disorders, is a question that must be addressed empirically, and databases that have relied on assessments that employ these early exits falsely inform nosological analyses, whether for latent class, prevalence, or other analyses. Muthén (see Chapter 1, "Should Substance Use Disorders Be Considered as Categorical or Dimensional?," in this volume) and others[9,10] have addressed these issues with various model-testing methodologies.

Additionally, each criterion should ideally be assessed independently. For example, when individual withdrawal symptoms are not asked about for each drug, or withdrawal relief questions are skipped if withdrawal symptoms are positive, the overlap between withdrawal symptoms and relief cannot be assessed. Although such a strategy takes more time, the data are needed to understand the overlap of criteria.

Data sets should also be collected with instruments that follow the nomenclature regarding descriptors, symptoms, and drugs. In the absence of more specificity in DSM, diagnostic assessments and algorithms used should be transparent regarding the operationalization of descriptors such as "frequent," "persistent," "markedly," and "often." These words are not defined consistently: some investigators accept several times, others accept more than once, and still others leave definitions of words such as "often" and "persistent" up to the respondent. When the respondent is allowed to choose, inconsistencies arise, resulting in poor reliability and ultimately biased associations.

Finally, assessments should carefully operationalize the DSM criteria regarding specific drugs in each drug category. Some erroneously combine the consequences of anesthetic gases and short-acting vasodilators such as amyl nitrite with the aliphatic, aromatic, and halogenated hydrocarbons, which makes comparisons of rates and consequences from inhalants difficult. Because inhalant criteria are not complete, with regard to withdrawal, for example, studies that combine all inhalants together cannot inform DSM regarding abuse and dependence.

THERE SHOULD BE FLEXIBILITY REGARDING REARRANGEMENTS OF SCORING ALGORITHMS

Early in the DSM-IV process, two options for dependence were presented—one that closely resembled DSM-III-R with a physiological subtype of tolerance or withdrawal, and a second option that required tolerance and withdrawal. If studies had used an assessment instrument that skipped tolerance if withdrawal was positively endorsed, or skipped withdrawal if tolerance was positively endorsed, the workgroup would have had no empirical data on which to base decisions. Similarly, social consequences, such as legal, family, and work issues, need to be evaluated separately to determine overlap among substances.[1] After treatment history was controlled for, factor analyses were conducted, and advisors in the field were consulted, it was decided that each criterion should remain separate, and that unfulfilled role obligations and legal problems should be moved out of the dependence category and into the abuse category. If early skips had been taken, such analyses would not have been possible. In addition, because the assessment ascertained separately the DSM-III-R compound items of unfulfilled role obligations and hazardous use, it was possible for investigators to determine the independence of the two items. Abuse in DSM-IV now represents problems with substance use in the absence of compulsive use, impaired control, and/or tolerance/withdrawal. Further, analyses that allow for flexibility in scoring of individual criteria, as well as in making diagnoses, such as allowing both abuse and dependence, dependence without abuse, abuse without dependence, or neither, will be most useful to the committee.

ASSESSMENTS SHOULD EVALUATE EACH SUBSTANCE INDIVIDUALLY

An ongoing debate in the field is whether if there is not time to assess all substances individually in a study, it is acceptable to consolidate all illicit substances, such as cocaine, stimulants, inhalants, cannabis, and sedatives, to make one generic drug dependence or abuse diagnosis. The decision to make a generic diagnosis of "drug abuse or dependence," rather than making individual abuse and dependence diagnoses, was agreed upon for the WMH-CIDI. Unfortunately, because each substance has its own age at onset, clinical correlates and course, heritability, abuse and dependence liability, and individual withdrawal criteria, one cannot determine the relevance of diagnoses made generically.

Additionally, such an assessment strategy allows us to understand the relevance of the cookie-cutter approach for all substances, for teenagers, or for users from nonwestern cultures. Only data sets that have used assessments such as the Substance Abuse Module (SAM), the Structured Clinical Interview for DSM-IV Axis I Disorders (SCID), the Diagnostic Interview Schedule (DIS), and the Alcohol Use Disorder and Associated Disabilities Interview Schedule (AUDADIS), which have disaggregated the substances and their resultant criteria, are informative on this issue. Other contributions to this series address this issue for cannabis and for teens (see Chapter 13, "Adolescents and Substance-Related Disorders"; Chapter 14, "Are Specific Dependence Criteria Necessary for Different Substances"; and Chapter 15, "Should Criteria for Drug Dependence Differ Across Drugs?" in this volume), among others.

ASSESSMENTS THAT RETAIN FORMER VERSIONS OF THE CRITERIA ARE MOST HELPFUL

In order to review the rationale that some addictive behaviors listed in DSM-III or DSM-III-R should be reintroduced into the next version, only data sets that have been surveyed with multiple systems can address this issue. Although the interview time is expanded when assessments elicit all data necessary to cover multiple diagnostic systems (ICD and DSM) and different versions of these diagnostic manuals (such as DSM-III, DSM-III-R, DSM-IV), the effort decidedly compares the performance of each system to determine how widely or narrowly the diagnostic nets are cast. The Composite International Diagnostic Interview–Substance Abuse Module (CIDI-SAM) is one such assessment that has maintained former and current criteria for all substances. It does this by using one or more criteria for more than one system and version.[11,12] However, when a slightly different version of a question is necessary for a newer system (such as the change from one or more unsuccessful efforts to cut down or control to unsuccessful efforts), instruments such as the SAM include both in order to test the effect of the change. This strategy elucidates the implications of changing criteria and diagnostic definitions of substance abuse and dependence for each substance.[1,12]

SHORTENED SCREENER VERSIONS ARE NOT USEFUL

Data that were collected with shortened so-called screener versions of an interview, rather than full versions in which all questions are asked, are largely uninformative for deciding whether to include or exclude certain criteria for nosological purposes. Because screener versions make a diagnosis in the quickest time possible, by definition they skip respondents out of a section as soon as a positive diagnosis is made, or as soon as knowing that the addition of one or more positive items could not change the diagnosis from negative to positive. Although these methods generate categorical diagnoses, they fail to inform critical criterion-level analyses, because all criterion possibilities have not been posed to the respondents.

Recently, the literature has evolved on the issue of diagnostic orphans, or subthreshold cases. Data sets collected with screener versions do not allow for a delineation between subthreshold cases and the full-blown subtype.[13,14] The studies listed in Tables 18–1 and 18–2, as well as NESARC, will add critical data on cut points and thresholds.

DIVERSE SAMPLES ARE MOST INFORMATIVE

DSM-IV decisions were criticized for relying on a lack of heterogeneity in the samples of users assessed.[15] As shown in Tables 18–1 and 18–2, a large collection of samples is now amassed for the DSM-V and ICD-11 endeavor. Samples span the range of general population and treatment settings, all diagnostic systems and versions, lifetime and current comorbid conditions, full substance abuse histories (including club drugs, steroids, and caffeine), a variety of assessment instruments (including clinical and lay interviews, semistructured and structured) and multiple study designs. In fact, there are test–retest studies and clinical validation strategies with a resolution of discrepancies, multiple probability designs, multisite collaborative designs, hair and urine testing, complementary functional magnetic resonance imaging (fMRI), collateral designs with multiple informants, and genetic linkage. Various cultures have also been included in studies, allowing for comparisons of data from Israel, Australia, Europe, and Taiwan with data from the United States. With individuals of all ages and ethnicities and with both lifetime and current drug use histories ascertained, investigators will have numerous opportunities to help the workgroups test the myriad hypotheses generated that could be relevant to revisions or additions to substance use disorder criteria and definitions.

Regardless of the samples collected, the conditional prevalence of each criterion item (i.e., the rate among users of that substance) will be evaluated, as was conducted in the DSM-IV Committee, to minimize biased rates based on non–drug users.

ALGORITHMS THAT ASSESS DIAGNOSES SHOULD BE ACCESSIBLE AND TRANSPARENT FOR REVIEW

Investigators must eventually evaluate one another's interpretation of the diagnostic nosology, often referred to as the *operationalization of criteria*, or the scoring algorithms. Such a review can be conducted through the sharing of diagnostic scoring programs and/or question labels, showing data users which questions pertain to which criteria, along with detailed descriptions of the operationalizations. This full disclosure model is important for each data set, whether it is a public use data set or one that was collected individually. Such transparency helps users by making them aware of the decisions made by the co-authors of the scoring program. As discussed in a review article on faithfulness of interviews to the nosologies,[24] methods for devising scoring programs are mainly trusted by users without checking. Errors, if found at all, are discovered only when a data set is released for public use. However, program authors should develop errors before the programs are disseminated to other researchers. One strategy for completing this task is to allow multiple checkers to enter different behavior patterns and score the data. Test cases can also be run, by means of either sample cases or randomized responses, so that rare combinations can be tested. Finally, rules for indeterminate diagnoses must be written and tested so that a false negative does not ensue from a collection of responses that were missed. That is, if questions are refused or responses not given, instead of the person being assigned negative for the disorder, after *x* combinations of positive, missing, and negative responses, the diagnosis would be indeterminate.

MIXED METHODS AND CONTEXTUAL DATA ARE USEFUL TO A DIMENSIONAL DIAGNOSTIC APPROACH

With many teams of investigators using interdisciplinary approaches to their scientific endeavors, the data sets that will be used to make DSM-V decisions will be influenced by many perspectives. Sources of information, in addition to questionnaire data, will include biological markers for linking behavioral traits with DNA for example, or to validate self-report (via hair and urine analyses; collateral informants); and fMRI or other neurobiological data to understand commonalities in functioning due possibly to substances.

Research plans are under way to prepare for how all of these data can be combined for dimensional rather than dichotomous scores, as outlined in the article by Helzer et al. (see Chapter 2). Criteria could include family history, onset of use, biomarkers, and other experimental data useful for discovering altogether new typologies or underlying determinants (see Chapter 11, "Subtypes of Substance Dependence and Abuse," in this volume).[17–19] Data sets that have blended contextual and biological data in the investigation of drug and alcohol use will be able to determine alternative phenotypes for substance use disorders by providing a stronger genetic "signal" in molecular genetics studies. This could be accomplished via comorbidity, or even subtypes sharing genetic and environmental pathways. The indices could also be used to find subtypes for genetic linkage and association studies to eventually uncover individual genes that influence risk for addictive behaviors.[20]

Mixed method designs have also been utilized in several studies (Cottler and Ridenour studies in Table 18–1), incorporating both ethnographic and epidemiological methods. Study designs with multiple sources of data help to confirm the strength of an association. For example, arguments in favor of MDMA as a separate drug class may be made by presenting data on the consequences of MDMA, stimulants, and hallucinogens separately among users of both classes of drugs, along with fMRI results and clinical impressions on the diagnoses. This is achievable because MDMA is assessed separately from hallucinogens and stimulants. Preliminary self-report data have already shown high rates of preoccupation and continuing to use despite harm. Withdrawal symptoms from MDMA are high as well.[21,22] Although the data have been corroborated by two other data collection sites, more work needs to be carried out to evaluate the evidence that MDMA should be separate. In order to add credence to the results, ethnographic studies have been conducted where users with and without specific criteria, such as withdrawal, are interviewed and queried about the consequences of MDMA.

ASSESSMENTS SHOULD BE RELIABLE AND VALID

Many of the assessments of the early 1970s were designed to be administered by clinicians. In the 1980s a new approach emerged that has remained popular in the field—assessing behaviors by nonclinical interviewers. Proper training and supervision of the diagnostic interviewers is mandatory in order to realize the full reliability and validity potential of the assessment and/or method of assessment. Several of the studies listed in Table 18–1 aimed specifically to assess the test–retest reliability and validity of substance use disorder criteria and/or diagnoses by using clinical reappraisals, collateral informants, biological confirmatory testing of hair or urine, and other methods. Those that used stringent methods such as independent, blinded raters for each interview are most informative. The field is united in its belief that assessments should be reliable and valid, yet it has overlooked a test of the reliability and validity of the criteria themselves. Unlike hypertension and diabetes, addiction has no gold standard or biomarker. Additionally, a generic "drug abuse/dependence diagnosis" does not exist—rather, criteria must be met for each individual substance. As Rounsaville et al. stated,[17] substance use disorder diagnoses can never fully be validated because DSM and ICD classificatory systems are descriptive. The most interesting tests are yet to come—those that are nosologically and therapeutically meaningful: that is, those that provide information on prognosis, response to interventions, course of illness over time, neurobiological findings, and comorbidity.

Recognizing that the field has some way to go before it reaches the saturation point in conducting reliability and validity studies, we highlight several more approaches to psychometric investigations, including analyses of reasons why respondents' self-reports of substance use, and its consequences, may be unreliable and invalid. Specifically, the use of this approach is warranted when the focus is on the concordance between the assessor and the self-reported reasons for observed discrepancies. With the discrepancy protocol, the interviewer asks respondents what they feel the best answer might be, as well as the perceived meaning of the question. These techniques have been used successfully in test–retest studies among substance users.[23] Such techniques provide useful information for improving the nomenclature.

DATA SETS SHOULD ALLOW FOR NEW DISCOVERIES

Usually, studies have no time to devote to the surveillance of new drug use disorders, new withdrawal criteria, and new combinations of criteria; however, that is precisely what is needed during the time that the DSM-V and ICD-11 workgroups are preparing for their revisions. Queries might include quantity and frequency questions for each substance used, in order to evaluate the possibility of including them as criterion items for a diagnosis of substance abuse or dependence. The difficulty in describing heavy drinking, which has been the subject of many analyses, is minimal compared with that of describing quantity and frequency for all other drugs, in view of the different routes of administration and dosages of specific substances. Data sets that have collected detailed data on quantity/frequency of alcohol and drug use will be able to shed light on the variability of such answers.

The workgroup will also address the considerable evidence amassed to include a cannabis withdrawal syndrome in DSM (see Chapter 14, "Are Specific Dependence Criteria Necessary for Different Substances," in this volume). Similar reviews might be tackled as well for hallucinogen, phencyclidine (PCP), and inhalant withdrawal. Studies that include numerous potential withdrawal symptoms for these substances, such as some of those listed in Table 18–1 (Cottler, Ridenour, Hasin), allow surveillance of undetermined syndromes; studies that utilize test–retest designs with clinicians and nonclinicians allow for validity and reliability data for these new concepts. Data sets that involve exploratory questions of potential new classifications of drug categories will also be useful. Several such candidates include MDMA abuse/dependence, caffeine abuse/dependence, and steroid abuse. Proposals funded by NIDA's recent Request for Applications will yield promising data on these candidate drugs of abuse and dependence.[21]

Summary and Recommendations

In this chapter, we have outlined the important characteristics of nosologically informative data sets for addressing the salient issues facing the DSM-V and ICD-11 workgroups. Fortunately, the data sets listed in Tables 18–1 and 18–2 are available immediately to assist the workgroups in their deliberations. These data sets and others will also provide an opportunity for investigators to simultaneously address critical questions regarding the key concepts at conferences and workshops in the DSM-V prelude phase, which is currently under way. Replication across data sets may lead ultimately to changes in diagnostic definitions of substance use disorders, as in DSM-IV.

Investigators involved in randomized clinical trials (RCTs) abide by a Consolidated Standards of Reporting Trials (CONSORT)[24] statement that describes their findings, sample participants, and other characteristics in a standardized manner. A checklist and flowchart help other investigators evaluate the findings from the RCTs. Such a statement could be constructed for the DSM-V and ICD-11 substance use disorders workgroups, as well as all other workgroups, for any data set that would be used for revisions to the diagnostic criteria. Similar to CONSORT, the data set statement could result in an evidence-based approach to ultimately increase the quality of the reports to the workgroups. Also similar to CONSORT, the data set statement could be available in several languages and endorsed by the American Psychiatric Association, as well as prominent journals such as *Archives of General Psychiatry, Journal of Clinical Psychiatry, Addiction, Drug and Alcohol Dependence,* and *Journal of Studies on Alcohol,* among others. The value added would be the acknowledgment that the data used for revisions met the highest standards—that is, had met an optimal number of methodological requirements to make it informative for nosological research. It would also offer a standard method for investigators to report information on the algorithms, whether there were skipouts, as well as all of the other characteristics that are ideally informative for nosological purposes.

Some years ago, Babor et al.[25] suggested that continuing to operationalize key concepts yields more clear definitions and a more informed debate on the critical issues. Along the same lines, Gordis[26] stated over 25 years ago that "[n]o scientific discipline can be any better than the quality of its raw data." It seems that our discipline (the substance use field) is in pretty good shape. In fact, the criticisms that were leveled against the DSM-IV process should not be issues for the DSM-V and ICD-11 revision process, with the multitude of nosologically informative data sets at hand.

References

1. Cottler LB, Schuckit MA, Helzer JE, et al: The DSM-IV field trial for substance use disorders: major results. Drug Alcohol Depend 38:59–69, 1995.
2. Grant BF, Moore TC, Kaplan K: Source and Accuracy Statement: Wave 1 National Epidemiologic Survey on Alcohol and Related Conditions (NESARC). Bethesda, MD, National Institute on Alcohol Abuse and Alcoholism, 2003.
3. Demyttenaere K, Bruffaerts R, Posada-Villa J, et al, for the WHO World Mental Health Survey Consortium: Prevalence, severity, and unmet need for treatment of mental disorders in the World Health Organization World Mental Health Surveys. JAMA 291:2581–2590, 2004.
4. Kessler RC, Üstün TB: The World Mental Health (WMH) Survey Initiative version of the World Health Organization (WHO) Composite International Diagnostic Interview (CIDI). Int J Methods Psychiatr Res 13:93–121, 2004.
5. Kessler RC, McGonagle KA, Zhao S, et al: Lifetime and 12-month prevalence of DSM-III-R psychiatric disorders in the United States: results from the National Comorbidity Survey. Arch Gen Psychiatry 51:8–19, 1994.
6. Insel TR, Fenton WS: Psychiatric epidemiology: it's not just about counting anymore. Arch Gen Psychiatry 62:590–592, 2005.
7. Hasin DS, Grant BF: The co-occurrence of DSM-IV alcohol abuse and DSM-IV alcohol dependence: results from the National Epidemiologic Survey on Alcohol and Related Conditions on heterogeneity that differ by population subgroup. Arch Gen Psychiatry 61:891–896, 2004.
8. Hasin DS, Hatzenbueler M, Smith S, et al: Co-occurring DSM-IV drug abuse in DSM-IV drug dependence: results from the National Epidemiologic Survey on Alcohol and Related Conditions. Drug Alcohol Depend 80:117–123, 2005.
9. Hasin DS, Schuckit MA, Martin CS, et al: The validity of DSM-IV alcohol dependence: what do we know and what do we need to know? Alcohol Clin Exp Res 27:244–252, 2003.
10. Schuckit MA, Smith TL, Danko GP, et al: Prospective evaluation of the four DSM-IV criteria for alcohol abuse in a large population. Am J Psychiatry 16:350–360, 2005.

11. Langenbucher JW, Morgenstern J, Miller K: DSM-III, DSM-IV and ICD-10 as severity scales for drug dependence. Drug Alcohol Depend 39:139–150, 1995.
12. Cottler LB: Comparing DSM-III-R and ICD-10 substance use disorders. Addiction 88:689–696, 1993.
13. Sarr M, Bucholz KK, Phelps DL: Using cluster analysis of alcohol use disorders to investigate "diagnostic orphans": subjects with alcohol dependence symptoms but no diagnosis. Drug Alcohol Depend 60:295–302, 2000.
14. Hasin D, Paykin A: Dependence symptoms but no diagnosis: diagnostic "orphans" in a 1992 national sample. Drug Alcohol Depend 53:215–222, 1999.
15. Grant B: The DSM-IV field trial for substance use disorders: major results (brief commentary). Drug Alcohol Depend 38:71–75, 1995.
16. Robins L, Cottler LB: Making a structured psychiatric diagnostic interview faithful to the nomenclature. Am J Epidemiol 160:808–813, 2004.
17. Rounsaville B, Petry N, Carroll K: Single vs. multiple drug focus in substance abuse clinical trials research. Drug Alcohol Depend 70:117–125, 2003.
18. Alterman AI, Cacciolo J, Mulvaney F, et al: Alcohol dependence and abuse in three groups at varying familial alcoholism risk. J Consult Clin Psychol 70:336–342, 2002.
19. Glowinski A, Madden P, Bucholz K, et al: Genetic epidemiology of self-reported lifetime DSM-IV major depressive disorder in a population based twin sample of female adolescents. J Child Psychol Psychiatry 44:988–996, 2003.
20. Beseler C, Jacobson KC, Kremen WS, et al: Is there heterogeneity among syndromes of substance use disorder for illicit drugs? Addict Behav 31:929–947, 2006.
21. Cottler LB, Womack SB, Compton WM, et al: Ecstasy abuse and dependence among adolescents and young adults: applicability and reliability of DSM-IV criteria. Hum Psychopharmacol 16:599–606, 2001.
22. Cottler LB, Hoffer L: The Club Drug Study: St. Louis, Miami, and Sydney, Australia—(CD-SLAM). National Institute on Drug Abuse (NIDA) Epidemiology Trends in Drug Abuse. Proceedings of the Community Epidemiology Work Group, II. Bethesda, MD, National Institute on Drug Abuse, 2003, pp 341–343.
23. Cottler LB, Compton WM, Brown L, et al: The Discrepancy Interview Protocol: a method for evaluating and interpreting discordant survey responses. Int J Methods Psychiatr Res 4:173–182, 1994.
24. Moher D, Schulz KF, Altman D, et al: The CONSORT Statement: revised recommendations for improving the quality of reports of parallel-group randomized trials 2001. Explore (NY) 1:40–45, 2005.
25. Babor T, Lauerman RJ, Cooney NL: In search of the alcohol dependence syndrome: a cross national study of its structure and validity, in Cultural Studies on Drinking and Drinking Problems (Report on a Conference, No. 176). Edited by Paakkanen P, Sulkunen P. 1987.
26. Gordis L: Assuring the quality of questionnaire data in epidemiologic research. Am J Epidemiol 109:21–24, 1979.

19

EMPIRICAL BASIS OF SUBSTANCE USE DISORDERS DIAGNOSIS

Research Recommendations for DSM-V

Marc A. Schuckit, M.D.
John B. Saunders, M.D., F.R.C.P.

The research questions and issues presented in this chapter represent the outcome of a consultation process that started at the DSM-V Launch Conference in February 2004. For the substance use disorders field, the key event was a consultation conference, "Diagnostic Issues in Substance Use Disorders: Refining the Research Agenda," which took place at the U.S. National Institutes of Health in February 2005 (see "Introduction" in this volume). Questions raised at the meeting that were of potential interest to the development of DSM-V were recorded, and an abbreviated list of these items was shared with participants at the end of the meeting. This large and unedited group of questions was then considered by the core workgroup and steering committee, and subsequently refined further.

The more focused list presented here was created by eliminating redundancy among questions and placing the items into four categories: 1) questions that could be

---

Reprinted from Schuckit MA, Saunders JB: "Empirical Basis of Subsyance Use Disorders: Diagnosis Research Recommendations for DSM-V." *Addiction* 101 (suppl 1):170–173, 2006. Used with permission of the Society for the Study of Addiction.

addressed immediately through secondary analyses of existing data sets; 2) items likely to require position papers to propose criteria or more focused questions with a view to subsequent analyses of existing data sets; 3) issues that could be proposed for literature reviews, but with a lower probability that these might progress to a data-analytical phase; and 4) suggestions or comments that might not require immediate action but that should be considered by the DSM-V Committee as part of its deliberations, and potentially by the committee charged with producing the next revision of the ICD.

Research Questions

QUESTIONS THAT COULD BE ADDRESSED BY ANALYSIS OF EXISTING DATA SETS

A. Can latent class analyses or similar approaches help select diagnostic items most relevant for substance abuse versus dependence and potential subsyndromal entities such as hazardous use?

B. Do substance abuse, dependence, and subsyndromal entities (e.g., hazardous use) fit into a single dimension?

C. Is there a core set of dependence items that can be used for all drugs of abuse? Are there specific additional items (beyond the core) that should be added for nicotine dependence and other items that should be added for cannabis dependence and for other substances?

D. How can severity be best defined? Should dependence criteria be weighted? Should a simple count of the number of dependence or abuse items endorsed be used? Must a threshold be established? Is severity separate from level of impairment? Once severity is established, are the criteria applicable across cultures?

E. What are the implications when more than one dependence syndrome occur together? How does this co-occurrence relate to clinical course, reliability, and validity of the diagnostic criteria?

F. If categories are created for substance abuse and dependence (or alternative diagnostic entities), how are diagnostic orphans best handled? What are the cross-sectional and longitudinal implications of any approach proposed to deal with diagnostic orphans?

G. How is the concept of polysubstance dependence best handled? Should the emphasis be on two or more substances (not three or more as currently in DSM) among individuals who do not meet criteria for any one drug dependence?

H. What are the cross-sectional and longitudinal implications of encouraging researchers and clinicians to diagnose substance abuse when it is present, even when there is coexisting dependence on the same drug?

I. Can the validity and reliability of current substance abuse and dependence criteria (or new criteria if they are developed) be improved through relatively simple clarifications in wording and avoidance of compound diagnostic criterion items?

J. Does the general approach for substance abuse and dependence criteria need to be modified in adolescents? Can this be simply carried out through alternative wording of existing criteria? Can the same criteria for remission and severity be used in adolescents?
K. What are the developmental trajectories for different substance use disorders in adolescents? Does this have any implications on the criteria or thresholds to be used for young subjects?
L. How well does the dimensional approach suggested by Helzer et al. (see Chapter 2, "Should There Be Both Categorical and Dimensional Criteria for the Substance Use Disorders in DSM-V?," in this volume) perform cross-sectionally and longitudinally regarding different drugs of abuse?
M. Can reliable and clinically useful criteria for remission be developed? Are these likely to be the same across all substances of abuse? How well do such criteria predict the course of a substance use disorder or response to treatment?
N. What are the optimal criteria for cannabis withdrawal? What do existing data sets teach us about cross-sectional and longitudinal performance of these criteria?
O. What do longitudinal and cross-sectional data tell us regarding the optimal criteria for caffeine withdrawal? caffeine abuse? caffeine dependence?
P. What are the optimal criteria (if any) for nicotine abuse? What do the current data sets tell us about the cross-sectional and longitudinal performance of such criteria?
Q. What do existing data tell us regarding the existence of a persisting (permanent?) schizophrenia-like psychosis among individuals with heavy use of stimulants (amphetamines or cocaine)?
R. Are modifications needed for valid diagnosis of opioid use disorders in patients who are compliant with prescribed opioid treatment for chronic pain? Are modifications needed 1) at the level of syndrome definition? 2) in the threshold for diagnosis? 3) by inclusion of additional or modified criteria? or 4) by expanded definitions or examples of current criteria?

This list could be addressed in the order any of the researchers with available databases prefer. Another determinant might be the priority a funding agency would be likely to apply.

QUESTIONS LIKELY TO REQUIRE POSITION PAPERS TO PROPOSE CRITERIA OR MORE SPECIFIC QUESTIONS WITH A VIEW TO SUBSEQUENT DATA ANALYSIS

A. What is the quality of the data supporting the existence of a protracted abstinence syndrome? What are the drugs most likely to be appropriate for such a diagnosis? What are the optimal criteria? Do these need to be different across different types of drugs?

B. How might the concept of craving be best defined? Can craving be introduced as a specific criterion item in DSM?

C. How can the concept "loss of control" be best defined? Should this concept be considered for inclusion in DSM?

D. What guidelines are available regarding which (if any) subtypes of dependence should be proposed for DSM-V? Possibilities include age at onset, comorbid diagnoses, and more continuous versus "binge" use of the substance.

E. Are there any biological markers that are useful in identifying diagnosis, subtypes, adolescent onset, and other key parameters? This question is reviewed by Koob in Chapter 3 ("Neurobiology of Addiction") of this volume, but an additional position paper examining additional markers may be useful.

F. Can potentially useful criteria for prodromal syndromes be developed and tested with existing data sources? What are the assets and liabilities of labeling someone (especially an adolescent) as in a prodromal phase or "at risk" category for any substance-related diagnosis? If such labels are developed, would they be best placed in the Z codes?

G. Can a systematic way be developed and tested for evaluating thresholds for diagnostic criteria across different cultures?

H. What criteria should be used to make the decision of whether to broaden the current substance use disorders section? What alternative approaches are available—for example, using a "compulsive disorders" or "harmful behavior disorders" heading for these additional conditions rather than combining them with the current substance use disorders? A broad-based and systematic position paper should address the pros and cons of expanding the substance use disorders to include a broad range of "compulsive" or "addictive" disorders. If the substance use disorders category is broadened, should it include all "compulsive-like" behaviors? If not, which of the behaviors (e.g., regarding sexuality, shopping, exercising, computer use) should be used, and what criteria can be invoked to systematically make these decisions? This paper should be structured to ask specific questions that might be amenable for systematic analyses using existing data sets if at all possible.

I. Should a full diagnostic syndrome (e.g., the criteria for a major depressive episode or for panic disorder) be required for someone to be diagnosed with a substance-induced condition when the syndrome only occurs in the context of substance use or withdrawal? Should the criteria for a substance use disorder more directly state that the onset must be within 1 month of intoxication or withdrawal? A paper needs to highlight such specific questions regarding comorbidities.

J. Is there a way to develop (and test) the relative assets and liabilities of a dimensional versus categorical approach to comorbid conditions?

K. What are the assets and liabilities of developing specific wording for interviews and questionnaires for each of the diagnostic items for abuse, dependence, and withdrawal as relevant to each drug category? A position paper should consider the assets and liabilities of developing specific wording for interviews (face-to-face) and questionnaires (paper and pencil instruments) for each of the diagnostic items for abuse, dependence, withdrawal and so on as relevant to each category of drugs. Such a listing might be used as an addendum to DSM-V for researchers. If a compendium of appropriate diagnostic items can be developed, these would, optimally, be pilot tested as part of the DSM-V preparation process.

QUESTIONS LIKELY TO BE APPROPRIATE FOR LITERATURE REVIEWS, BUT WITH A LOWER PROBABILITY OF PROGRESSION TO A DATA-ANALYTICAL PHASE

A. Can all drugs of abuse fit into existing diagnostic categories (e.g., γ-hydroxybutyrate [GHB] as a depressant and 3,4-methylenedioxymethamphetamine [MDMA] as either a stimulant or a hallucinogen), or is it necessary to develop new categories of drugs?
B. Should special consideration be given to the impact that nicotine might have on the development and course of dependence on other drugs of abuse?
C. Is there a need to develop separate diagnostic criteria for anabolic steroids?
D. Are there sufficient data from the literature to help establish the validity and reliability of the substance abuse and dependence criteria across different groups (African, African American, different types of Latino groups, South Asian and East Asian populations)?
E. Are there "natural experiments" available in the literature to address DSM research questions? A review paper might look to see if there are "natural experiments" available that might be used to help address a variety of research questions. These include looking at the joint impact of nicotine dependence and pathological gambling by evaluating changes in gambling practices once no-smoking laws were instituted, and similar natural experiments that might be useful to the DSM-V process.

ISSUES AND COMMENTS THAT COULD BE CONSIDERED BY THE DSM-V COMMITTEE IN ITS DELIBERATIONS

A. Avoid compound diagnostic items whenever possible.
B. Try to use as few criterion items as possible for each entity to optimize clinical usefulness.
C. Consider whether it is or is not appropriate to define a syndrome by its consequences.

D. If subtypes are developed, be certain that they are simple enough for clinicians to use, while improving communication, inferring prognosis, and demonstrating validity and reliability.
E. Consider the optimal words to use for syndromes. This process includes striking a balance between not changing names of conditions unless absolutely essential, and being certain that any new word or name inserted has more assets than liabilities. For example, should *substance-induced* be replaced with *co-occurring* or *substance-related*? Is there a better term than *abuse*? Should *dependence* be replaced by *addiction*?
F. What is the best definition for a persisting disorder?
G. When results across studies differ, does the confusion reflect different methodologies rather than truly different results?
H. Clearly distinguish between steps used to improve research criteria and those optimally appropriate for clinical criteria.
I. Should clinical vignettes be used as part of the diagnostic manual? As part of a research-oriented manual?
J. Can any changes be made in the ICD numbering approach to place drugs of abuse in a more prominent place within the ICD? Can numbering reflect more commonsense rules that will be easier to remember?

Furthering the Research Agenda

We invite readers of the chapters in this book to submit proposals and write with suggestions to the co-chairs of the DSM-V Substance Use Disorders Workgroup, Marc Schuckit and John Saunders, as to how the current list might be enhanced. Readers may wish to do this on their own or through group discussions among colleagues. An additional important approach is to consider proposing seminars and presentations at local, national, and international meetings to discuss the list and offer suggestions.

Some readers of the contributions on which this book is based have the opportunity of addressing the research questions by using existing data sets. We would very much encourage these activities, and we hope that readers will send the co-chairs copies of any posters or papers that address any issues relevant to the DSM-V process for these conditions. Similarly, it is hoped that others might write literature-based review papers or develop research protocols that will help us address the important issues outlined within the articles presented here.

Index

Page numbers printed in **boldface** *type refer to tables or figures.*

www.ingramcontent.com/pod-product-compliance
Ingram Content Group UK Ltd.
Pitfield, Milton Keynes, MK11 3LW, UK
UKHW021845100926
8556IPUK00019B/1067

9 780890 422991